D0948785

FUTURE OF EMERGENCY CARE

EMERGENCY CARE FOR CHILDREN
GROWING PAINS

Committee on the Future of Emergency Care
in the United States Health System

Board on Health Care Services

INSTITUTE OF MEDICINE
OF THE NATIONAL ACADEMIES

THE NATIONAL ACADEMIES PRESS
Washington, D.C.
www.nap.edu

THE NATIONAL ACADEMIES PRESS   500 Fifth Street, N.W.   Washington, DC 20001

NOTICE: The project that is the subject of this report was approved by the Governing Board of the National Research Council, whose members are drawn from the councils of the National Academy of Sciences, the National Academy of Engineering, and the Institute of Medicine. The members of the committee responsible for the report were chosen for their special competences and with regard for appropriate balance.

This study was supported by Contract No. 282-99-0045 between the National Academy of Sciences and the U.S. Department of Health and Human Services' Agency for Healthcare Research and Quality (AHRQ); Contract No. B03-06 between the National Academy of Sciences and the Josiah Macy, Jr. Foundation; and Contract No. HHSH25056047 between the National Academy of Sciences and the U.S. Department of Health and Human Services' Health Resources and Services Administration (HRSA) and Centers for Disease Control and Prevention (CDC), and the U.S. Department of Transportation's National Highway Traffic Safety Administration (NHTSA). Any opinions, findings, conclusions, or recommendations expressed in this publication are those of the author(s) and do not necessarily reflect the view of the organizations or agencies that provided support for this project.

Library of Congress Cataloging-in-Publication Data

Emergency care for children : growing pains / Committee on the Future of Emergency Care in the United States Health System, Board on Health Care Services.
   p. ; cm. — (Future of emergency care series)
 ISBN-13: 978-0-309-10171-4 (hardback)
 ISBN-10: 0-309-10171-9 (hardback)
 1. Pediatric emergencies. 2. Pediatric intensive care. 3. Children—Wounds and injuries—Treatment. 4. Emergency medical services. I. Institute of Medicine (U.S.). Committee on the Future of Emergency Care in the United States Health System. II. Series.
 [DNLM: 1. Emergency Medical Services—organization & administration—United States. 2. Child—United States. 3. Child Health Services—organization & administration—United States. 4. Infant—United States. WS 205 E527 2007]
RJ370.E4487 2007
618.92′0025—dc22

2007002800

Additional copies of this report are available from the National Academies Press, 500 Fifth Street, N.W., Lockbox 285, Washington, DC 20055; (800) 624-6242 or (202) 334-3313 (in the Washington metropolitan area); Internet, http://www.nap.edu.

For more information about the Institute of Medicine, visit the IOM home page at: www.iom.edu.

The serpent has been a symbol of long life, healing, and knowledge among almost all cultures and religions since the beginning of recorded history. The serpent adopted as a logotype by the Institute of Medicine is a relief carving from ancient Greece, now held by the Staatliche Museen in Berlin.

"Knowing is not enough; we must apply.
Willing is not enough; we must do."
—Goethe

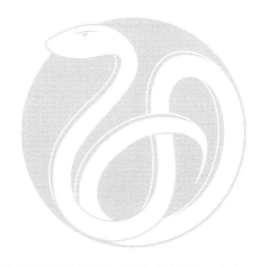

INSTITUTE OF MEDICINE
OF THE NATIONAL ACADEMIES

Advising the Nation. Improving Health.

THE NATIONAL ACADEMIES
Advisers to the Nation on Science, Engineering, and Medicine

The **National Academy of Sciences** is a private, nonprofit, self-perpetuating society of distinguished scholars engaged in scientific and engineering research, dedicated to the furtherance of science and technology and to their use for the general welfare. Upon the authority of the charter granted to it by the Congress in 1863, the Academy has a mandate that requires it to advise the federal government on scientific and technical matters. Dr. Ralph J. Cicerone is president of the National Academy of Sciences.

The **National Academy of Engineering** was established in 1964, under the charter of the National Academy of Sciences, as a parallel organization of outstanding engineers. It is autonomous in its administration and in the selection of its members, sharing with the National Academy of Sciences the responsibility for advising the federal government. The National Academy of Engineering also sponsors engineering programs aimed at meeting national needs, encourages education and research, and recognizes the superior achievements of engineers. Dr. Wm. A. Wulf is president of the National Academy of Engineering.

The **Institute of Medicine** was established in 1970 by the National Academy of Sciences to secure the services of eminent members of appropriate professions in the examination of policy matters pertaining to the health of the public. The Institute acts under the responsibility given to the National Academy of Sciences by its congressional charter to be an adviser to the federal government and, upon its own initiative, to identify issues of medical care, research, and education. Dr. Harvey V. Fineberg is president of the Institute of Medicine.

The **National Research Council** was organized by the National Academy of Sciences in 1916 to associate the broad community of science and technology with the Academy's purposes of furthering knowledge and advising the federal government. Functioning in accordance with general policies determined by the Academy, the Council has become the principal operating agency of both the National Academy of Sciences and the National Academy of Engineering in providing services to the government, the public, and the scientific and engineering communities. The Council is administered jointly by both Academies and the Institute of Medicine. Dr. Ralph J. Cicerone and Dr. Wm. A. Wulf are chair and vice chair, respectively, of the National Research Council.

www.national-academies.org

Reviewers

This report has been reviewed in draft form by individuals chosen for their diverse perspectives and technical expertise, in accordance with procedures approved by the National Research Council's Report Review Committee. The purpose of this independent review is to provide candid and critical comments that will assist the institution in making its published report as sound as possible and to ensure that the report meets institutional standards for objectivity, evidence, and responsiveness to the study charge. The review comments and draft manuscript remain confidential to protect the integrity of the deliberative process. We wish to thank the following individuals for their review of this report:

JOEL J. ALPERT, Professor and Chairman Emeritus, Department of Pediatrics and Professor Emeritus, Public Health Law, Boston University School of Medicine, Massachusetts

ARTHUR COOPER, Trauma and Pediatric Surgical Services, Harlem Hospital Center, New York, NY

PETER J. CUNNINGHAM, Center for Studying Health System Change, Washington, DC

SANDRAL HULLETT, Jefferson Health System, Birmingham, Alabama

DAVID M. JAFFE, Department of Pediatrics, Division of Emergency Medicine, Washington University School of Medicine, St. Louis, Missouri

JOSEPH P. ORNATO, Department of Emergency Medicine, Virginia Commonwealth University/ Medical College of Virginia, Richmond

RITU SAHNI, Department of Emergency Medicine, Oregon Health &
Science University, Portland
MICHAEL W. SHANNON, Children's Hospital, Boston, Harvard Medical
School, Massachusetts
SCOTT D. WILLIAMS, Chief Medical Officer, HCA Mountain Division,
Salt Lake City, Utah

Although the reviewers listed above have provided many constructive
comments and suggestions, they were not asked to endorse the conclusions
or recommendations nor did they see the final draft of the report before
its release. The review of this report was overseen by **Enriqueta C. Bond,**
Burroughs Wellcome Fund, and **Thomas F. Boat,** Children's Hospital Research Foundation and Department of Pediatrics, University of Cincinnati.
Appointed by the National Research Council and Institute of Medicine,
they were responsible for making certain that an independent examination
of this report was carried out in accordance with institutional procedures
and that all review comments were carefully considered. Responsibility for
the final content of this report rests entirely with the authoring committee
and the institution.

Foreword

The state of emergency care affects every American. When illness or injury strikes, Americans count on the system to respond with timely and high-quality care. Yet today, the emergency and trauma care that Americans receive can fall short of what they expect and deserve.

Emergency care is a window on health care, revealing both what is right and what is wrong with our delivery system. Americans rely on hospital emergency departments in growing numbers because of the skilled specialists and advanced technologies they offer. At the same time, the increasing use of the emergency care system also represents failures of the larger health care system—the growing numbers of uninsured Americans, the limited alternatives available in many communities, and the inadequate preventive care and chronic care management received by many. These demands can degrade the quality of emergency care and hinder its ability to provide urgent and lifesaving care to seriously ill and injured patients wherever and whenever they need it.

The Committee on the Future of Emergency Care in the United States Health System, ably chaired by Gail Warden, set out to examine the emergency care system in the United States; explore its strengths, limitations, and future challenges; describe a desired vision of the emergency care system; and recommend strategies required to achieve that vision. Their efforts build on past contributions of the National Academies, including the landmark National Research Council report *Accidental Death and Disability: The Neglected Disease of Modern Society* in 1966, *Injury in America: A Continuing Health Problem* in 1985, and *Emergency Medical Services for Children* in 1993.

The committee's task in the present study was to examine the full scope of emergency care, from 9-1-1 and medical dispatch to hospital-based emergency and trauma care. The three reports produced by the committee—*Hospital-Based Emergency Care: At the Breaking Point*, *Emergency Medical Services at the Crossroads*, and *Emergency Care for Children: Growing Pains*—provide three different perspectives on the emergency care system. The series as a whole unites the often fragmented prehospital and hospital-based systems under a common vision for the future of emergency care.

As the committee prepared its reports, federal and state policy makers were turning their attention to the possibility of an avian influenza pandemic. Americans are asking whether we as a nation are prepared for such an event. The emergency care system is on the front lines of surveillance and treatment. The more secure and stable our emergency care system is, the better prepared we will be to handle any possible outbreak. In this light, the recommendations presented in these reports take on increased urgency. The guidance they offer can assist all of the stakeholders in emergency care—the public, policy makers, providers, and educators—to chart the future of emergency care in the United States.

Harvey V. Fineberg, M.D., Ph.D.
President, Institute of Medicine
June 2006

Preface

Emergency care has made important advances in recent decades: emergency 9-1-1 service now links virtually all ill and injured Americans to immediate medical response; organized trauma systems transport patients to advanced, lifesaving care within minutes; and advances in resuscitation and lifesaving procedures yield outcomes unheard of just two decades ago. Yet just under the surface, a growing national crisis in emergency care is brewing. Emergency departments (EDs) are frequently overloaded, with patients sometimes lining hallways and waiting hours and even days to be admitted to inpatient beds. Ambulance diversion, in which overcrowded EDs close their doors to incoming ambulances, has become a common, even daily problem in many cities. Patients with severe trauma or illness are often brought to the ED only to find that the specialists needed to treat them are unavailable. The transport of patients to available emergency care facilities is often fragmented and disorganized, and the quality of emergency medical services (EMS) is highly inconsistent from one town, city, or region to the next. In some areas, the system's task of caring for emergencies is compounded by an additional task: providing nonemergent care for many of the 45 million uninsured Americans. Furthermore, the system is ill prepared to handle large-scale emergencies, whether a natural disaster, an influenza pandemic, or an act of terrorism.

This crisis is multifaceted and impacts every aspect of emergency care—from prehospital EMS to hospital-based emergency and trauma care. The American public places its faith in the ability of the emergency care system to respond appropriately whenever and wherever a serious illness or injury occurs. But while the public is largely unaware of the crisis, it is real and growing.

The Institute of Medicine's Committee on the Future of Emergency Care in the United States Health System was convened in September 2003 to examine the emergency care system in the United States, to create a vision for the future of the system, and to make recommendations for helping the nation achieve that vision. The committee's findings and recommendations are presented in the three reports in the *Future of Emergency Care* series:

- *Hospital-Based Emergency Care: At the Breaking Point* explores the changing role of the hospital ED and describes the national epidemic of overcrowded EDs and trauma centers. The range of issues addressed includes uncompensated emergency and trauma care, the availability of specialists, medical liability exposure, management of patient flow, hospital disaster preparedness, and support for emergency and trauma research.
- *Emergency Medical Services at the Crossroads* describes the development of EMS over the last four decades and the fragmented system that exists today. It explores a range of issues that affect the delivery of prehospital EMS, including communications systems; coordination of the regional flow of patients to hospitals and trauma centers; reimbursement of EMS services; national training and credentialing standards; innovations in triage, treatment, and transport; integration of all components of EMS into disaster preparedness, planning, and response actions; and the lack of clinical evidence to support much of the care that is delivered.
- *Emergency Care for Children: Growing Pains* describes the special challenges of emergency care for children and considers the progress that has been made in this area in the 20 years since the establishment of the federal Emergency Medical Services for Children (EMS-C) program. It addresses how issues affecting the emergency care system generally have an even greater impact on the outcomes of critically ill and injured children. The topics addressed include the state of pediatric readiness, pediatric training and standards of care in emergency care, pediatric medication issues, disaster preparedness for children, and pediatric research and data collection.

THE IMPORTANCE AND SCOPE OF EMERGENCY CARE

Each year in the United States approximately 114 million visits to EDs occur, and 16 million of these patients arrive by ambulance. In 2002, 43 percent of all hospital admissions in the United States entered through the ED. The emergency care system deals with an extraordinary range of patients, from febrile infants, to business executives with chest pain, to elderly patients who have fallen.

EDs are an impressive public health success story in terms of access to care. Americans of all walks of life know where the nearest ED is and understand that it is available 24 hours a day, 7 days a week. Trauma systems also represent an impressive achievement. They are a critical component of the emergency care system since approximately 35 percent of ED visits are injury-related, and injuries are the number one killer of people between the ages of 1 and 44. Yet the development of trauma systems has been inconsistent across states and regions.

In addition to its traditional role of providing urgent and lifesaving care, the emergency care system has become the "safety net of the safety net," providing primary care services to millions of Americans who are uninsured or otherwise lack access to other community services. Hospital EDs and trauma centers are the only providers required by federal law to accept, evaluate, and stabilize all who present for care, regardless of their ability to pay. An unintended but predictable consequence of this legal duty is a system that is overloaded and underfunded to carry out its mission. This situation can hinder access to emergency care for insured and uninsured alike, and compromise the quality of care provided to all. Further, EDs have become the preferred setting for many patients and an important adjunct to community physicians' practices. Indeed, the recent growth in ED use has been driven by patients with private health insurance. In addition to these responsibilities, emergency care providers have been tasked with the enormous challenge of preparing for a wide range of emergencies, from bioterrorism to natural disasters and pandemic disease. While balancing all of these tasks is difficult for every organization providing emergency care, it is an even greater challenge for small, rural providers with limited resources.

Improved Emergency Medical Services: A Public Health Imperative

Since the Institute of Medicine (IOM) embarked on this study, concern about a possible avian influenza pandemic has led to worldwide assessment of preparedness for such an event. Reflecting this concern, a national summit on pandemic influenza preparedness was convened by Department of Health and Human Services Secretary Michael O. Leavitt on December 5, 2005, in Washington D.C., and has been followed by statewide summits throughout the country. At these meetings, many of the deficiencies noted by the IOM's Committee on the Future of Emergency Care in the United States Health System have been identified as weaknesses in the nation's ability to respond to large-scale emergency situations, whether disease outbreaks, naturally occurring disasters, or

continued

acts of terrorism. During any such event, local hospitals and emergency departments will be on the front lines. Yet of the millions of dollars going into preparedness efforts, a tiny fraction has made its way to medical preparedness, and much of that has focused on one of the least likely threats—bioterrorism. The result is that few hospital and EMS professionals have had even minimal disaster preparedness training; even fewer have access to personal protective equipment; hospitals, many already stretched to the limit, lack the ability to absorb any significant surge in casualties; and supplies of critical hospital equipment, such as decontamination showers, negative pressure rooms, ventilators, and intensive care unit beds, are wholly inadequate. A system struggling to meet the day-to-day needs of the public will not have the capacity to deal with a sustained surge of patients.

FRAMEWORK FOR THIS STUDY

This year marks the fortieth anniversary of the publication of the landmark National Academy of Sciences/National Research Council report *Accidental Death and Disability: The Neglected Disease of Modern Society.* That report described an epidemic of automobile-related and other injuries, and harshly criticized the deplorable state of trauma care nationwide. The report prompted a public outcry, and stimulated a flood of public and private initiatives to enhance highway safety and improve the medical response to injuries. Efforts included the development of trauma and prehospital EMS systems, creation of the specialty in emergency medicine, and establishment of federal programs to enhance the emergency care infrastructure and build a research base. To many, the 1966 report marked the birth of the modern emergency care system.

Since then, the National Academies and the Institute of Medicine (IOM) have produced a variety of reports examining various aspects of the emergency care system. The 1985 report *Injury in America* called for expanded research into the epidemiology and treatment of injury, and led to the development of the National Center for Injury Prevention and Control within the Centers for Disease Control and Prevention. The 1993 report *Emergency Medical Services for Children* exposed the limited capacity of the emergency care system to address the needs of children and contributed to the expansion of the EMS-C program within the Department of Health and Human Services. It has been 10 years, however, since the IOM examined any aspect of emergency care in depth. Furthermore, no National Academies report has ever examined the full range of issues surrounding emergency care in the United States.

That is what this committee set out to do. The objectives of the study were to (1) examine the emergency care system in the United States; (2) explore its strengths, limitations, and future challenges; (3) describe a desired vision for the system; and (4) recommend strategies for achieving this vision.

STUDY DESIGN

The IOM Committee on the Future of Emergency Care in the United States Health System was formed in September 2003. In May 2004, the committee was expanded to comprise a main committee of 25 members and three subcommittees. A total of 40 main and subcommittee members, representing a broad range of expertise in health care and public policy, participated in the study. Between 2003 and 2006, the main committee and subcommittees met 19 times; heard public testimony from nearly 60 speakers; commissioned 11 research papers; conducted site visits; and gathered information from hundreds of experts, stakeholder groups, and interested individuals.

The magnitude of the effort reflects the scope and complexity of emergency care itself, which encompasses a broad continuum of services that includes prevention and bystander care; emergency calls to 9-1-1; dispatch of emergency personnel to the scene of injury or illness; triage, treatment, and transport of patients by ambulance and air medical services; hospital-based emergency and trauma care; subspecialty care by on-call specialists; and subsequent inpatient care. Emergency care's complexity can be also be traced to the multiple locations, diverse professionals, and cultural differences that span this continuum of services. EMS, for example, is unlike any other field of medicine—over one-third of its professional workforce consists of volunteers. Further, EMS has one foot in the public safety realm and one foot in medical care, with nearly half of all such services being housed within fire departments. Hospital-based emergency care is also delivered by an extraordinarily diverse staff—emergency physicians, trauma surgeons, critical care specialists, and the many surgical and medical subspecialists who provide services on an on-call basis, as well as specially trained nurses, pharmacists, physician assistants, nurse practitioners, and others.

The division into a main committee and three subcommittees made it possible to break down this enormous effort into several discrete components. At the same time, the committee sought to examine emergency care as a comprehensive system, recognizing the interdependency of its component parts. To this end, the study process was highly integrated. The main committee and three subcommittees were designed to provide for substantial overlap, interaction, and cross-fertilization of expertise. The committee concluded that nothing will change without cooperative and visionary leadership at many levels and a concerted national effort among the principal stakeholders—federal, state, and local officials; hospital leadership; physicians, nurses, and other clinicians; and the public.

The committee hopes that the reports in the *Future of Emergency Care* series will stimulate increased attention to and reform of the emergency care system in the United States. I wish to express my appreciation to the members of the committee and subcommittees and the many panelists who provided input at the meetings held for this study, and to the IOM staff for their time, effort, and commitment to the development of these important reports.

Gail L. Warden
Chair

Acknowledgments

The *Future of Emergency Care* series benefited from the contributions of many individuals and organizations. The Committee and Institute of Medicine (IOM) staff take this opportunity to recognize and thank those who helped in the development of the reports in the series.

A large number of individuals assembled materials that helped the committee develop the evidence base for its analyses. The committee appreciates the contributions of experts from a variety of organizations and disciplines who gave presentations during committee meetings or authored papers that provided information incorporated into the series of reports. The full list of presenters is provided in Appendix C. Authors of commissioned papers are listed in Appendix D.

Committee members and IOM staff conducted a number of site visits throughout the course of the study to gain a better understanding of certain aspects of the emergency care system. We appreciate the willingness of staff from the following organizations to meet with us and respond to questions: Beth Israel Deaconess Medical Center, Boston Medical Center, Children's National Medical Center, Grady Memorial Hospital, Johns Hopkins Hospital, Maryland Institute for EMS Services Systems, Maryland State Police Aviation Division, Richmond Ambulance Association, and Washington Hospital Center.

We would also like to express appreciation to the many individuals who shared their expertise and resources on a wide range of issues: Karen Benson-Huck, Linda Fagnani, Carol Haraden, Lenworth Jacobs, Tom Judge, Nadine Levick, Ellen MacKenzie, Dawn Mancuso, Rick Murray, Ed

Racht, Dom Ruscio, Carol Spizziri, Caroline Steinberg, Rosemary Stevens, Peter Vicellio, and Mike Williams.

This study received funding from the Josiah Macy, Jr. Foundation, the National Highway Traffic Safety Administration (NHTSA), and three agencies within the Department of Health and Human Services: the Agency for Healthcare Research and Quality (AHRQ), the Centers for Disease Control and Prevention (CDC), and the Health Resources and Services Administration (HRSA). We would like to thank the staff from those organizations who provided us with information, documents, and insights throughout the project, including Drew Dawson, Laurie Flaherty, Susan McHenry, Gamunu Wijetunge, and David Bryson of NHTSA; Dan Kavanaugh, Christina Turgel, and David Heppel from HRSA; Robin Weinick and Pam Owens from AHRQ; Rick Hunt and Bob Bailey from the CDC National Center for Injury Prevention and Control; and many other helpful members of their staffs.

Important research and writing contributions were made by Molly Hicks of Keene Mill Consulting, LLC. Karen Boyd, a Christine Mirzayan Science and Technology Fellow of the National Academies, and two student interns, Carla Bezold and Neesha Desai, developed background papers. Also, our thanks to Rona Briere, who edited the reports, and to Alisa Decatur, who prepared them for publication.

Contents

Summary

Children represent a special challenge for emergency and trauma care providers, in large part because they have unique medical needs in comparison with adults. Respiratory rates, heart rates, and blood pressure levels all change as children grow, so vital signs that would be normal for an adult patient may signal distress in a child. Special care is necessary when providers intubate a child to accommodate a shorter trachea and higher larynx. Medication doses must be carefully calculated specifically for each pediatric patient based on his or her weight. Providers must also know how to handle children's emotional reactions to illness and injury, which vary by age. Children may not be old enough to communicate what is wrong with them or how they became injured, making triage more difficult. It is not surprising, then, that many emergency providers feel stress and anxiety when caring for pediatric patients.

For decades, policy makers and providers have recognized the special needs of children, but the emergency and trauma care system has been slow to develop an adequate response to those needs. This shortcoming is due in part to inadequacies of the broader system. The emergency and trauma care system is highly fragmented, with little coordination among prehospital emergency medical services (EMS), hospital services, and public health. Use of emergency departments (EDs) has grown considerably even as many EDs have closed, contributing to crowded conditions in those that remain open. Ambulance diversion has become a daily occurrence in many cities around the country. Key specialists needed to treat emergency and trauma patients are increasingly difficult to find, resulting in longer waits and more distant prehospital transport for critically injured patients. Emergency care providers on the front lines of safety net care encounter patients with intractable

1

social problems. Much of the service provided to these difficult patients is compensated poorly or not at all. This situation places tremendous financial pressure on safety net hospitals, some of which have closed or are in danger of closing as a result.

The problems faced by children in the current emergency care system are even more daunting. Although children represent 27 percent of all ED visits, many hospitals are not well prepared to handle pediatric patients. For example:

- Only about 6 percent of EDs in the United States have all of the supplies deemed essential for managing pediatric emergencies; only half of hospitals have at least 85 percent of those supplies.
- Of the hospitals that lack the capabilities to care for pediatric trauma patients, only half have written transfer agreements with other hospitals.
- Although pediatric skills deteriorate quickly without practice, continuing education in pediatric care is not required or is extremely limited for many prehospital emergency medical technicians (EMTs).
- Many medications prescribed for children are "off label," meaning they have not been adequately tested or approved by the U.S. Food and Drug Administration (FDA) for use in pediatric populations.
- Disaster preparedness plans often overlook the needs of children, even though their needs during a disaster differ from those of adults.
- Evidence indicates that pediatric treatment patterns vary widely among emergency care providers, that many of these providers do not properly stabilize seriously injured or ill children, that many undertreat children in comparison with adults, and that many fail to recognize cases of child abuse.
- These shortcomings are often exacerbated in rural areas, where dedicated, well-intentioned prehospital and ED providers often make do without the specialized pediatric training and resources that most of us would expect to be in place.

As a result of the above problems, many children with an emergency medical condition do not receive appropriate care under the current system. Many urban areas have children's hospitals or hospitals with pediatric EDs staffed by pediatric emergency medicine specialists and equipped with the latest technologies for the care and treatment of children. However, the vast majority of ED visits made by children are not to children's hospitals or those with a pediatric ED, but to general hospitals, which are less likely to have pediatric expertise, equipment, and policies in place.

The Institute of Medicine's (IOM) Committee on the Future of Emergency Care in the United States Health System was formed in September 2003 to examine the emergency care system in the United States; explore its strengths, limitations, and future challenges; describe a desired vision of the system; and recommend strategies for achieving that vision. The committee was also tasked with taking a focused look at the state of pediatric emergency care, prehospital emergency care, and hospital-based emergency and trauma care. This report is one in a series of three that presents the committee's findings and recommendations in these areas. Summarized below are the committee's findings and recommendations for improving pediatric emergency and trauma care. In addition, this report serves as a follow-up to the 1993 IOM report *Emergency Medical Services for Children*, which represented the first comprehensive look at pediatric emergency care in the United States. That report, which documented shortcomings in a number of areas, received considerable attention from emergency care providers, professional organizations, policy makers, and the public. Over the past 13 years, the federal Emergency Medical Services for Children (EMS-C) program, a grant program that assists states in dealing with pediatric deficiencies within their emergency care systems, has been actively addressing the shortcomings identified in that report. The committee's findings and recommendation regarding the EMS-C program are summarized below as well.

ACHIEVING THE VISION OF A 21st-CENTURY EMERGENCY CARE SYSTEM

As noted above, emergency care for children cannot be improved until some of the long-standing problems within the overall emergency care system are addressed. To that end, the committee developed a vision for the future of emergency care that centers around three goals: coordination, regionalization, and accountability. Many elements of this vision have been advocated previously; however, progress toward achieving these elements has been derailed by deeply entrenched political interests and cultural attitudes, as well as funding cutbacks and practical impediments to change. Concerted, cooperative efforts at all levels of government—federal, state, regional, local—and the private sector are necessary to finally break through and achieve optimum emergency care.

Coordination

One of the most long-standing problems with the emergency care system is that services are fragmented. EMS, hospitals, trauma centers, and public health have traditionally worked in silos. For example, public safety and EMS agencies often lack common radio frequencies and protocols for communicating with each other during emergencies. Similarly, emergency care providers lack access to patient medical histories that could be useful in decision making. Only about half of hospitals have pediatric interfacility transfer agreements. Moreover, planning is fragmented; often pediatric concerns are overlooked entirely, or planning for adult and pediatric care occurs independently.

The committee envisions a system in which patients of all ages and in all communities receive well-planned and coordinated emergency care services. Dispatch, EMS, ED providers, public safety, and public health should be fully interconnected and united in an effort to ensure that each patient receives the most appropriate care, at the optimal location, with the minimum delay. From the standpoint of the patient and parents, delivery of emergency care services should be seamless. Inclusion of pediatric concerns during planning can help the system meet the needs of children to the best of its ability.

Regionalization

Because not all hospitals within a community have the personnel and resources to support the delivery of high-level emergency care, critically ill and injured patients should be directed specifically to those facilities with such capabilities. That is the goal of regionalization. There is substantial evidence that the use of regionalization of services to direct such patients to designated hospitals with greater experience and resources improves outcomes and reduces costs across a range of high-risk conditions and procedures. A few states have taken steps to regionalize pediatric emergency care, allowing advanced life support ambulances to bring such patients only to hospitals designated as having pediatric capabilities. However, a state-by-state analysis shows that many states still have not formally regionalized pediatric intensive or trauma care.

Thus the committee supports further regionalization of emergency care services. However, use of this approach requires that EMTs, as well as parents and caregivers, be clear on which facilities have the necessary resources. Just as trauma centers are categorized according to their capabilities (i.e., level I–level IV/V), a standard national approach to the categorization of EDs that reflects both their adult and pediatric capabilities is needed so that the categories will be clearly understood by providers and the public across all states and regions of the country. To that end, the committee recommends that **the Department of Health and Human Services and the National Highway Traffic Safety Administration, in partnership with professional organizations, convene a panel of individuals with multidisciplinary expertise to develop evidence-based categorization systems for emergency medical services, emergency departments, and trauma centers based on adult and pediatric service capabilities (3.1).**[1]

---

[1]The committee's recommendations are numbered according to the chapter of the main report in which they appear. Thus, for example, recommendation 3.1 is the first recommendation in Chapter 3.

This information, in turn, could be used to develop protocols that would guide EMTs in the transport of patients. However, more research and discussion are needed to determine under what circumstances patients should be brought to the closest hospital for stabilization and transfer instead of being transported directly to the facility with the highest level of care if that facility is farther away. Debate also continues over what procedures are effective for the care of children in the field. Therefore, the committee also recommends that **the National Highway Traffic Safety Administration, in partnership with professional organizations, convene a panel of individuals with multidisciplinary expertise to develop evidence-based model prehospital care protocols for the treatment, triage, and transport of patients, including children (3.2).**

Accountability

Without accountability, participants in the emergency care system need not accept responsibility for failures and can avoid making changes to improve the delivery of care. Accountability has failed to take hold in emergency care to date because responsibility is dispersed across many different components of the system, so it is difficult even for policy makers to determine where system breakdowns occur and how they can subsequently be addressed. When hospitals lack pediatric transfer agreements, when providers receive no continuing pediatric education, and when pediatric specialists and on-call specialists are not available, no one party is to blame—it is a system failure.

To build accountability into the system, the committee recommends that **the Department of Health and Human Services convene a panel of individuals with emergency and trauma care expertise to develop evidence-based indicators of emergency and trauma care system performance, including the performance of pediatric emergency care (3.3).** Because of the need for an independent, national process with the broad participation of every component of emergency care, the federal government should play a lead role in promoting and funding the development of these performance indicators. The indicators developed should include structure and process measures, but evolve toward outcome measures over time. These performance measures should be nationally standardized so that statewide and national comparisons can be made. Measures should evaluate the performance of individual providers within the system, as well as that of the system as a whole. Measures should also be sensitive to the interdependence among the components of the system; for example, EMS response times may be related to EDs going on diversion.

Using the measures developed through such a national, evidence-based, multidisciplinary effort, performance data should be collected at regular intervals from all hospitals and EMS agencies in a community. Public dissemination of performance data is crucial to driving the needed changes in the delivery of emergency care services. Dissemination can take various forms, including public report cards, annual reports, and state public health reports. Because of the potential sensitivity of performance data, they should initially be reported in the aggregate rather than at the level of the individual provider organization. However, individual provider organizations should have full access to their own data so they can understand and improve their performance, as well as their contribution to the overall system. Over time, performance information on individual provider organizations should become an important part of the public information on the system.

Achieving the Vision

States and regions face a variety of different situations with respect to emergency and trauma care, including the level of development of adult and pediatric trauma systems; the effectiveness of state EMS offices and regional EMS councils; and the degree of coordination among fire departments, EMS, hospitals, trauma centers, and emergency management. Thus no single approach to enhancing emergency care systems will accomplish the three goals outlined above, and it will be necessary to explore and evaluate a number of different avenues for achieving the committee's vision. The committee therefore recommends that **Congress establish a demonstration program, administered by the Health Resources and Services Administration, to promote coordinated, regionalized, and accountable emergency care systems throughout the country, and appropriate $88 million over 5 years to this program (3.4).** Grants should be targeted at states, which could develop projects at the state, regional, or local level; cross-state collaborative proposals would also be encouraged. Over time and over a number of controlled initiatives, such a process should lead to important insights about what strategies work under different conditions. These insights would provide best-practice models that could be widely adopted to advance the nation toward the committee's vision for efficient, high-quality emergency and trauma care. It will be essential for the federal granting agency and grant recipients to consider explicitly the implications of proposed projects for both adult and pediatric patients.

Furthermore, the fragmented responsibility for emergency care at the federal level must be reduced. Responsibility is widely dispersed among multiple federal agencies within the Department of Health and Human Services (DHHS), the Department of Transportation (DOT), and the Department of Homeland Security (DHS). The scattered nature of federal responsibility for emergency care makes it difficult for the public to identify a clear point of contact, limits the visibility necessary to secure and maintain funding, and creates overlaps and gaps in program funding. The committee recommends that Congress establish a lead agency for emergency and trauma care within 2 years of the release of this report. The lead agency should be housed in the Department of Health and Human Services, and should have primary programmatic responsibility for the full continuum of emergency medical services and emergency and trauma care for adults and children, including medical 9-1-1 and emergency medical dispatch, prehospital emergency medical services (both ground and air), hospital-based emergency and trauma care, and medical-related disaster preparedness. Congress should establish a working group to make recommendations regarding the structure, funding, and responsibilities of the new agency, and develop and monitor the transition. The working group should have representation from federal and state agencies and professional disciplines involved in emergency and trauma care (3.6).

ADDRESSING SPECIFIC PEDIATRIC CONCERNS

In addition to the above reforms to the broader emergency care system, the delivery of optimum pediatric emergency care will require addressing a number of concerns specific to pediatric populations. It will be necessary to strengthen the capabilities of the emergency care workforce to treat pediatric patients, improve patient safety, exploit advances in medical and information technology, foster family-centered care, enhance disaster preparedness, and improve the evidence base.

Strengthening the Workforce

Ideally, because of the unique way in which pediatric patients should be triaged and treated, all children should be served by emergency care providers with formal training and experience in pediatric emergency care. In reality, providers' levels of pediatric emergency care training vary considerably. Residency programs, medical schools, nursing schools, states, EMS agencies, and hospitals have varying requirements for initial and continuing pediatric emergency care education and training. In some cases, the training is intensive; however, emergency medicine or pediatrics training often represents only a small part of a provider's total training time. Of particular concern are emergency care providers who rarely encounter pediatric patients, making it difficult for them to maintain pediatric skills. This is a long-standing problem that has improved somewhat over time, but naturally has led to continued concern about the ability of the emergency care workforce to care properly for pediatric patients. To reduce the consequences of illness and injury, the workforce must have the knowledge and skills necessary to provide appropriate pediatric emergency care. The committee believes all emergency care providers should possess a certain level of competency to deliver emergency care to children. Therefore, the committee recommends that **every pediatric- and emergency care–related health professional credentialing and certification body define pediatric emergency care competencies and require practitioners to receive the level of initial and continuing education necessary to achieve and maintain those competencies (4.1).**

Treatment patterns of providers in emergency care for pediatric patients differ not only because of differences in training, but also because of the lack of evidence-based clinical practice guidelines for many different types of conditions. This is troubling since the use of such guidelines has been shown to improve the quality of care. The committee recommends that **the Department of Health and Human Services collaborate with professional organizations to convene a panel of individuals with multidisciplinary expertise to develop, evaluate, and update clinical practice guidelines and standards of care for pediatric emergency care (4.2).** The committee believes these guidelines should be evidence-based, developed through an evidence evaluation process. That process should include individuals from different disciplines and different types of emergency care organizations to promote consensus and uniformity.

Simply recommending more training and the development of guidelines is not enough, however. Someone must be responsible at the provider level for ensuring that continuing education opportunities are available and exploited. Similarly, the development of clinical guidelines is useless without widespread adoption by providers. Thus the committee believes that pediatric leadership is needed in each provider organization. The committee recommends that **emergency medical services agencies appoint a pediatric emergency coordinator, and that hospitals appoint two pediatric emergency coordinators—one a physician—to provide pediatric leadership for the organization (4.3).** The pediatric coordinator position would not be a full-time position, but a shared role. Still, the coordinators would have a number of responsibilities, including ensuring adequate skill and knowledge among fellow ED or EMS providers, overseeing pediatric care quality improvement initiatives, and ensuring the availability of pediatric medications, equipment, and supplies.

Improving Patient Safety

Emergency care services are delivered in an environment where the need for haste, the distraction of frequent interruptions, and clinical uncertainty abound, thus posing a number of potential threats to patient safety. Children are, of course, at great risk under these circumstances because of their physical and developmental vulnerabilities, as well as their need for care that may be atypical for providers used to treating adult patients.

The committee recommends that **hospitals and emergency medical services agencies implement evidence-based approaches to reducing errors in emergency and trauma care for children (5.3).** There is, however, a paucity of high-quality data on the epidemiology of medical errors among children, particularly within the emergency care system. Instead, there have been only a few, typically small studies demonstrating that care delivered to children is compromised at several points during prehospital EMS care or an ED visit. Thus continued research is needed to determine the best strategies for improving patient safety in prehospital and ED pediatric care. At the same time, however, various hospitals and EMS agencies have had some success with several promising strategies that could be replicated by other organizations.

One category of medical errors well documented to be common in both the EMS and ED environments is those that occur during the prescribing, dispensing, and administration of medications. To address this problem for pediatric patients, the committee recommends that **the Department of Health and Human Services and the National Highway Traffic Safety Administration fund the development of medication dosage guidelines, formulations, labeling guidelines, and administration techniques for the emergency care setting to maximize effectiveness and safety for infants, children, and adolescents. Emergency medical services agencies and hospitals should incorporate these guidelines, formulations, and techniques into practice (5.2).**

Perhaps the foremost problem associated with pediatric medication in the emergency care setting is the above-noted prescribing of medications for children off label. Medications designed for adults may not be suitable for children, yet once a drug has been approved by the FDA, further studies to determine its safety and efficacy in infants and children are rarely conducted. Moreover, emergency care professionals have few evidence-based guidelines and little information to assist them in the prescribing of medications for pediatric patients. As a result, emergency providers must prescribe medications for children without a full understanding of their risks, benefits, or implications for these patients. Therefore, the committee recommends that **the Department of Health and Human Services fund studies of the efficacy, safety, and health outcomes of medications used for infants, children, and adolescents in emergency care settings in order to improve patient safety (5.1).**

Exploiting Advances in Medical and Information Technology

Technology is likely to advance the way care is delivered in the prehospital and ED settings. New technologies designed to accelerate diagnosis and workflow—advanced imaging modalities, rapid diagnostic tests, laboratory automation, EMS technologies, patient tracking tools, and new triage models—are likely to be adopted. As these new technologies are introduced, it is critical to consider how they can help (and whether they may bring harm to) pediatric patients. While this may appear to be an obvious consideration, there have been many examples of medical technologies originally developed for adults but used on children with unintended consequences.

A market for products designed specifically for pediatric patients has not been well developed. To this end, the committee recommends that **federal agencies and private industry fund research on pediatric-specific technologies and equipment for use by emergency and trauma care personnel (5.4).** To stimulate demand for pediatric-appropriate technologies, emergency providers should be made aware of the potential shortcomings of products designed for adults and adapted for children. Federal agencies and private industry also need to take a close look at technologies already in place and available for use on pediatric patients that have not been adequately tested for potentially harmful effects on these patients.

A similar issue exists in the development of information technologies. Hospitals, EMS systems, and government entities are beginning to make substantial investments in information technologies that may improve the quality and efficiency of emergency care delivery. Yet the safety, impact, and risks of these systems for pediatric patients have received little attention. Specific consideration of pediatric needs during the design of such systems is critical to ensure that they are appropriate for the pediatric patient. For example, electronic health records must be designed so that providers can record measurements with a granularity appropriate for newborns and infants, and computerized physician order entry tools must incorporate pediatric-specific dosing tables.

Fostering Family-Centered Care

One of the six aims for health care quality improvement proposed by the IOM in its 2001 landmark report *Crossing the Quality Chasm: A New Health System for the 21st Century* was patient-centeredness, meaning that care should encompass the qualities of compassion; empathy; and responsiveness to the needs, values, and preferences of the individual patient. Parents are recognized as a pediatric patient's primary source of strength and support and play an integral role in the child's health and well-being. Increasing recognition of both the importance of meeting the psychosocial and developmental needs of children and the role of families in promoting the health and well-being of their children has led to the concept of family-centered care.

There are several definitions of family-centered care, but they all essentially recognize that providers should acknowledge and make use of the family's presence, skills, and knowledge of their child's condition when caring for the child. Indeed, a growing body of research demonstrates the importance of ensuring the involvement of patients and families in their own health care decisions, better informing families of treatment options, and improving patients' and families' access to information. A number of studies have found some evidence that family-centered care is associated with improved health outcomes, patient and family satisfaction, and provider satisfaction. Unfortunately, few EMS agencies and EDs have written policies or guidelines for family-centered care in place, and few providers are trained in family-centered approaches. Because such approaches to care can mutually benefit the patient, family, and provider, the committee recommends that **emergency medical services agencies and hospitals integrate family-centered care into emergency care practice (5.5).**

Enhancing Disaster Preparedness

As noted earlier, because of their anatomical, physiological, developmental, and emotional differences, children are generally more vulnerable than adults in the event of a disaster. They also require specialized equipment and different approaches to treatment during such an event. For example, adult decontamination units cannot be used because rescuers need to be able to adjust water temperature and pressure to suit the needs of children (e.g., provide high-volume, low-pressure, heated water). Children also require different antibiotics and different dosages to counter many chemical and biological agents. As with the development of the emergency care system, however, the needs of children have traditionally been overlooked in disaster planning. A 1997 Federal Emergency Management Agency (FEMA) survey found that none of the states had incorporated pediatric components into their disaster plans.

Hurricane Katrina, which struck as this report was being written, highlighted the shortcomings of the nation's disaster planning at many levels. Katrina was extreme in its scope and impact, but even small disasters can present enormous challenges to a system that struggles to meet day-to-day patient needs. Though it is still too early to compile all of the lessons learned from Hurricane Katrina, we have learned enough from this and other disasters to recognize that improved planning for disasters is necessary, and that children must be a particular focus of such efforts. The committee recommends that **federal agencies (the Department of Health and Human Services, the National Highway Traffic Safety Administration, and the Department of Homeland Security), in partnership with state and regional planning bodies and emergency care providers, convene a panel with multidisciplinary expertise to develop strategies for addressing pediatric needs in the event of a disaster.** This effort should encompass the following:

• Development of strategies to minimize parent–child separation and improved methods for reuniting separated children with their families.

• Development of strategies to improve the level of pediatric expertise on Disaster Medical Assistance Teams and other organized disaster response teams.

• Development of disaster plans that address pediatric surge capacity for both injured and noninjured children.

• Development of and improved access to specific medical and mental health therapies, as well as social services, for children in the event of a disaster.

• Development of policies to ensure that disaster drills include a pediatric mass casualty incident at least once every 2 years (6.1).

Improving the Evidence Base

Pediatric emergency care is a young field; even in the late 1970s, there were no pediatric emergency medicine textbooks or journals. Although the amount of research conducted in pediatric emergency care has increased considerably over the past 25 years, a significant information gap remains. Indeed, basic questions about the structure of the pediatric emergency care system and patient outcomes remain unanswered. Many of the treatments and management strategies that are widely practiced today are not supported by scientific evidence. A national commitment to emergency care research for children is needed.

Lack of adequate data and limited research funding are among the most important barriers to the advancement of research in pediatric emergency care. No single hospital or EMS agency is likely to have access to sample sizes large enough to answer important questions about critically ill or injured children. The use of research networks, in which researchers from different institutions pool data, has proven to be successful in addressing such challenges. The large number of patients included in the networks allows researchers to carry out trials designed to evaluate rare conditions or complications. If these networks receive the funding needed for sustainability, they not only generate important findings, but also help train and support the development of young investigators.

Since emergency care research is often not based on a single disease entity, a key characteristic of much of this research is its tendency to cut across multiple specialty domains. This has made it difficult for researchers in the field to obtain training grants from the siloed funding structure of the National Institutes of Health, the largest single source of support for biomedical research in the world. The committee recommends that **the Secretary of Health and Human Services conduct a study to examine the gaps and opportunities in emergency care research, including pediatric emergency** care, and recommend a strategy for the optimal organization and funding of the research effort. This study should include consideration of the training of new investigators, development of multicenter research networks, involvement of emergency and trauma care researchers in the grant review and research advisory processes, and improved research coordination through a dedicated center or institute. Congress and federal agencies involved in emergency and trauma care research (including the Department of Transportation, the Department of Health and Human Services, the Department of Homeland Security, and the Department of Defense) should implement the study's recommendations (7.1).

Focused research attention is needed on pediatric injury, the leading cause of death and disability in children beyond the first year of life. National and state trauma registries, which are used to collect, store, and retrieve data on trauma patients, allow researchers to study the etiologic factors, demographic characteristics, diagnoses, treatments, and clinical outcomes of pediatric trauma patients. However, no single trauma registry currently provides accurate estimates of the scope and characteristics of pediatric trauma. The American College of Surgeons' National Trauma Data Bank constitutes the world's largest repository of pediatric trauma data, but continued steps are needed to expand its pediatric capacity. The committee recommends that **administrators of state and national trauma registries include standard pediatric-specific data elements and provide the data to the National Trauma Data Bank. Additionally, the American College of Surgeons should establish a multidisciplinary pediatric specialty committee to continuously evaluate pediatric-specific data elements for the National Trauma Data Bank and identify areas for pediatric research** (7.2).

THE EMERGENCY MEDICAL SERVICES
FOR CHILDREN PROGRAM

Despite its modest annual appropriation, the EMS-C program boasts many accomplishments. It has initiated hundreds of injury prevention programs; provided thousands of hours of training to EMTs, paramedics, and other emergency medical care providers; developed educational materials covering every aspect of pediatric emergency care; and established a pediatric research network. Still, as discussed earlier, certain segments of the emergency care system continue to be poorly prepared to care for children, and the work of the program continues to be relevant and vital.

Addressing some of the long-standing problems in pediatric emergency care, as well as the new concerns raised in this report, will require the leadership of a well-recognized, well-respected entity not just within pediatrics, but within the broader emergency care system. The EMS-C program, with its long history of working with federal partners, state policy makers, researchers, providers, and professional organizations across the spectrum of emergency care, is well positioned to assume this leadership role. But additional resources are necessary so the program will have the capacity to rapidly address the deficiencies in the pediatric emergency care system for children. The committee recommends that **Congress appropriate $37.5 million per year for the next 5 years to the Emergency Medical Services for Children program (3.7).**

The proposed 5-year period is not intended as a limit on federal funding dedicated to improving pediatric emergency care; indeed, there will always be a need to monitor and study pediatric emergency care. However, the hope is that the various components of leadership in emergency care at the federal level will be better integrated in the future. Pediatric emergency care will always remain an important piece of that federal leadership, but may not require a separate, stand-alone program. After 5 years, it will be necessary to reevaluate how best to identify and fund pediatric emergency care objectives at the federal level. Future funding levels for the EMS-C program must also be reevaluated.

CONCLUDING REMARKS

The quality of the U.S. emergency care system is of critical importance to all Americans. Regardless of income, insurance status, race, ethnicity, geography, or age, everyone relies on the emergency care system to provide needed care in the event of a critical illness or injury. Although the current system operates poorly in many respects, a more reliable system is achievable. Change must be stimulated quickly, however, as millions of Americans continue to access this flawed system each week.

As reforms to the broader emergency care system are accomplished, policy makers at the federal, state, and local levels must not repeat mistakes made in previous decades by neglecting the special needs of pediatric patients. Consideration of those needs must be fully integrated into all aspects of emergency care planning. Individual providers (physicians, nurses, EMTs, and others), as well as provider organizations, also have an important role to play in stimulating improvements in pediatric emergency care. Indeed, they have a responsibility to ensure that care delivered to children meets the highest possible standards of quality.

1

Introduction

In 2002, children under age 19 made more than 29 million visits to emergency departments (EDs) in the United States (2002 National Hospital Ambulatory Medical Care Survey [NHAMCS] data, calculations by Institute of Medicine [IOM] staff). Approximately 20 percent of children make one or more visits to an ED each year; 7 percent make two or more visits (National Center for Health Statistics, 2005). Despite this heavy reliance on the emergency care system, the public typically gives little thought to the adequacy of the system for children. Yet they have lofty expectations. Parents and caregivers expect emergency and trauma care providers to deliver high-quality care to their children when it is needed. They expect the system to be agile, able to respond quickly at any hour of the day or night and handle any type of pediatric emergency appropriately (Harris Interactive, 2004). In reality, however, the public knows little about how well local emergency care and trauma systems perform, both absolutely and in comparison with other systems. In particular, there is little understanding of the major shortcomings of the emergency care system in the United States today.

Emergency care systems are largely local in nature, and they vary accordingly. State and local prevention laws, the training of prehospital emergency medical technicians (EMTs), and the availability of hospitals and pediatric emergency medicine physicians are but a few examples of such variations—key elements that have an important impact on the functioning of the emergency care system. Some areas of the country, particularly urban settings, have children's hospitals and hospitals with pediatric EDs staffed by pediatric emergency specialists and equipped with the latest technologies for the care and treatment of children. In other areas, however, pediatric-specific resources are highly limited. Dedicated, well-intentioned prehospital emergency medical services (EMS) and ED providers make do without the resources that most would expect to be available for the care of children. For example:

- Only about 6 percent of hospitals have available all the pediatric supplies deemed essential by the American Academy of Pediatrics and American College of Emergency Physicians for managing pediatric emergencies, although about half of hospitals have at least 85 percent of those supplies (Middleton and Burt, 2006).
- Of hospitals that do not have a separate pediatric inpatient ward, only about half have written transfer agreements with other hospitals (Middleton and Burt, 2006), which are necessary in case a critically ill or injured child arrives at a hospital that lacks pediatric expertise.
- Although research shows that pediatric skills deteriorate after a short time without practice (Su et al., 2000; Wolfram et al., 2003), pediatric continuing education is not required or is extremely limited for many prehospital providers (Glaeser et al., 2000).
- Many medications prescribed and administered to children in the ED are "off label," meaning they have not been adequately tested in pediatric populations and therefore are not approved for use in children by the U.S. Food and Drug Administration (FDA).
- Disaster preparedness plans largely overlook the needs of children, even though children's needs in the event of a disaster often differ from those of adults (Dick et al., 2004; NASEMSD, 2004).

The lack of preparedness carries a cost: many children with an emergency medical condition do not receive appropriate care under the current system. This conclusion is clear from a recent mock drill conducted in 35 of North Carolina's EDs, including 5 trauma centers. Nearly all of the EDs in the study failed to stabilize seriously injured children properly during trauma simulations. Almost all failed to administer dextrose properly to a child in hypoglycemic shock (a life-threatening drop in blood sugar), correctly warm a hypothermic child, or order proper administration of intravenous (IV) fluids (Hunt et al., 2006). Ongoing research suggests that these problems are not unique to North Carolina EDs. While data on pediatric emergency care outcomes are largely unavailable, data on practice patterns indicate shortcomings in the treatment and care of pediatric patients. Examples include high rates of pediatric medication errors (Selbst et al., 1999; Hubble and Paschal, 2000; Kozer et al., 2002; Fairbanks, 2004; Marcin et al., 2005), low rates of pain management for pediatric patients (Brown et al., 2003), and many missed cases of child abuse (Petrack and Christopher, 1997;

Saade et al., 2002; Kunen et al., 2003; Trokel et al., 2006). Studies also indicate wide variation in practice patterns in the care of children (Glaser et al., 1997; Isaacman et al., 2001; Hampers and Faries, 2002; Davis et al., 2005), as well as an undertreatment of children in comparison with adults (Su et al., 1997; Gausche et al., 1998; Orr et al., 2006).

Providing quality pediatric emergency and trauma care is not just about having the right training and equipment. Indeed, the delivery of care should be built on a strong foundation in which emergency care is well planned and coordinated, care is based on scientific evidence, data are collected so providers can learn from past experience, and system performance is monitored to ensure quality. Moreover, since preventing an injury or illness is almost always better and more cost-effective than even the best emergency care, the emergency care system should promote prevention through surveillance, research, and patient education. Unfortunately, today's emergency care system generally does not function in this way.

STUDY CONTEXT

The Current Emergency Care System

While not new, the problems facing the nation's emergency care system that are reviewed in this report have been growing and have become more visible to the public. Critical stories have increasingly been appearing in the media regarding slow EMS response, ambulance diversions, trauma center closures, the medical malpractice crisis, ground and air ambulance crashes, and the alarming decline in on-call specialist coverage. The events of September 11, 2001, and more recent disasters, such as the train bombings in Madrid, the bus and train bombings in London, and Hurricane Katrina, have heightened the visibility of the issue. Although emergency care is a vital component of the nation's health system, to date there has been no comprehensive study of emergency care in the United States.

A study of the emergency care system is a logical extension of previous work conducted by the National Academy of Sciences and the IOM. In 1966, the National Academy of Sciences (NAS) and the National Research Council (NRC) produced the landmark report *Accidental Death and Disability: The Neglected Disease of Modern Society* (NAS and NRC, 1966), which helped focus attention on the lack of adequate trauma care in the United States and is widely recognized as the impetus for the development of the prehospital EMS system in place today. Other reports, such as *Emergency Medical Services at Midpassage* and *The Emergency Department: A Regional Medical Resource* (NAS and NRC, 1978), have also had a major impact in shaping the development of the emergency care system. More recently, several IOM studies on injury and disability have emphasized the need for skilled emergency care to limit the adverse consequences of illness and injury. Additionally, in 1993 the IOM produced the report *Emergency Medical Services for Children* (IOM, 1993), which focused a great deal of attention on the subject.

The emergency care system has reached a critical point in its development. The specialty of emergency medicine has achieved a substantial level of maturity; the capabilities of EMS have expanded dramatically; trauma systems in a few states are beginning to attain full development; technology offers the potential to revolutionize emergency care services; and the events of September 11, 2001, and subsequent disasters have lent new public visibility and urgency to emergency care planning. In contrast to these advances, the organization and delivery, regulation, and financing of emergency care remain in an outdated, politically entrenched mode that is resistant to change. As emergency care providers become increasingly stressed, timely access to quality emergency care is jeopardized for everyone.

Overview of Pediatric Emergency Care

Nearly 30 percent of all ED visits are made by children (see Figure 1-1). While the majority of pediatric ED visits involve children over age 5, there are 96.2 ED visits per 100 infants, more than twice the rate for all children under age 15 of 40.8 ED visits per 100 (see Figure 2-2 in Chapter 2) (McCaig and Burt, 2005). The most frequent diagnoses for young children (under age 10) in the ED are upper respiratory infection and otitis media (ear infection). Among older children (ages 10–17), the most common diagnoses are superficial injury/contusion and sprains and strains (2002 State Emergency Department Database [SEDD] data supplied by Agency for Healthcare Re-

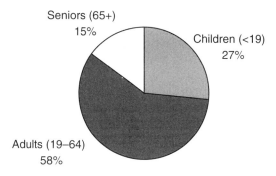

FIGURE 1-1 Emergency department visits by age, 2002.
SOURCE: 2002 NHAMCS data, calculations by IOM staff.

search and Quality [AHRQ] staff). Only 4 percent of all pediatric ED visits result in a hospital admission (2002 NHAMCS data, calculations by IOM staff; 2002 SEDD data supplied by AHRQ staff). Just 1 percent of children who visit the ED are transferred to another hospital (2002 NHAMCS data, calculations by IOM staff), presumably a higher-level facility.

Children's hospitals are an important source of pediatric emergency care. They are the most specialized centers of care for children in the United States, and because they are focused solely on the care of children, they are the hospitals that tend to be best prepared for emergency pediatric visits in terms of expertise and pediatric resources (Gausche-Hill et al., 2004). However, children's hospitals represent only about 5 percent of all U.S. hospitals (NACHRI, 2005). According to one estimate, only 7 percent of ED visits made by children are to a children's hospital (Gausche-Hill et al., 2004). Some non-children's hospitals have a separate pediatric ED. Like children's hospitals, they tend to be better prepared for pediatric emergency visits in terms of pediatric expertise, equipment, and policies and procedures (Gausche-Hill et al., 2004). Taken together, it is estimated that only 18 percent of all pediatric visits are to pediatric EDs at either a children's or a general hospital (2002 NHAMCS data, calculations by IOM staff).

Thus, the vast majority of pediatric ED visits are made to general hospitals that treat adults and children in the same department. The quality of emergency care provided to children at these EDs is of concern because, as noted, they tend be less well prepared for pediatric emergencies than dedicated pediatric EDs. While data on outcomes by facility type are largely unavailable, studies indicate that pediatric trauma patients treated at children's hospitals have lower mortality rates, lengths of stay, and charges than those treated at adult hospitals (Densmore et al., 2006). EDs that treat both children and adults are unlikely to have a pediatric emergency medicine physician on staff, and many lack basic pediatric equipment and supplies (Gausche-Hill et al., 2004; Middleton and Burt, 2006). Even more concerning, between 19 and 26 percent of all pediatric ED visits are to hospitals in rural and remote areas (Gausche-Hill et al., 2004; 2002 NHAMCS data, calculations by IOM staff). Many of those hospitals lack around-the-clock physician coverage, have relatively few pediatric visits, and lack a separate pediatric inpatient ward. Having a low volume of pediatric patients, lacking a separate pediatric ward, and being located in a rural area are hospital characteristics independently associated with lower levels of preparedness for pediatric ED patients (Gausche-Hill et al., 2004; Middleton and Burt, 2006).

While children make nearly 30 percent of all ED visits, their use of prehospital services is relatively limited (see Figure 1-2); in fact, children represent only 5–10 percent of all EMS calls (Seidel et al., 1984; Federiuk et al., 1993). The low proportion of pediatric EMS volume represents a

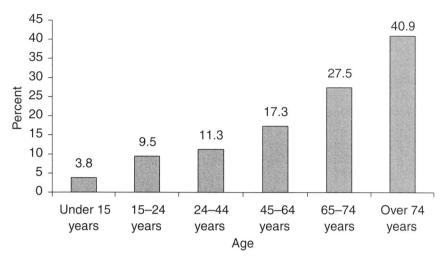

FIGURE 1-2 Percentage of patients that arrive at the emergency department by ambulance.
SOURCE: McCaig, 2005.

challenge because it is difficult for EMTs to maintain pediatric skills when they encounter critically ill or injured pediatric patients so infrequently. In contrast to the situation with adults, about half of prehospital calls for children are for injuries, the other half for medical problems (Seidel et al., 1991). Similar to ED visits, medical complaints are more common in children under 5, while older children are more likely to be transported for injuries (Sapien et al., 1999). While the majority of pediatric EMS transports are appropriate (Foltin et al., 1998), many are medically unnecessary (Camasso-Richardson et al., 1997; Kost and Arruda, 1999; Hamilton et al., 2003).

NEED FOR A SEPARATE REPORT
ON PEDIATRIC EMERGENCY CARE

The statement "children are not little adults" is often used to convey the fact that children have unique medical needs relative to adults. In fact, the anatomical, physiological, developmental, and emotional attributes of children impact not only their susceptibility to illness and injury, but also the ways in which providers need to assess and treat them (see Table 1-1). Caring for sick and injured children requires that providers have specialized training and skills, as well as access to specialized equipment and supplies. However, the initial development of the nation's emergency system largely

TABLE 1-1 Examples of Differences Between Children and Adults and Implications for Care

	Pediatric Characteristic	Implications for Illness and Injury	Implications for Care
Anatomical Differences	Greater surface area relative to body volume.	Greater risk of excessive loss of heat and fluids; children are affected more quickly and easily by toxins that are absorbed through the skin.	Increased body surface area makes children more susceptible to greater heat loss when they are exposed during resuscitation; the higher percentage of body surface area devoted to the head relative to the lower extremities must be taken into account when determining the percentage of body surface area involved in burn injuries.
	Smaller airways; tongue is large relative to the oropharynx; larynx is higher and more anterior in the neck; vocal cords are at a more anterocaudal angle; epiglottis is soft and shaped differently from that in adults.	A right main stem intubation can lead to iatrogenic complications; more susceptible to respiratory distress due to airway swelling from infection or inflammation.	Special equipment and training are needed for intubation; appropriately sized endotracheal intubation tubes, stylettes, and laryngoscope blades are necessary. A child's airway is more difficult to maintain and intubate. Children are at higher risk for a right mainstem bronchus intubation.
	Less protective muscle around internal organs.	Internal organs are more susceptible to traumatic forces.	Recognition of internal injury requires a high degree of suspicion, and such injury should not be ruled out based on the absence of external signs of trauma.
	Small size.	More vulnerable to exposure and toxicity from agents that are heavier than air, such as sarin gas and chlorine, and that accumulate closer to the ground.	

continued

TABLE 1-1 Continued

	Pediatric Characteristic	Implications for Illness and Injury	Implications for Care
	Less fat, less elastic connective tissue, and closer proximity of chest and abdominal organs.	Higher frequency of multiple organ injury.	
	Head is proportionally larger and heavier in children.	Head injury is common in young children.	Head size also makes children more susceptible to greater heat loss when they are exposed during resuscitation.
	More pliable skeleton; thoracic cage of a child does not provide as much protection of organs as that of adults.	More susceptible to fracture and other injuries from blunt trauma.	Orthopedic injuries with subtle symptoms are easily missed; hepatic or splenic injuries can go unrecognized and produce significant blood loss, leading to shock.
Physiological Differences	Respiratory and heart rates vary with age.	More susceptible to air pollutants.	Knowledge of normal and abnormal rates based on age is required; normal vital signs differ for children and adults. An increased heart rate is often the first sign of shock in a pediatric patient, versus blood pressure in an adult. Children maintain heart rate during the early phases of hypovolemic shock, creating a false impression of normalcy.
	Higher metabolic rates.	More susceptible to contaminants in food or water; greater risk for increased loss of water when ill or stressed.	Medication doses must be carefully calculated based on the child's weight and body size.

TABLE 1-1 Continued

	Pediatric Characteristic	Implications for Illness and Injury	Implications for Care
	Lower blood pressure levels than adults; levels vary with age.		Indicators of serious illness may not appear until the child is near collapse. Vital signs are less reliable indicators of serious illness than in adults. Respiratory arrest is more common than cardiac arrest; cardiopulmonary arrest is signaled by respiratory arrest or shock, rather than by cardiac arrhythmias.
	Immature immunological systems.	Greater risk of infection; less herd immunity from infections such as smallpox.	
Developmental Differences	Communication barriers may exist in all pediatric age groups, but the nature of the barrier varies by age (infants and young children cannot articulate symptoms).		Assessment tools need to be tailored to reflect age-appropriate responses.
Emotional Differences	Greater, varying emotional needs based on developmental level.		Need for family-centered policies and a family-friendly environment in EDs. Depending on age, children require or prefer the presence of a parent during treatment.
	Higher sensitivity to environmental factors during treatment.	Age and developmental level of child, characteristics of event, and parental reactions play significant roles in determining the child's reactions and recovery.	Providers must manage the mental health needs of pediatric patients and parents' reactions.

overlooked the unique needs of children. The system was originally directed by physicians trained in adult medical specialties, many of whom had little experience with pediatric patients and the unique features of pediatric care. As a result, pediatric emergency care did not advance as quickly as adult emergency care, and performance and outcomes for children trailed those for adults (Seidel et al., 1984; Mishark et al., 1992; Boswell et al., 1995; Doran et al., 1995).

The committee's vision for the future, outlined in Chapter 3 of this report, is that of a fully integrated emergency care system that appropriately meets the needs of both adult and pediatric patients. Under this system, pediatric concerns are included in all aspects of emergency care planning, research, and evaluation. The committee's hope is that a separate report outlining basic shortcomings in the emergency care system's ability to meet the needs of pediatric patients will not be necessary in the future. Today, however, the key shortcomings reviewed below stand as impediments to the future system envisioned by the committee, and must be acknowledged and addressed if that vision is to be realized.

System Planning

No organization or individual is responsible for overseeing the operation or ensuring the quality of the nation's emergency care system. At the federal and state levels, the current system is largely fragmented and uncoordinated. This fragmentation is a particularly critical problem for pediatric emergency care because EMS agencies and hospitals tend to vary in capability, commitment, and training standards for pediatric emergency care. In many states, hospitals are not categorized according to their ability to care for critically ill and injured children. In the absence of such categorization, it is difficult for EMTs, much less parents, to identify which hospitals are most appropriate for a critically ill or injured child. Another example of the lack of planning is the absence of transfer agreements between hospitals (Middleton and Burt, 2006).

Provider Training

Table 1-1 shows some examples of the specialized pediatric knowledge required of emergency care providers when they encounter a sick or injured child. Emergency care providers who lack pediatric training, experience, and treatment protocols may find it difficult to distinguish a critically ill or injured child from other children with less serious conditions. They may also have difficulty determining the proper course of treatment or deciding whether a higher level of care is needed. It is not surprising that emergency

providers generally feel more stress and anxiety caring for pediatric patients than for adults (Federiuk et al., 1993; Glaeser et al., 2000; Frush and
Hohenhaus, 2004). Despite its importance, many emergency physicians
have little formal training in pediatric emergency medicine (Moorhead et al.,
2002). Additionally, studies have shown that knowledge and skills gained
through education and training deteriorate fairly quickly if not practiced
and reinforced regularly. Yet continuing education requirements in pediatrics for EMTs vary from community to community and do not exist in many
areas (Glaeser et al., 2000).

Disaster Preparedness

Children suffer disproportionately in the event of a disaster. For example, they are more vulnerable to a biological or chemical attack because
they take more breaths per minute, and their breathing zone is closer to
the ground. They also have thinner skin, which provides less protection
and allows greater absorption of chemicals (AAP, 2002). Moreover, some
antidotes available for the treatment of adults in the event of such an attack are not currently available for children (Markenson, 2005). Children
are often more vulnerable to biological agents, as well as naturally occurring diseases, that produce vomiting and/or diarrhea because they have less
fluid reserve than adults and can become dehydrated more rapidly (Illinois
EMS-C, 2005). If children sustain burns, they have a greater likelihood of
life-threatening fluid loss and susceptibility to infection (Shannon, 2004).
If they sustain injuries that cause massive blood loss, they develop irreversible shock more quickly (AAP, 2002). Additionally, children are dependent
on adults for everyday care; in the event that they are separated from their
caregiver(s) in a disaster, they lose their support system.

As noted above, initial efforts at disaster planning did not incorporate
the needs of children. Even today, many states do not address pediatric issues in their disaster plans (NASEMSD, 2004), and disaster drills frequently
lack a realistic pediatric component (Mace and Bern, 2004; Dick et al.,
2004; Maniece-Harrison, 2005). As a result, most communities are not
as prepared as they should be for pediatric care in the event of a disaster.
Moreover, local disaster plans often fail to address specific pediatric needs
in the event of mass decontamination, sheltering, or evacuation.

Research Base

Pediatric emergency care is a relatively young field, so its research base
is limited. Some significant advances have occurred in the research infrastructure in the field, including the development of a Pediatric Emergency

Care Applied Research Network (PECARN) and two national databases (National Hospital Ambulatory Medical Care Survey and Healthcare Cost and Utilization Project) that allow for analyses of pediatric emergency care in the ED. Nonetheless, many of the triage methods, treatment patterns, and prevention initiatives used for pediatric populations in the EMS and ED environments are not supported by scientific evidence. Additionally, little is known about patient outcomes and system performance. In the case of prehospital care, the knowledge gap is even greater. Some of the most basic questions, including how many children are served by the EMS system and what services are provided to pediatric patients, remain unanswered.

Quality of Care

Haste, uncertainty, and interruptions abound in the EMS and ED environments, increasing the risk of errors and adverse events for patients of all ages. Delivering care to children presents added challenges to quality care delivery: some children are preverbal and cannot self-report their symptoms; many children have multiple caregivers, which increases the likelihood that emergency care providers will be given an incomplete, inaccurate, or conflicting medical and medication history; and children are likely to be accompanied by parents suffering from great anxiety, which requires staff to attend to the parents while also staying focused on the needs of the child (Chamberlain et al., 2004).

Providing high-quality emergency care services to children requires an infrastructure designed to support care to pediatric patients. However, many of the advances made in emergency care have not been appropriate or well designed for pediatric emergency care. For example, studies to determine the safety and efficacy of emergency care medications for children are rarely conducted; thus, as noted above, medication is often prescribed for children off label (Rapkin, 1999). New medical technologies often are not designed with children in mind, but nevertheless are used on pediatric patients, sometimes with unintended consequences. One example is the infusion pump, which delivers medications and fluids intravenously; the original design of the pumps contributed to pediatric dosing errors (Reves, 2003). Information systems and provider decision-support systems that lack pediatric dosing information or those that prohibit providers from entering data on a scale small enough for children are of little benefit to pediatric patients. Additionally, despite the clear evidence on the effectiveness of family-centered care, an approach to health care delivery that promotes the inclusion of family members in the child's care, many EMS agencies and EDs lack policies that support and implement such approaches to care in emergency settings (Loyacono, 2001; MacLean et al., 2003).

STUDY OBJECTIVES AND FRAMEWORK

The IOM's study of the future of emergency care in the U.S. health system was initiated in September 2003. Support for the study was provided by the Josiah Macy, Jr. Foundation, the National Highway Traffic Safety Administration (NHTSA), AHRQ within the U.S. Department of Health and Human Services (DHHS), the Centers for Disease Control and Prevention (CDC), and the Health Resources and Services Administration (HRSA). The study was designed to build on previous work in the field by bringing together all of the key components of emergency care—prehospital EMS, hospital-based emergency care, trauma care, and injury prevention and control. The committee was charged with assessing the current emergency care system, identifying its strengths and weaknesses, creating a vision for the future system, and making policy recommendations for achieving that vision.

The committee was structured to balance the desire for a highly integrated systems approach to the study with an interest in focusing attention on pediatric, EMS, and hospital-based emergency care issues. The result was a main committee and three subcommittees representing those three focus areas (see Figure 1-3).

The main committee guided the overall study process. The three subcommittees examined the unique challenges associated with the provision of emergency services to children, issues related to prehospital EMS, and issues related to hospital-based emergency and trauma care. The charge to the pediatric subcommittee is shown in Box 1-1. The membership of the main committee and subcommittees overlapped—the 11-member pediatric subcommittee, for example, included 5 members from the main committee. Subcommittees met both separately, reporting their discussions and findings to the main committee, and in combined session with the main committee. Altogether, 40 individuals served on one or more of the four committees.[1] See Appendixes A and B, respectively, for a listing of all committee and subcommittee members and for biographical information on members of the main committee and the subcommittee on pediatric emergency care. Three reports covering each of the three subject areas were developed. The present report presents the committee's findings with regard to pediatric emergency care. The recommendations from all three reports appear in Appendix E.

A total of 17 main committee and subcommittee meetings were held between February 2004 and October 2005. The committee commissioned 11 technical papers (see Appendix D) and heard testimony from a wide

---

[1]One committee member, Henri R. Manasse, Jr., resigned from the original 41-member body during the course of the study.

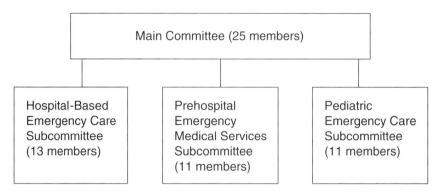

FIGURE 1-3 Committee and subcommittee structure.

range of experts (see Appendix C). Staff and committee members met with a variety of stakeholders and interested individuals, conducted site visits, and participated in public meetings sponsored by stakeholder groups and the study sponsors.

BOX 1-1
Subcommittee on Pediatric Emergency Care Services:
Statement of Task

The objectives of this study are to: (1) examine the emergency care system in the United States; (2) explore its strengths, limitations, and future challenges; (3) describe a desired vision of the emergency care system; and (4) recommend strategies required to achieve that vision. In this context, the Subcommittee on Pediatric Emergency Care Services will examine the unique challenges associated with the provision of emergency services to children and families, and evaluate progress since the publication of *Emergency Medical Services for Children* (IOM, 1993). The subcommittee will consider:

- the role of pediatric emergency services as an integrated component of the overall health system;
- system-wide pediatric emergency care planning, preparedness, coordination, and funding;
- embedded pediatric training in professional education; and
- health services and clinical research.

KEY TERMS AND DEFINITIONS

To ensure clarity and consistency, the following terminology is used throughout this study's three reports. *Emergency medical services*, or *EMS*, denotes prehospital emergency medical services, such as 9-1-1 and dispatch, emergency medical response, field triage and stabilization, and transport by ambulance or helicopter to a hospital or between facilities. *EMS system* refers to the organized delivery system for EMS within a specified geographic area—local, regional, state, or national—as indicated by the context.

Emergency care is broader than *EMS*, and encompasses the services involved in emergency medical care, including EMS, hospital-based ED and trauma care, and on-call specialty care. *Emergency care system* refers to the organized delivery system for emergency care within a specified geographic area. It is important to note that the committee's definitions of emergency care and the emergency care system may be narrower than other definitions, such as those used by the federal Emergency Medical Services for Children (EMS-C) program, which also encompass injury prevention and rehabilitation services.

Trauma care is the care received by a victim of trauma in any setting, while a *trauma center* is a hospital specifically designated to provide trauma care; some trauma care is provided in settings other than a trauma center. *Trauma system* refers to the organized delivery system for trauma care at the local, regional, state, or national level. Because trauma care is an essential component of emergency care, it is always assumed to be encompassed by the terms *hospital-based* or *inpatient emergency care*, *emergency care system*, and *regional emergency care system*.

The term *pediatric emergency medical services* denotes prehospital care for children, while *pediatric emergency care* refers to the full continuum of services involved in emergency medical care for children. Note that the terms *emergency medical services for children* are used only in reference to the EMS-C program.

From a development perspective, there is no precise age at which childhood ends and adulthood begins. EMS agencies and hospitals use different age ranges to define pediatric patients. For the purposes of this report, however, a *child* is someone aged 18 or younger, while an *infant* is a child who is under age 1.

ORGANIZATION OF THE REPORT

This report presents the committee's findings and recommendations regarding pediatric emergency care.

Chapter 2 provides a brief history of the development of pediatric emergency care, as well as a look at the state of emergency care for children in 2006. The chapter examines some of the threats to children's health, as well as children's use of emergency care services. It also looks at the quality of those services and some of the funding challenges associated with delivering pediatric emergency care.

Chapter 3 sets forth the committee's vision for the emergency care system of the future, which encompasses three goals: improving the coordination of emergency care, expanding regionalization of emergency care services, and introducing accountability into the system. The chapter also offers a number of recommendations for achieving this vision.

Chapter 4 examines workforce issues. It describes the training that emergency care workers receive in pediatric emergency care and notes deficiencies. The importance of skill maintenance is emphasized since, as noted above, many emergency providers encounter critically ill or injured children infrequently.

Chapter 5 reviews the threats to pediatric patient safety in the prehospital and ED environments and the resources needed to address some of those threats. The chapter also describes new initiatives in pediatric emergency care, such as the promotion of family-centered approaches and the development of information technologies and medical devices designed with the needs of children in mind.

Chapter 6 addresses a particularly timely topic—the special needs of children in the event of a disaster. The discussion includes a look at children's medical and nonmedical needs after a major disaster, such as Hurricane Katrina, and suggests areas in which federal agencies and regional authorities could direct their attention to meet those needs.

Finally, Chapter 7 focuses on research needs in pediatric emergency care. It reviews the progress the field has made to increase its research base and suggests the steps that should be taken to expand that base.

REFERENCES

AAP (American Academy of Pediatrics). 2002. *The Youngest Victims: Disaster Preparedness to Meet the Needs of Children.* Washington, DC: AAP.

Boswell W, McElveen N, Sharp M, Boyd CR, Frantz EI. 1995. Analysis of prehospital pediatric and adult intubation. *Air Medical Journal* 14:125–127.

Brown J, Klein E, Lewis C, Johnston B, Cummings P. 2003. Emergency department analgesia for fracture pain. *Annals of Emergency Medicine* 42(2):197–205.

Camasso-Richardson K, Wilde J, Petrack E. 1997. Medically unnecessary pediatric ambulance transports: A medical taxi service? *Academic Emergency Medicine* 4(12):1137–1141.

Chamberlain J, Slonim A, Joseph J. 2004. Reducing errors and promoting safety in pediatric emergency care. *Ambulatory Pediatrics* 4(1):55–63.

Davis DH, Localio AR, Stafford PW, Helfaer MA, Durbin DR. 2005. Trends in operative management of pediatric splenic injury in a regional trauma system. *Pediatrics* 115(1):89–94.

Densmore JC, Lim HJ, Oldham KT, Guice KS. 2006. Outcomes and delivery of care in pediatric injury. *Journal of Pediatric Surgery* 41(1):92–98.

Dick RM, Liggin R, Shirm SW, Graham J. 2004. EMS preparedness for mass casualty events involving children. *Academic Emergency Medicine* 11(5):559.

Doran JV, Tortella BJ, Drivet WJ, Lavery RF. 1995. Factors influencing successful intubation in the prehospital setting. *Prehospital and Disaster Medicine* 10(4):259–264.

Fairbanks T. 2004. *Human Factors and Patient Safety in Emergency Medical Services. Science Forum on Patient Safety and Human Factors Research.* Rochester, NY: University of Rochester.

Federiuk CS, O'Brien K, Jui J, Schmidt TA. 1993. Job satisfaction of paramedics: The effects of gender and type of agency of employment. *Annals of Emergency Medicine* 22(4):657–662.

Foltin G, Pon S, Tunik M, Fierman A, Dreyer B, Cooper A, Welborne, Treiber M. 1998. Pediatric ambulance utilization in a large American city: A systems analysis approach. *Pediatric Emergency Care* 14(4):453–454.

Frush K, Hohenhaus S. 2004. *Enhancing Pediatric Patient Safety Grant.* Durham, NC: Duke University Health System.

Gausche M, Tadeo R, Zane M, Lewis R. 1998. Out-of-hospital intravenous access: Unnecessary procedures and excessive cost. *Academic Emergency Medicine* 5(9):878–882.

Gausche-Hill M, Lewis R, Schmitz C. 2004. *Survey of U.S. Emergency Departments for Pediatric Preparedness: Implementation and Evaluation of Care of Children in the Emergency Department: Guidelines for Preparedness.* Unpublished results.

Glaeser P, Linzer J, Tunik M, Henderson D, Ball J. 2000. Survey of nationally registered emergency medical services providers: Pediatric education. *Annals of Emergency Medicine* 36(1):33–38.

Glaser NS, Kuppermann N, Yee CK, Schwartz DL, Styne DM. 1997. Variation in the management of pediatric diabetic ketoacidosis by specialty training. *Archives of Pediatrics & Adolescent Medicine* 151(11):1125–1132.

Hamilton S, Adler M, Walker A. 2003. Pediatric calls: Lessons learned from pediatric research. *JEMS: Journal of Emergency Medical Services* 28(7):56–63.

Hampers LC, Faries SG. 2002. Practice variation in the emergency management of croup. *Pediatrics* 109(3):505–508.

Harris Interactive. 2004. *Trauma Care: Public's Knowledge and Perception of Importance.* Rochester, NY: The Coalition for American Trauma Care.

Hubble MW, Paschal KR. 2000. Medication calculation skills of practicing paramedics. *Prehospital Emergency Care* 4(3):253–260.

Hunt EA, Hohenhaus SM, Luo X, Frush KS. 2006. Simulation of pediatric trauma stabilization in 35 North Carolina emergency departments: Identification of targets for performance improvement. *Pediatrics* 117(3):641–648.

Illinois EMS-C (Illinois Emergency Medical Services for Children). 2005. *Pediatric Disaster Preparedness Guidelines.* Chicago, IL: Illinois Department of Public Health and Loyola University Medical Center.

IOM (Institute of Medicine). 1993. *Emergency Medical Services for Children.* Washington, DC: National Academy Press.

Isaacman DJ, Kaminer K, Veligeti H, Jones M, Davis P, Mason JD. 2001. Comparative practice patterns of emergency medicine physicians and pediatric emergency medicine physicians managing fever in young children. *Pediatrics* 108(2):354–358.

Kost S, Arruda J. 1999. Appropriateness of ambulance transportation to a suburban pediatric emergency department. *Prehospital Emergency Care* 3(3):187–190.

Kozer E, Scolnik D, Macpherson A, Keays T, Shi K, Luk T, Koren G. 2002. Variables associated with medication errors in pediatric emergency medicine. *Pediatrics* 110(4):737.

Kunen S, Hume P, Perret JN, Mandry CV, Patterson TR. 2003. Underdiagnosis of child abuse in emergency departments. *Academic Emergency Medicine* 10(5):546-a.

Loyacono TR. 2001. Family-centered prehospital care. *Emergency Medical Services* 30(6):83.

Mace SE, Bern A. 2004. Needs assessment of current pediatric guidelines for use by disaster medical assistance team members in response to disaster and shelter care. *Annals of Emergency Medicine* 44(4):S35.

MacLean S, Guzzetta C, White C, Fontaine D, Eichhorn D, Meyers T, Desy P. 2003. Family presence during cardiopulmonary resuscitation and invasive procedures: Practices of critical care and emergency nurses. *Journal of Emergency Nursing* 29(3):208–221.

Maniece-Harrison B. 2005. *Training.* Unpublished document of the National Advisory Committee on Children and Terrorism. [Online]. Available: http://www.bt.cdc.gov/children/word/working/training.doc [accessed October 2005].

Marcin JP, Seifert L, Cho M, Cole SL, Romano PS. 2005. *Medication Errors among Acutely Ill and Injured Children Presenting to Rural Emergency Departments.* Presentation at the Pediatric Academic Societies Meeting, Washington, DC.

Markenson D. 2005. *Model Pediatric Components for State Disaster Plans and Additional Resources.* Presentation at the 2005 EMSC Annual Grantee Meeting, Washington, DC. Maternal and Child Health Bureau.

McCaig LF, Burt CW. 2005. *National Hospital Ambulatory Medical Care Survey: 2003 Emergency Department Summary.* Hyattsville, MD: National Center for Health Statistics.

Middleton KR, Burt CW. 2006. *Availability of Pediatric Services and Equipment in Emergency Departments: United States, 2002-03.* Hyattsville, MD: National Center for Health Statistics.

Mishark KJ, Vukov LF, Gudgell SF. 1992. Airway management and air medical transport. *The Journal of Air Medical Transport* 11(3):7–9.

Moorhead JC, Gallery ME, Hirshkorn C, Barnaby DP, Barsan WG, Conrad LC, Dalsey WC, Fried M, Herman SH, Hogan P, Mannle TE, Packard DC, Perina DG, Pollack CV Jr, Rapp MT, Rorrie CC Jr, Schafermeyer RW. 2002. A study of the workforce in emergency medicine: 1999. *Annals of Emergency Medicine* 40(1):3–15.

NACHRI (National Association of Children's Hospitals and Related Institutions). 2005. *FAQs on Children's Hospitals.* [Online]. Available: http://www.childrenshospitals.net/Template.cfm?Section=FAQs_on_Childrens_Hospitals&Template=/TaggedPage/TaggedPageDisplay.cfm&TPLID=91&ContentID=14286 [accessed December 6, 2005].

NAS, NRC (National Academy of Sciences, National Research Council). 1966. *Accidental Death and Disability: The Neglected Disease of Modern Society.* Washington, DC: National Academy of Sciences.

NAS, NRC. 1978. *Emergency Medical Services at Midpassage.* Washington, DC: National Academy of Sciences.

NASEMSD (National Association of State EMS Directors). 2004. *Pediatric Disaster and Terrorism Preparedness.* Falls Church, VA: NASEMSD.

National Center for Health Statistics. 2005. *Health, United States, 2005 with Chartbook on Trends in the Health of Americans.* Hyattsville, MD: Public Health Service.

Orr RA, Han YY, Roth K. 2006. Pediatric transport: Shifting the paradigm to improve patient outcome. In: Fuhrman B, Zimmerman J, eds. *Pediatric Critical Care* (3rd edition). Mosby, Elsevier Science Health. Pp. 141–150.

Petrack EM, Christopher NC. 1997. Pain management in the emergency department: Patterns of analgesic utilization. *Pediatrics* 99(5):711.

Rapkin K. 1999. Pediatric "off-label" prescribing: What every APN should know. *The Internet Journal of Advanced Nurse Practice* 3(1).

Reves JG. 2003. "Smart pump" technology reduces errors. *Anesthesia Patient Safety Foundation* 18(1).

Saade DN, Simon HK, Greenwald M. 2002. Abused children: Missed opportunities for recognition in the ED. *Academic Emergency Medicine* 9(5):524.

Sapien RE, Fullerton L, Olson LM, Broxterman KJ, Sklar DP. 1999. Disturbing trends: The epidemiology of pediatric emergency medical services use. *Academic Emergency Medicine* 6(3):232–238.

Seidel JS, Hornbein M, Yoshiyama K, Kuznets D, Finklestein JZ, St Geme JW Jr. 1984. Emergency medical services and the pediatric patient: Are the needs being met? *Pediatrics* 73(6):769–772.

Seidel JS, Henderson DP, Ward P, Wayland BW, Ness B. 1991. Pediatric prehospital care in urban and rural areas. *Pediatrics* 88(4):681.

Selbst SM, Fein JA, Osterhoudt K, Ho W. 1999. Medication errors in a pediatric emergency department. *Pediatric Emergency Care* 15(1):1–4.

Shannon M. 2004. *Addressing Pediatric and School-based Surge Capacity in a Mass Casualty Event*. Rockville, MD: AHRQ.

Su E, Mann NC, McCall M, Hedges JR. 1997. Use of resuscitation skills by paramedics caring for critically injured children in Oregon. *Prehospital Emergency Care* 1(3):123–127.

Su E, Schmidt TA, Mann NC, Zechnich AD. 2000. A randomized controlled trial to assess decay in acquired knowledge among paramedics completing a pediatric resuscitation course. *Academic Emergency Medicine* 7(7):779–786.

Trokel M, Wadimmba A, Griffith J, Sege R. 2006. Variation in the diagnosis of child abuse in severely injured infants. *Pediatrics* 117(3):722–728.

Wolfram RW, Warren CM, Doyle CR, Kerns R, Frye S. 2003. Retention of pediatric advanced life support (PALS) course concepts. *Journal of Emergency Medicine* 25(4):475–479.

2

History and Current State
of Pediatric Emergency Care

Before setting forth a vision for emergency care in the future, it is important to understand the system that exists today and how it evolved. This chapter describes the development and current state of the emergency care system with respect to children.

The first part of the chapter provides a historical overview of pediatric emergency care. The field is surprisingly young and has trailed the development of the broader emergency care system by a decade or two. In this review, attention is focused on two important topics: (1) the creation, activities, and achievements of the Emergency Medical Services for Children (EMS-C) program, a federal program that aims to ensure essential emergency medical care for ill or injured children and adolescents, and (2) the 1993 Institute of Medicine (IOM) report *Emergency Medical Services for Children*, which represented the first comprehensive look at the need for and effectiveness of pediatric emergency care services in the United States. An understanding of the development of pediatric emergency care provides a sense of progress, as well as greater insight into the system's resources, challenges, successes, and failures. In fact, many of the challenges facing the system today are the same ones that existed more than a decade ago.

The second part of the chapter focuses in detail on pediatric emergency care in 2006. It begins with an overview of illness and injury in children based on the most recent national data available. This is followed by a discussion of trends in emergency care use by children.

The chapter continues with an assessment of how well the emergency care system works today. The committee concludes that while considerable progress has been made over the past two decades, the system falls short of consistently providing quality emergency care to children, and that continued efforts are needed to address its deficiencies.

The chapter concludes with a look at the financing of pediatric emergency care services. This review highlights a number of issues surrounding reimbursement for pediatric services and/or reimbursement at children's hospitals that have become a growing problem for some providers.

DEVELOPMENT OF EMERGENCY CARE FOR CHILDREN

1940s–1960s: The Beginning of the Modern Emergency Care System

The modern emergency room developed at a time when the specialization of medical practice swept the nation after World War II. As the number of house calls from general physicians declined, patients increasingly turned to the local hospital for treatment. This trend was reinforced by the development of private insurance plans, which geared payments toward hospitals and away from home visits (Rosen, 1995). The development of the emergency room also reflects the passage of the Hill-Burton Act of 1946, which gave states federal grants to build hospitals provided that the states met a variety of conditions, including a community service obligation. Among other things, the community service obligation required hospitals that received the federal funding to maintain an emergency room. This requirement applies to the vast majority of nonprofit U.S. hospitals in operation today (Rosenblatt et al., 2001).

Emergency care as a field advanced as the result of several forces that drew attention to emergency care in the 1950s and 1960s. One was new knowledge about the value of prompt prehospital treatment and transport derived from military experience in Korea. During that conflict, technical innovations such as the creation of battalion aid stations and rapid transport by helicopter to mobile field hospitals were introduced and resulted in dramatically improved survival rates for battle-wounded soldiers. Experience in Vietnam led to advances in trauma care. Surgeons returning to the United States from Korea and Vietnam recognized that the systems developed by the Army for triage, transport, and field surgery could surpass anything available to civilians at home (Rosen, 1995), and they believed that similar innovations could and should be applied to civilian care. Around the same time, advances in cardiac care, such as the creation of "mobile coronary care units," improved the survival rate of patients prior to reaching the hospital (Pantridge and Geddes, 1967).

Another major turning point was the publication of the landmark National Academy of Sciences (NAS)/National Research Council (NRC) report *Accidental Death and Disability: The Neglected Disease of Modern Society* in 1966 (NAS and NRC, 1966). The report described the epidemic of injuries and deaths from automobile crashes and other causes in the United States and lamented the deplorable system for treating those injuries nationwide. In 1966, prehospital and hospital services were largely inadequate or nonexistent. Although a few communities were providing ambulance services through their fire or police departments, it is estimated that morticians provided about half of such services. No specific training was required for ambulance attendants. Most emergency rooms could offer only advanced first aid, and only a few hospitals appeared to have the infrastructure necessary to provide complete care for the critically ill and injured.

The 1970s: Rapid Development of EMS Systems

The 1966 NAS/NRC report stimulated a flood of public and private initiatives designed to enhance highway safety and improve the medical response to accidental injuries. These initiatives included the development of the national trauma system, the creation of the specialty of emergency medicine, and the establishment of federal programs to enhance the nation's emergency care infrastructure and research base. Perhaps most significant was passage of the Emergency Medical Services Systems (EMSS) Act of 1973 (P.L. 93-154), which created a categorical grant program that led to the nationwide development of about 300 regional EMS systems (IOM, 1993). Despite these achievements, the need to treat pediatric emergencies in a unique way was not fully appreciated at the time. The EMSS Act led to the development of systems that were focused primarily on adult trauma and adult cardiac care. Specialized pediatric needs received little attention; indeed, only limited expertise in pediatric emergency medicine existed (Foltin and Fuchs, 1991).

Nonetheless, some initial efforts were made in the 1970s in certain geographic areas to incorporate the needs of children into emergency medicine and EMS systems. Dedicated pediatric emergency departments (EDs) began to develop, staffed by pediatricians who were willing to devote their full attention to emergency care. Also, some hospitals established pediatric intensive care units (PICUs) and began conducting research on pediatric emergency care. In 1975, Maryland established a regional pediatric trauma center, one of the first in the country. Physicians in Los Angeles, along with local professional societies and the county EMS agency, developed a pediatric-focused training curriculum for paramedics and management guidelines for pediatric emergency care (IOM, 1993). The level of sophistication of emergency rooms generally improved during this time, and the term shifted from "emergency room" to "emergency department" as emergency services began to constitute a full department within hospitals.

The 1980s: Pediatric Emergency Care in Its Infancy

The burgeoning EMS system suffered a setback in 1981 when Congress passed legislation that indirectly resulted in a sharp loss of funding for state EMS activities. Categorical federal funding that had been dedicated to EMS was replaced by the Preventive Health and Health Services Block Grant, which essentially shifted responsibility for EMS from the federal to the state level. Because the states were given greater discretion regarding the use of funds and EMS was a relative newcomer without a significant political constituency, most states chose to spend the money in other areas of need. The immediate impact of the shift to block grants was a considerable reduction in total funding allocated to EMS (Office of Technology Assessment, 1989).

Conversely, attention to pediatric emergency care grew dramatically throughout the 1980s as initial data on this domain of care became available. For example, studies indicated that children represented about 10 percent of all ambulance runs (Seidel et al., 1984); that young children were likely to suffer from respiratory distress, whereas older children were likely to need trauma care (Fifield et al., 1984); and that up to half of pediatric deaths due to trauma might be preventable (Ramenofsky et al., 1984). Studies also indicated that children's outcomes, given the same severity of injury, tended to be worse than those of adults (Seidel et al., 1984; Seidel, 1986a). For example, a study of 88 general acute care hospitals in Los Angeles County found nearly twice as many deaths among children with serious traumatic injuries as among adults with similar injuries (Seidel et al., 1984). Most of the deaths occurred in areas lacking pediatric tertiary care centers. The studies also revealed that prehospital personnel generally had little training in pediatric care. Also, most lacked the equipment needed to treat children (Seidel, 1986b).

Findings of these early studies led to recognition of the need to address pediatric emergency care and of the existence of a distinct body of knowledge that should be applied in so doing. This recognition stimulated action on several fronts. First, there were advances in resources for care. In the 1980s, several cities designated pediatric trauma centers. Advocates for pediatric emergency care in Los Angeles developed a new two-tiered approach for organizing such care. Under this system, seriously ill or injured children were to be treated only at hospitals that had been certified as meeting a certain set of requirements and capabilities for pediatric care. Perhaps the most significant development for pediatric emergency care was the establishment in 1984 of the federal EMS-C program, a grant program that assists states in addressing pediatric deficiencies within their emergency care systems. The first federal funding for EMS-C was made available in 1985, and later appropriation acts continued to increase funding for the program. The EMS-C program is discussed in detail later in the chapter.

Second, there were advances in resources for information. In the early 1980s, the U.S. Department of Education, through the National Institute of Disability and Rehabilitation Research, funded the development of the National Pediatric Trauma Registry. The registry enabled researchers to identify the demographics of pediatric trauma. Data from the registry revealed that automobile crashes were the primary source of pediatric trauma, that injuries were most often blunt, and that an injured child stood a 3 percent chance of dying from trauma. Data from the registry were also used to develop the Pediatric Trauma Score, a system used to help EMTs determine the facility to which an injured child should be transported (Harris, 1987).

Third, professional societies began to give greater attention to pediatric emergency care. In the late 1970s, pediatricians who worked in EDs began to discuss issues in pediatric emergency care; the result was the formation of a section on pediatric emergency medicine within the American Academy of Pediatrics (AAP) in 1981 (Pena and Snyder, 1995; AAP, 2000). In 1983, the American College of Emergency Physicians (ACEP) held an interspecialty conference on childhood emergencies that led to the establishment of a joint AAP/ACEP Task Force on Pediatric Emergency Medicine the following year (AAP, 2000). ACEP also formed a member section on pediatric emergency medicine in 1998 (Pena and Snyder, 1995). In 1985, a Provisional Committee on Pediatric Emergency Medicine was created within AAP; it became a full committee in 1998 (AAP, 2000). Both the Emergency Nurses Association (ENA) and the National Association of EMS Physicians (NAEMSP) had established pediatric sections by the end of the 1980s (IOM, 1993).

Fourth, there were important advances in pediatric emergency medicine. By the early 1980s, many physicians had recognized that emergency care for children was not as well advanced as that for adults and that specialized resources for the training of providers in pediatric emergency care was needed. The longest-running pediatric emergency medicine fellowship was established in 1980 (Pena and Snyder, 1995; Macias, 2005). Early experts in the field began to synthesize knowledge in the area and make it more widely available. The first pediatric emergency care textbook was published in 1983, and the first journal devoted to pediatric emergency care was launched in 1985.

A number of training courses were developed as well. In 1988, the American Heart Association and the AAP initiated the Pediatric Advanced Life Support (PALS) course. The AAP and ACEP joint task force developed and sponsored the Advanced Pediatric Life Support (APLS) manual, published in 1989. Some courses were also developed locally. An example is the Pediatric Emergency Medical Services Training Program (PEMSTP) at Children's National Medical Center in Washington, D.C., which prepared EMT instructors to teach pediatric aspects of emergency care. Progress continued in the early 1990s when the ENA developed standardized training for emergency nurses with its Emergency Nursing Pediatric Course (ENPC). All of these efforts helped develop an emergency care workforce with enhanced pediatric skills.

Finally, injury prevention efforts, which had gained momentum in the 1970s, expanded greatly in the 1980s. The Poison Prevention Packaging Act of 1970 required manufacturers of toxic, corrosive, or irritative substances to use child-resistant closures (Harborview Injury Prevention and Research Center, 2006). The first state law requiring the use of child safety seats was enacted by Tennessee in 1978; by 1985, however, all states had passed such legislation (Traffic Safety Center, 2002). Additionally, state and local laws were passed to establish requirements for the installation of smoke detectors, window guards, and pool fencing. Concern about the prevention of injury and illness was reflected in national health promotion and disease prevention goals first published in 1980 and updated in 1990 and 2000 (DHHS, 1980, 1990, 2000). The 1985 IOM report *Injury in America* highlighted the heavy toll of injuries and called for more research in prevention and improved care. Much as the NAS/NRC report *Accidental Death and Disability* led to the passage of the EMSS Act of 1973, *Injury in America: A Continuing Health Problem* led to the creation of an injury prevention program at the Centers for Disease Control and Prevention (CDC), which later became CDC's National Center for Injury Prevention and Control (IOM, 1993).

Today, the incidence of sudden infant death syndrome (SIDS) and pediatric cardiac arrest has declined as parents have learned the proper sleep position for infants (AAP, 1992; Willinger, 1995). Injury prevention efforts, such as the poison prevention packaging law, bicycle helmet requirements, child passenger restraint requirements, smoke detector promotion programs, and drowning prevention programs, are beginning to decrease morbidity and mortality due to injury in children (Clarke and Walton, 1979; Rivara et al., 1997; Stenklyft, 1999; Haddix et al., 2001; Macpherson and MacArthur, 2002; Mittelstaedt and Simon, 2004). Many of these prevention efforts were spearheaded by programs such as the National Safe Kids Campaign, founded in 1987.

In addition to injury, prevention efforts targeted reducing pediatric illness. In 1980, for example, Starko and colleagues (1980) produced a study indicating that the use of aspirin may be associated with the onset of Reye's syndrome, a deadly disease most common in children that affects all organs of the body and occurs after a viral infection, such as the flu or chickenpox (National Institute of Neurological Disorders and Stroke, 2006). As parents learned of the link between aspirin and Reye's syndrome, there was a decline in both the use of children's aspirin and the number of Reye's syndrome cases reported to CDC (Arrowsmith et al., 1987; Belay et al., 1999).

Prevention efforts have successfully changed the scope of pediatric illness seen in the ED. For example, the *Hemophilus influenzae* (Hib) vaccine, introduced in 1990, has nearly eliminated epiglottitis in children and markedly decreased the incidence of meningitis, sepsis, and septic shock (Subedar and Rathore, 1995; Stenklyft, 1999). And the introduction of the PCV7 vaccine has reduced the number of invasive pneumococcal infections among children (Kaplan et al., 2004).

The 1990s: Birth of a New Subspecialty

The number of pediatric emergency medicine fellowships had begun to increase, although most of these had been developed at children's hospitals under the leadership of pediatricians. In the late 1980s, representatives from the American Board of Emergency Medicine (ABEM) and the American Board of Pediatrics collaborated to ensure that such fellowships would be accessible to both pediatricians and emergency medicine physicians. Together, the two organizations submitted a proposal to the American Board of Medical Specialties that pediatric emergency care be a recognized subspecialty (Pena and Snyder, 1995). The proposal was approved, and in 1992, the first subspecialty certifying exam in pediatric emergency medicine was administered (Stenklyft, 1999). In 1998, pediatric emergency medicine fellowships became accredited. Most fellowship programs are now 3 years in duration and include a research component (Stenklyft, 1999). By 1999, the nation had approximately 1,000 board-certified subspecialists in pediatric emergency medicine.

In 1993, the IOM released findings from its comprehensive study on the need for and effectiveness of pediatric emergency care (IOM, 1993). Despite the advances in pediatric emergency care that had occurred through the 1980s and early 1990s, the study identified gaps in several major areas, including education and training; appropriate equipment and supplies; communications; funding; and planning, evaluation, and research. In response to these findings, the Maternal and Child Health Bureau (MCHB) within the Health Resources and Services Administration (HRSA) and the National Highway Traffic Safety Administration (NHTSA) published a 5-year plan for pediatric emergency care in 1995. That plan was revised and updated in 2000 (DHHS et al., 2000), and a new plan was published in 2001 (DHHS et al., 2001). Additionally, ACEP and the AAP published recommended equipment guidelines for prehospital units and emergency departments (Guidelines for Pediatric Equipment, 1996; AAP, 2001).

Pediatric Emergency Care in 2006

If there is one word to describe pediatric emergency care in 2006, it is uneven. As mentioned in Chapter 1, the specialized resources available to treat seriously ill or injured children vary greatly based on location. Some children have access to children's hospitals and hospitals with separate pe-diatric inpatient capabilities, which tend to be well prepared for pediatric emergencies; others must rely on hospitals with limited pediatric medical expertise and equipment (Middleton and Burt, 2006). Requirements for pediatric continuing medical education for EMTs vary greatly across states. Some states and communities have organized trauma systems and designat-ed pediatric facilities, while others do not. As a result, not all children have access to the same quality of care. While data on system performance are not routinely collected, it appears that where a child lives has an important impact on whether the child can survive a serious illness or injury.

The day-to-day presentation of pediatric patients is challenging enough for emergency care systems in some areas; addressing new and emerging threats to children's health may be beyond the capabilities of the current system. Experience has shown that the outbreak and management of con-tagious diseases, such as new strains of influenza and severe acute respira-tory syndrome (SARS), can cause a major disruption in the emergency care system (Augustine et al., 2004). The effect of these new health threats on children is not yet well understood. Several case studies of SARS have been published, but most of the clinical, laboratory, and radiological information available is based on adult patients (Bitnun et al., 2003). Some case studies suggest that while children are susceptible to SARS, symptoms of the disease may be milder in young children as compared with adolescents and adults (Fong et al., 2004; Leung et al., 2004). However, these studies are based on a very small sample. The efficacy of pediatric treatment for SARS requires additional evaluation; indeed, no pediatric treatment regime for SARS cur-rently exists (Leung et al., 2004).

Avian influenza is another emerging threat that could put children at particular risk. Children may be more susceptible to the disease because of their increased proximity to one another at schools and day care centers. They may also be more likely to come into contact with poultry or bird fecal matter while playing. It is unknown whether immunity differences in children have any significance in their susceptibility to avian influenza, since it is presumed that the vast majority of humans have no immunity against the H5N1 virus, the strain of greatest concern (U.S. Department of State, 2006).

Development of Pediatric Trauma Care

Trauma represents a particular kind of medical emergency. It is typi-cally defined as having a physical wound caused by force or impact, such as a fall or automobile accident; burns and other severe wounds are also deemed a form of trauma. Other life-threatening medical conditions caused by preexisting conditions are generally not considered trauma. Trauma care is distinguished from care received in a general ED by the specialized diagnostic and treatment procedures necessary to care for the traumatically injured patient. Trauma centers are designed to meet the complex surgical demands of critically ill patients immediately. To qualify as a trauma center, a hospital must have a number of capabilities, including a resource-intensive ED, a high-quality intensive care ward, and an operating room that is functional at all times. Ideally, traumatically injured children are cared for in a pediatric trauma center, a facility with the personnel, equipment, space, and other resources required to provide the necessary care 24 hours a day, 7 days a week (Ramenofsky, 2006). The American College of Surgeons' (ACS) Committee on Trauma has defined the term "pediatric trauma center" in its categorization of trauma centers into levels based on their capabilities. A level I pediatric trauma center, the highest level, is a children's hospital or an adult center with pediatric expertise (Ramenofsky, 2006).

Given that the development of pediatric emergency care has lagged behind that of adult emergency care, it is surprising that the first pediatric trauma center was established in 1962—5 years before the first adult trauma center was established (Ramenofsky, 2006). In 1970, the American Pediatric Surgical Association (APSA) was founded; 2 years later, one of the members requested greater emphasis on trauma, and the association established a Committee on Trauma, which continues today. Also in 1972, the APSA joined the American Medical Association, the ACS, the American Academy of Orthopedic Surgeons, and the American Association for the Surgery of Trauma in sponsoring the American Trauma Society (ATS) (Personal communication, M. Stanton, March 12, 2006). The ATS, established in the late 1960s, was an advocate for the EMSS Act of 1973. Today it works to promote trauma care and prevention, serving as an advocate for trauma victims and their families and for optimal care for all trauma victims (ATS, 2006).

However, advanced resources for the care of pediatric trauma patients were largely unavailable until the 1980s. In 1982, the *Journal of Trauma* published the first description of resources necessary to treat the injured child. Others followed. In 1984, the ACS Committee on Trauma included an appendix on pediatric trauma care in its standards manual, which was the first document to define the standards of care necessary to treat trauma patients. A chapter on pediatric trauma appeared in the ACS resource manual in 1987 (Ramenofsky, 2006).

Today, most regions have dedicated trauma facilities, board-certified surgeons have training and experience in trauma care and pediatric surgery, and most states have organized trauma systems. Injuries are no longer viewed as "accidents" but as predictable events that can be prevented through the application of harm reduction strategies (Cooper, 2006). As detailed later in the chapter, however, unintentional injury continues to be the leading cause of death in children over age 1 and an important source of

ED visits. While this report is focused on the emergency care system and the pediatric component of that system, the committee emphasizes that greater effort is needed to build a comprehensive injury control strategy or system to reduce injuries among both children and adults.

The Emergency Medical Services for Children Program

The creation of the federal EMS-C program in 1984 grew at least in part out of policy makers' personal experiences with the pediatric emergency care system. Several congressional staff members had had disturbing experiences with the emergency care system's ability to care for their children. Their experiences highlighted serious shortcomings of a typical ED's capacity to care for children in crisis. Around the same time, emergency physicians began approaching federal lawmakers to tell them that children were arriving at the ED in worse condition than adults. As a result, Senators Daniel Inouye (D-HI), Orrin Hatch (R-UT), and Lowell Weicker (R-CT) sponsored the creation of the EMS-C demonstration grant program under the Health Services, Preventive Health Services, and Home Community Based Services Act of 1984 (IOM, 1993; CPEM, 2001).

The goal of the EMS-C program is to reduce child and youth morbidity and mortality resulting from severe illness or trauma by supporting injury prevention programs and improvements in the quality of medical care received by children. The program aims to ensure (1) that state-of-the-art emergency medical care is available for ill or injured children and adolescents; (2) that pediatric services are well integrated into an EMS system backed by optimal resources; and (3) that the entire spectrum of emergency services—including illness and injury prevention, acute care, and rehabilitation—is provided to children and adolescents as well as adults (Perez, 1998). While this report is focused on pediatric EMS and hospital-based pediatric emergency care, the EMS-C program covers a broader continuum of care, from illness and injury prevention to bystander care, dispatch, prehospital EMS, definitive hospital care, rehabilitation, and return to the community (see Figure 2-1). The EMS-C program is the only federal program that specifically supports essential emergency medical care for ill or injured children and adolescents. The program is administered by HRSA with support from NHTSA.

The program initially focused on providing grants to states and accredited schools of medicine for needs assessments and demonstration projects (Advocates for EMS, 2004; Krug and Kuppermann, 2005). Its original authorization provided $2 million in funding for fiscal year 1985 (IOM, 1993). That funding supported four state partnership demonstration projects that created some of the first strategies for addressing important pediatric emergency care issues, such as disseminating education programs for pre-

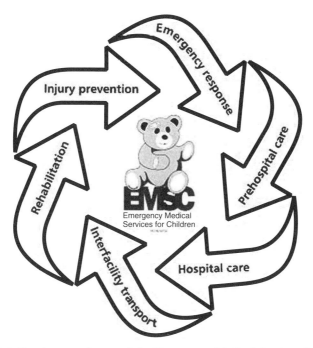

FIGURE 2-1 Continuum of care of the Emergency Medical Services for Children program.

hospital and hospital-based providers, establishing data collection processes to identify significant pediatric issues in the EMS system, and developing tools for assessing critically ill or injured children (CPEM, 2001).

Growth of the EMS-C Program

Funding for the EMS-C program has grown since its inception, as have the number and types of initiatives funded. Reauthorization of the program in 1988 lifted the initial limit of four grants per year and provided funding of $3 million for fiscal year 1989, $4 million for fiscal year 1990, and $5 million for fiscal year 1991 (IOM, 1993).

The program underwent several changes in 1991. First, the focus of the state grants shifted from demonstration to implementation projects (IOM, 1993). The objective of implementation projects is to put into place what is known to work (HRSA, 1994). Second, the program introduced new Targeted Issues Grants. These grants target specific issues related to the development of pediatric emergency care capacity, with the intent of providing potential national models. Examples of such grants awarded to date are an investigation of the psychosocial impact of emergencies on children and the development of new pediatric information systems (IOM, 1993).

States that receive EMS-C grants are expected to share ideas or products with other interested states, and the EMS-C National Resource Center was created to assist with such knowledge sharing. As states create new programs, the center provides technical assistance with strategic planning, program development, problem solving, identification of national resources, and program evaluation. The center also promotes understanding of pediatric issues in the EMS system through the development of reports and special materials for the states. Its library contains more than 1,000 products that address illness and injury prevention, patient care training and safety, equipment guidelines, medical direction, and public policy. Additionally, the National EMSC Data Analysis Resource Center (NEDARC) in Salt Lake City, Utah, specializes in providing grantees with technical assistance in data collection and analysis (Perez, 1998).

The program continued to expand and mature in the mid-1990s. In response to the recommendations of the 1993 IOM report *Emergency Medical Services for Children*, HRSA and NHTSA sponsored a meeting to help translate those recommendations into objectives and specific actions. The result was the EMS-C 5-Year Plan, a comprehensive, long-range strategy for the EMS-C program for 1995–2000 (DHHS et al., 1995). That plan was updated in 2000 and continued to guide the program through 2005 (DHHS et al., 2001). The program has partnered with a number of professional organizations to address the objectives in the plan (Krug and Kuppermann, 2005).

In recent years, the EMS-C program has also supported the infrastructure for pediatric emergency care research. In 2001, the program collaborated with the Research Branch of HRSA's MCHB to develop the Pediatric Emergency Care Applied Research Network (PECARN), the first federally funded multi-institutional network for research in pediatric emergency care. Funding for the infrastructure for PECARN has come through EMS-C program appropriations. PECARN consists of five cooperative agreements with academic medical centers. Its goal is to conduct meaningful and rigorous multi-institutional research on the prevention and management of acute illnesses and injuries in children and youths across the continuum of emergency medicine health care (PECARN, 2004). PECARN provides leadership and infrastructure to promote multicenter studies, support research collaboration among researchers in pediatric EMS, and encourage information exchanges between pediatric emergency care investigators and providers (DHHS, 2004).

Congress should be commended for recognizing the importance of the

EMS-C program and supporting its development.[1] Despite the program's growth, however, it continues to be funded at a relatively modest level. Fiscal year 2005 funding for the program was $19.86 million[2]; details on the program's expenditures are provided in Table 2-1. Note that administrative expenses are low in part because the two full-time staff overseeing the program at the national level are not funded from the program's budget, but from the MCHB's Program Management Fund.

Impact of the EMS-C Program

In 2005, the EMS-C program celebrated its twentieth anniversary. The program's accomplishments are numerous even with its modest level of appropriations. The program has broadly advanced the state of pediatric emergency care nationwide. It has improved the availability of child-size equipment in ambulances and EDs; initiated hundreds of programs to prevent injuries; and provided thousands of hours of training to EMTs, paramedics, and other emergency medical care providers. Educational materials covering every aspect of pediatric emergency care have been developed under the EMS-C program, and a formal partnership (the EMS-C Partnership for Children Stakeholder Group) has been forged with numerous national and professional organizations to help achieve the program's goals (MCHB, 2005a). Findings resulting from Targeted Issues Grants have enhanced the use of ketamine and analgesia for pediatric orthopedic emergencies (Graff et al., 1996) and led to improved understanding of pediatric intubation in the prehospital environment (Gausche-Hill et al., 2000) and pediatric airway management (MCHB, 2004b).

The EMS-C program's guidance and resources have led to important changes in pediatric emergency care at the state level. For example:

• Twelve states have adopted and disseminated pediatric guidelines that characterize acute care facilities (pediatric trauma care or critical care facilities or EDs approved for pediatrics) according to the equipment, drugs, trained personnel, and facilities necessary to provide varying levels of pediatric emergency care.

• Twenty states have pediatric emergency care statutes.

---

[1]Congress supported the continuation of funding for the EMS-C program even after the proposed elimination of the program in the President's budget for fiscal year 2006. The program is also eliminated in the President's budget for fiscal year 2007. As of this writing, Congress had not yet voted on the fiscal year 2007 appropriation for the program.

[2]The fiscal year 2005 appropriation for the EMS-C program was $19.86 million. However, the program is required to contribute approximately 1 percent of its appropriation to the Health Resources and Services Administration for administrative purposes, such as program accounting and evaluation. The EMS-C program had $19.66 million in real dollars for operations.

TABLE 2-1 EMS-C Program Expenditures for Fiscal Year (FY) 2005

Program Component	Description	Approximate FY 05 Funding
State Partnership Grants	• Grants to all states, the District of Columbia, and five territories to institutionalize pediatric EMS improvements • Grantees receive $100,000 to $115,000 per year	$5.6 million
Network Development Demonstration	• Infrastructure support for the Pediatric Emergency Care Applied Research Network (PECARN) • Five cooperative agreements at $700,000 each	$3.5 million
Targeted Issues Grants	• Grants to demonstrate the effectiveness of a model system that may be helpful to the field • 16 grants funded at $200,000 per year	$3.1 million
National Resource Center	• Contract with Children's National Medical Center in Washington, D.C., for establishment of a center to provide technical assistance to EMS-C grant recipients, prepare special reports and educational materials on EMS-C issues, plan national meetings, collect and disseminate EMS-C products and related resources, and encourage collaboration among national organizations to promote improvements in pediatric emergency care	$2.2 million
National EMSC Data Analysis Resource Center (NEDARC)	• Advises grantees and state EMS offices on data collection and analysis issues; conducts workshops in data analysis, grant writing, and other technical areas; assists with research design; and provides other types of technical assistance to grantees	$1.2 million
Interagency Agreements	• Funding to the Centers for Disease Control and Prevention for a pediatric emergency care data collection effort associated with the National Hospital Ambulatory Medical Care Survey • Funding to the National Highway Traffic Safety Administration to support projects that include the development of the National EMS Research Agenda and the National EMS Information System (NEMSIS) • Funding to the Indian Health Service for activities that include the training of EMS professionals among Native American and Alaskan populations	$800,000
Regional Symposia	• Grants to support the coordination, exchange, and dissemination of knowledge that leads to reductions in child and youth disability and death due to severe illness and injury • Six relatively small grants	$239,000
Other Activities	• One-time or irregular program expenditures, such as sponsoring a pediatric research workshop at the National Association of EMS Physicians Meeting, grants to support the development of clinical practice guidelines in two areas, and grants to the Maternal and Child Health Bureau Research Division	$3 million

- Twenty-seven states, tribal reservations, or federal territories have conducted a pediatric emergency care needs assessment within the last 5 years.
- Thirty-six of the 42 states having statewide computerized data collection systems now produce reports on pediatric EMS using statewide data.
- Forty-one states use pediatric guidelines for identification of acute care facilities, ensuring that children are transported to the right hospital in a timely manner.
- Forty-four states employ pediatric protocols for on-line medical direction of EMTs and paramedics at the scene of an emergency.
- Forty-eight states identify and require all essential pediatric EMS equipment on advanced life support (ALS) ambulances (Advocates for EMS, 2004; MCHB, 2005b).

While the program is focused on pediatric emergency care, many of its initiatives benefit patients of all ages. An example is an interagency agreement with NHTSA to support the development of the National EMS Research Agenda, the National EMS Information System, and the infrastructure for the National Association of State EMS Officials.

The 1993 IOM Report on Emergency Medical Services for Children

The activities of the EMS-C program were the subject of considerable congressional interest during the program's first decade. In response to this interest, in 1991 HRSA requested that the IOM undertake a study of pediatric EMS to examine the issues involved more broadly than was possible through the EMS-C program's individual demonstration projects (IOM, 1993). Previously the National Academy of Sciences, National Research Council, and IOM had conducted several other studies related to emergency care, but few had given much attention to pediatric emergency care. The findings and recommendations of the IOM study were published in the 1993 report *Emergency Medical Services for Children*. The report presented recommendations in five areas: education and training; essential tools; communication and 9-1-1 systems; planning, evaluation, and research; and federal and state agencies and funding. The report garnered considerable attention from emergency care providers, professional organizations, policy makers, and the public. Since its release, progress has been made in each of the recommendation areas, yet the issues raised have not been fully addressed. Examples are described below.

Education and Training

Concern in 1993 regarding emergency providers' knowledge about the proper care of pediatric patients remains salient today. Maintenance of skills is a challenge because many providers have infrequent contact with critically ill and injured children; only rarely do they perform ALS interventions on children. Surveys indicate that prehospital providers find the age group birth to 3 years most concerning and support increased continuing education in pediatric emergency care (Glaeser et al., 2000). Additionally, the majority of pediatric visits occur at general EDs (Gausche et al., 1995), which are less likely than specialized facilities to have providers specifically trained in pediatric emergency medicine. Anecdotal accounts of physicians expressing doubt about their skills to care for a critically ill or injured child are not uncommon (Frush and Hohenhaus, 2004). The abilities of emergency care providers to address the needs of children are discussed further in Chapter 4.

Essential Tools

The IOM committee that developed the 1993 report was concerned by reports that emergency providers lacked the equipment necessary to care properly for children and recommended that pediatric equipment and supplies be made more widely available. Since the release of the 1993 report, professional organizations have continued to update guidelines on essential and recommended equipment and supplies, and many states have used funding from the EMS-C program to purchase pediatric equipment. While some progress has been made, however, deficiencies in pediatric equipment and supplies remain a problem for some providers. The average ED has about 80 percent of the recommended pediatric supplies, and only 6 percent of the nation's EDs are fully equipped to care for children (Middleton and Burt, 2006). Some data indicate that there was no increase in the availability of pediatric equipment in EDs between 1998 and 2002 (Middleton, 2005).

Research on the availability of the pediatric supplies and equipment recommended for prehospital providers has been limited primarily to studies of regions or states, and no recent data are available. A 1993 study of EMS ambulance agencies in Oklahoma found that deficiencies in equipment needed for pediatric emergencies were common (Graham et al., 1993). A 1998 study of compliance with the guidelines of the Committee on Ambulance Pediatric Equipment and Supplies in Kansas revealed that only 5 percent of ambulance services reported having essential equipment on all vehicles; 92 percent of agencies failed to achieve compliance with the guidelines on any vehicle. The most frequently lacking pediatric basic life support (BLS) items were stethoscopes (58 percent), traction splints (53 percent), and nonrebreather masks (45 percent). The most frequently lacking pediatric ALS items were nasogastric tubes (75 percent), monitor electrodes (50 percent), and Magill forceps (41.7 percent) (Moreland et al., 1998). Again, there is scant evidence regarding the impact on patient outcomes of not having all essential pediatric equipment; however, having this equipment available is an essential element of preparedness.

The 1993 IOM report also recommended that states address the issue of categorization and regionalization in overseeing the development of pediatric emergency care. In many states, however, hospitals are not categorized based on their ability to care for critically ill or injured children. Additionally, many hospitals lack transfer agreements in case a critically ill or injured child arrives at a hospital that lacks pediatric expertise (Middleton and Burt, 2006). This issue is discussed further in the next chapter.

Planning, Evaluation, and Research

One of the great successes of the EMS-C program has been that all states now have an EMS-C coordinator, whose job it is to oversee grant funding received from the program. In many states, the coordinator position is full-time and involves other activities, including making sure that the state EMS system considers children's needs. However, there are still signs of deficiencies in trauma and disaster planning (MCHB, 2004a; NAEMSD, 2004). As mentioned earlier, about half of hospitals that lack a separate pediatric ward also lack written interfacility transfer agreements (Middleton and Burt, 2006). Moreover, although most state disaster plans address the need for pediatric equipment and medications at hospitals, only six states report that hospitals have those resources in place (NAEMSD, 2004).

Certainly there has been some expansion of pediatric emergency care research since 1993, but efforts to track patient outcomes have been hampered by the absence of an infrastructure for the systematic collection of a uniform set of data elements and by the inability to link datasets of different providers (prehospital, ED, others) as recommended in the 1993 IOM report. Research funding for pediatric emergency care is also highly limited. It is of note that the annual appropriation for the entire EMS-C program is less than the annual cost of some single large-scale National Institutes of Health (NIH) clinical trials (National Center for Complementary and Alternative Medicine, 2002; National Cancer Institute, 2005). As a result of the dearth of funding for emergency care research, many emergency medical interventions that are regularly provided to children have not been subjected to rigorous scientific trials. This issue is discussed further in Chapter 7.

PEDIATRIC EMERGENCY CARE IN 2006

This section describes the emergency care system for children in 2006. The focus is on the need for and use of pediatric emergency care.

Threats to Children's Health

Data from CDC's 2003 National Health Interview Survey indicate that children in the United States are generally in good health. Approximately 83 percent of parents described their children as being in "excellent" or "very good" health. Not surprisingly, children in two-parent families, families with higher incomes, and those covered by private insurance tended to be in better health than children living with their mothers only, children from poor families, and children without insurance (Dey and Bloom, 2005).

Threats to children's health and safety remain prevalent in our society. Injuries are the leading cause of death among those aged 1–19, and rates of childhood injury in the United States are considerably higher than those in other developed countries (United Nations Children's Fund, 2001; CDC, 2004). Illnesses, particularly asthma and infectious disease, impose a high burden on American children and their parents. In fact, approximately 20 million children in the United States suffer from at least one chronic condition, leaving them more susceptible to medical emergencies (AHRQ, 2002). Moreover, violence in our society remains prevalent; many children witness or are directly exposed to violence in their families and/or communities. The result is that millions of Americans rely on the emergency medical system to provide care for children when they need it most.

Injury

Statistics on childhood injury are available from a variety of sources, but perhaps the most comprehensive are from CDC's National Vital Statistics Reports and ACS's National Trauma Data Bank (NTDB). CDC collects data on injury deaths by cause; those data are displayed in Table 2-2, while data from the NTDB are shown in Table 2-3. The two datasets are somewhat different because the NTDB includes not just deaths, but all injured patients seen at one of the 474 participating trauma centers in 43 states (Fildes, 2005).

Both datasets show what has been known for many years: the most common cause of injury deaths and injury visits to trauma centers is motor vehicle crashes. According to NHTSA, more than half of children aged 0–14 who were killed in such crashes in 2003 were not restrained (CDC, 2005). More than a quarter of occupant deaths among children aged 0–14 involved a driver who was drinking (Shults, 2004).

Other threats to safety vary by age group. Young children aged 1–4 are at great risk of injury as they explore their environment. They are more likely than older children to fall into a pool and drown or swallow pills unintentionally. Indeed, drowning is the second leading cause of death in this age group. Young children also lack coordination, which makes them

TABLE 2-2 Number of Deaths from Selected Causes, by Age

Cause of Death	Age in Years				Total Deaths
	Under 1	1–4	5–14	15–24	
Injury					
Unintentional Injury	946	1,641	2,718	15,412	20,717
Motor Vehicle Accident	123	610	1,614	11,459	13,806
Accidental Poisoning/Exposure to Noxious Substances	26	31	43	1,679	1,779
Drowning	63	454	321	629	1,467
Exposure to Smoke, Fire, or Flames	36	221	253	193	703
Fall	16	37	42	247	342
Firearm Discharge	1	11	48	210	270
Assault (Homicide)	303	423	356	5,219	6,301
Suicide	NA	NA	264	4,010	4,274

SOURCE: National Center for Health Statistics, 2004.

TABLE 2-3 Percentage of Total Pediatric Patients Presenting at a Trauma Center, by Mechanism of Injury

Mechanism of Injury	Percentage of Total Patients
Motor Vehicle Traffic	43.3
Fall	19.7
Struck by, against	7.4
Transport, Other	6.4
Firearm	5.0
Pedal Cyclist, Other	3.7
Fire/Burn	3.1
Cut/Pierce	3.1
Natural/Environmental	1.3
Unspecified	1.2
Machinery	0.6
Pedestrian, Other	0.5
Drowning/Submersion	0.5
Poisoning	0.3
Overexertion	0.3
Suffocation	0.2
Other	3.4

NOTE: The data include patients that were seen at one of the 474 trauma centers in 43 states that participate in the National Trauma Data Bank.
SOURCE: ACS, 2004.

more susceptible to falls. Approximately 2.4 million cases of human poison exposures were reported to poison control centers in 2003; 44 percent of those cases occurred in children aged 1–4 (Watson et al., 2003). Additionally, these children may be at much higher risk of abuse (inflicted injuries) or neglect, particularly because of their dependency and their inability to communicate the abuse (National Center for Injury Prevention and Control, 2001).

Children aged 5–14 are often injured because of their impulsiveness and inability to judge the safety of a situation. They may run into the street without looking or give unwanted attention to animals (2.5 percent of children are bitten by dogs each year). They are also susceptible to bicycle crashes. In fact, 140,000 children are seen in the ED each year for traumatic brain injuries sustained while riding a bicycle; one-third of all bicyclists killed in crashes are children. Small size contributes to these children's risk of injury—motorists may not be able to see them in the road. The risk of violence, including child sexual abuse, is high in this age group. Emotional stress and social changes may contribute to the increased risk of suicide attempts and completed suicides involving adolescents (National Center for Injury Prevention and Control, 2001).

Teenagers and young adults between the ages of 15 and 19 are involved in violence more than any other age group. They are also at high risk for suicide. Developmental factors that result in impulsiveness and risk-taking behaviors may contribute to these risks. Motor vehicle crashes are most likely to occur among teenaged drivers, particularly during the first year behind the wheel; teenagers are more likely to speed, ride with an intoxicated driver, or drive after using alcohol or drugs than those in other age groups (National Center for Injury Prevention and Control, 2001).

Although the prevalence of childhood injury is high, trend data indicate improvement over time for unintentional injuries and some categories of intentional injuries. The unintentional injury death rate among children aged 0–14 declined 41 percent between 1987 and 2001; death rates fell for motor vehicle injury, bicycle injury, pedestrian injury, drowning, fire and burn injury, poisoning, and fall injury during the period (National Safe Kids Campaign, 2004). This improvement is likely the result of prevention efforts, such as laws and campaigns aimed at increased use of child safety seats, bicycle helmets, and smoke alarms.

Rates of intentional injury, homicide, suicide, and firearm-related fatality among teenagers all dropped from the mid-1990s through 2002 (the most recent year for which data are available). Between 1973 and 1993, the homicide rate for teenagers doubled from 8.1 to 20.7 deaths per 100,000, but the rate subsequently declined, falling to 9.3 in 2002. The rate of adolescent suicide also rose dramatically between 1970 and the mid-1990s (from

5.9 to 11.1 deaths per 100,000), but has since fallen to 7.4 (Child Trends Databank, 2004).

Trends in child abuse are more difficult to discern because of under-recognition and underreporting. There has been a slight increase in the number of child abuse cases reported to child protective services (Peddle and Wang, 2002) and in child abuse fatalities reported by the National Child Abuse and Neglect Data System (National Clearinghouse on Child Abuse and Neglect Information, 2004), but it is unclear whether these increases are a result of improved reporting or increased abuse. Regardless, child abuse and neglect remains a serious problem.

Illness

Children suffer from a myriad of illnesses, but not all types of illnesses are likely to lead to an experience with the emergency care system. For example, congenital abnormalities and birth-related conditions are among the leading causes of death among infants, yet they are rarely the reason for an ED visit (Table 2-4). Data from the Agency for Healthcare Research and Quality's (AHRQ) Healthcare Cost and Utilization Project (HCUP) State Emergency Department Database (SEDD) include the most frequent diagnoses for all pediatric ED visits in 12 states. Table 2-5 shows the primary diagnosis for treat and release ED visits for various pediatric age groups. Approximately 4 percent of all ED visits result in admission to the hospital (2002 NHAMCS data, calculations by IOM; 2002 SEDD data provided by AHRQ staff); Table 2-6 shows the primary diagnosis for such ED visits.

The illnesses most frequently responsible for an ED visit tend to be rather minor. Among children treated and released from the ED, the most common non-injury-related diagnosis for all age groups is upper respiratory infection (not including asthma, acute bronchitis, or pneumonia), which includes conditions such as the common cold, croup, and sinusitis. Otitis media, or ear infection, is another common illness responsible for many ED visits among younger children; three of four children experience this condition by the time they reach age 3 (National Institute on Deafness and Other Communication Disorders, 2002).

Among ED visits that result in hospital admission, the illnesses responsible vary considerably based on age group. Younger children tend to be hospitalized for serious upper respiratory infections, including acute bronchitis, pneumonia, and asthma. Infants and young children tend to have greater vulnerability to these illnesses than older children and nonelderly adults. Children whose parents or siblings smoke are especially susceptible to these three conditions (MayoClinic.com, 2005).

Of note, mood disorders are the most frequent diagnosis for children

TABLE 2-4 Ten Leading Causes of Death in Children and Number of Deaths, by Age Group (in years), 2002

	Less than 1	Ages 1–4	Ages 5–9	Ages 10–14	Ages 15–24
1.	Congenital anomalies 5,623	Unintentional injury 1,641	Unintentional injury 1,176	Unintentional injury 1,542	Unintentional injury 15,412
2.	Short gestation 4,673	Congenital anomalies 530	Malignant neoplasms 537	Malignant neoplasms 535	Homicide 5,219
3.	Sudden infant death syndrome (SIDS) 2,295	Homicide 423	Congenital anomalies 199	Suicide 260	Suicide 4,010
4.	Maternal pregnancy complications 1,708	Malignant neoplasms 402	Homicide 140	Congenital anomalies 218	Malignant neoplasms 1,730
5.	Placenta cord membranes 1,028	Heart disease 165	Heart disease 92	Homicide 216	Heart disease 1,022
6.	Unintentional injury 946	Influenza and pneumonia 110	Benign neoplasms 44	Heart disease 163	Congenital anomalies 492
7.	Respiratory distress 943	Septicemia 79	Septicemia 42	Chronic lower respiratory disease 95	Chronic lower respiratory disease 192
8.	Bacterial sepsis 749	Chronic lower respiratory disease 65	Chronic lower respiratory disease 41	Cerebrovascular disease 58	HIV 178
9.	Circulatory system disease 749	Complications of perinatal period 65	Influenza and pneumonia 38	Influenza and pneumonia 53	Cerebrovascular disease 171
10.	Intrauterine hypoxia 583	Benign neoplasms 60	Cerebrovascular disease 33	Septicemia 53	Diabetes mellitus 171

SOURCE: CDC, 2004.

TABLE 2-5 Ten Leading Primary Diagnoses for Treat and Release ED Cases in Selected States, by Age Group (in years)

	Less than 1	Ages 1–4	Ages 5–9	Ages 10–14	Ages 15–17
1.	Other upper respiratory infections (18%)	Other upper respiratory infections (14%)	Other upper respiratory infections (13%)	Superficial injury, contusion (12%)	Sprains and strains (13%)
2.	Otitis media (14%)	Otitis media (13%)	Superficial injury, contusion (9%)	Sprains and strains (11%)	Superficial injury, contusion (11%)
3.	Fever of unknown origin (8%)	Open wounds of head, neck, and trunk (8%)	Open wounds of head, neck, and trunk (7%)	Other upper respiratory infections (9%)	Other upper respiratory infections (6%)
4.	Viral infections (6%)	Superficial injury, contusion (6%)	Otitis media (6%)	Fracture of upper limb (7%)	Open wounds of extremities (5%)
5.	Acute bronchitis (5%)	Fever of unknown origin (6%)	Fracture of upper limb (5%)	Open wounds of extremities (6%)	Abdominal pain (4%)
6.	Noninfectious gastroenteritis (3%)	Viral infections (5%)	Open wounds of extremities (4%)	Other injuries due to external causes (5%)	Other injuries due to external causes (4%)
7.	Nausea and vomiting (3%)	Other injuries due to external causes (4%)	Other injuries due to external causes (4%)	Open wounds of head, neck, and trunk (4%)	Fracture of upper limb (3%)
8.	Other gastrointestinal disorders (3%)	Noninfectious gastroenteritis (3%)	Sprains and strains (4%)	Abdominal pain (3%)	Open wounds of head, neck, and trunk (3%)
9.	Other injuries due to external causes (3%)	Asthma (3%)	Viral infections (4%)	Asthma (3%)	Urinary tract infections (2%)
10.	Superficial injury, contusion (3%)	Pneumonia (2%)	Asthma (3%)	Otitis media (3%)	Headache, including migraines (2%)

SOURCE: Agency for Healthcare Research and Quality (AHRQ), Healthcare Cost and Utilization Project (HCUP), aggregate of 2002 State Emergency Department Databases from Connecticut, Georgia, Maine, Maryland, Massachusetts, Minnesota, Missouri, Nebraska, South Carolina, Tennessee, Utah, and Vermont (http://www.hcup-us.ahrq.gov). Percentages represent the proportion of discharges in each age group. Diagnostic groups listed are based on the Clinical Classifications Software (CCS) (http://www.hcup-us.ahrq.gov/tools.jsp). Data provided by AHRQ staff.

TABLE 2-6 Ten Leading Principal Diagnoses for Hospital Admissions That Begin in the ED in Selected States, by Age Group (in years)

	Less than 1	Ages 1–4	Ages 5–9	Ages 10–14	Ages 15–17
1.	Acute bronchitis (23%)	Pneumonia (15%)	Asthma (14%)	Appendicitis (13%)	Mood disorders (12%)
2.	Pneumonia (8%)	Asthma (15%)	Pneumonia (9%)	Mood disorders (8%)	Appendicitis (7%)
3.	Other perinatal conditions (8%)	Fluid and electrolyte disorders (10%)	Appendicitis (7%)	Asthma (7%)	Fracture of lower limb (4%)
4.	Fluid and electrolyte disorders (6%)	Acute bronchitis (6%)	Fluid and electrolyte disorders (5%)	Fracture of lower limb (4%)	Intracranial injury (4%)
5.	Fever of unknown origin (5%)	Epilepsy, convulsions (6%)	Fracture of upper limb (4%)	Pneumonia (3%)	Poisoning by other medications and drugs (3%)
6.	Urinary tract infection (4%)	Other upper respiratory infections (4%)	Epilepsy, convulsions (4%)	Diabetes mellitus with complications (3%)	Crushing injury or internal injury (3%)
7.	Viral infections (4%)	Intestinal infection (4%)	Fracture of lower limb (3%)	Fracture of upper limb (3%)	Asthma (3%)
8.	Other upper respiratory infections (3%)	Urinary tract infection (2%)	Urinary tract infections (3%)	Sickle cell anemia (3%)	Diabetes mellitus with complications (3%)
9.	Asthma (3%)	Noninfectious gastroenteritis (2%)	Skin and subcutaneous tissue infections (2%)	Intracranial injury (3%)	Urinary tract infections (2%)
10.	Intestinal infection (3%)	Skin and subcutaneous tissue infections (2%)	Sickle cell anemia (2%)	Abdominal pain (2%)	Other complications of pregnancy (2%)

SOURCE: Agency for Healthcare Research and Quality (AHRQ), Healthcare Cost and Utilization Project (HCUP), aggregate of 2002 state inpatient databases from Connecticut, Georgia, Maine, Maryland, Massachusetts, Minnesota, Missouri, Nebraska, South Carolina, Tennessee, Utah, and Vermont (http://www.hcup-us.ahrq.gov). All data are the proportion of discharges in each age group. Diagnostic groups listed are based on the Clinical Classifications Software (CCS) (http://www.hcup-us.ahrq.gov/tools.jsp). Data provided by AHRQ staff.

aged 15–17 admitted from the ED and the second most frequent diagnosis for those aged 10–14. Mood disorders encompass a wide variety of behavioral issues but generally fall into two categories: depression and bipolar (or manic-depressive) disorder (Beers and Berkow, 2005).

Certain types of illnesses, particularly asthma and diabetes, become exacerbated and result in hospital admission when children have health care needs that go unmet. Failure to obtain timely care can affect health status and functioning in the near and long terms and can influence the likelihood of seeking services at an ED. Data from the National Health Interview Survey for the mid-1990s indicate that unmet health care needs were prevalent among children. Near-poor and poor children were three times as likely to have unmet health care needs as nonpoor children, and uninsured children were three times as likely to have unmet needs as privately insured children (Newacheck et al., 2000).

Children with Mental Health Problems

Mental health disorders in children and adolescents deserve special mention because of their growing prevalence as causes for ED visits, as well as the difficulty that patients with mental illness pose to emergency care providers. It is estimated that 20 percent of U.S. children have a mental disorder with at least mild functional impairment; 5 to 9 percent of children aged 9–17 have a serious emotional disturbance (DHHS, 1999). These problems not only contribute to difficulties at home, at school, and in relationships with peers, but if untreated can lead to such consequences as failure in school, involvement in the juvenile or adult criminal justice system, and higher health care costs as adults, as well as suicide.

Based on extrapolation from National Electronic Injury Surveillance System (NEISS) data, more than 200,000 children present to the ED with mental health problems each year (Melese-d'Hospital et al., 2002), and research has shown that such ED visits are on the rise (Santucci et al., 2000; Sullivan and Rivera, 2000; Sills and Bland, 2002); at one pediatric ED, for example, mental health–related visits rose 59 percent between 1995 and 1999 (Santucci et al., 2000). Moreover, the patients involved are getting younger and younger; depression, bipolar disorder, and anxiety are now being identified in children of elementary school age (Scheck, 2006).

Studies have pointed to shortcomings in the effectiveness of the emergency care system in dealing with children with mental health problems. A mid-1990s survey of hospitals revealed that formal mental health services for children are unavailable in most EDs (U.S. Consumer Product Safety Commission, 1997). In a pilot study of pediatric mental health cases at 10 hospitals participating in the NEISS, researchers found that mental health evaluations of patients varied by presenting condition. Three-fourths of emotionally disturbed children received an evaluation by a mental health professional, compared with 69 percent who had attempted suicide and 35 percent categorized as having problems with drug and/or alcohol use (Melese-d'Hospital et al., 2002). Results of other studies indicate that proper management in the ED of adolescents who have attempted suicide is lacking. Although the importance of follow-up psychiatric treatment has been demonstrated, psychotherapy is recommended to fewer than half of adolescent suicidal patients evaluated in the ED (Piacentini et al., 1995). Additionally, adolescents with somatic complaints are infrequently screened for depression (Porter et al., 1997).

These findings should not be surprising considering that ED providers often lack the training, skills, and resources to deal effectively with mentally ill patients. Standardized psychiatric training is not required of residents in emergency medicine and pediatric emergency medicine. Fewer than one-quarter of emergency medicine residency programs provide formal psychiatric training (Santucci et al., 2003). Surveys of nurses—even those working in designated pediatric EDs—show that pediatric psychiatric emergencies are among the conditions they feel the least comfortable and knowledgeable in managing (Fredrickson et al., 1994). ED physicians may not have the time to perform a thorough mental health evaluation, and many rely on psychiatrists, psychologists, or social workers for the purpose. When that assistance is not available, patients may not receive an evaluation at all. The ED setting also makes it difficult to care for a mentally ill patient. The lack of privacy and the noisy, high-stimulus environment may make it uncomfortable for patients to participate in a mental health evaluation (Hoyle and White, 2003).

The psychiatric resources available within EDs vary greatly among hospitals. For example, teaching hospitals use psychiatric residents to provide consultations to patients with psychiatric problems. Other hospitals use a pool of mental health professionals, including clinical nurse specialists, to provide such services, although these professionals may not be available around the clock. Still, in some hospitals, nurses from inpatient units evaluate psychiatric patients in the ED (Falsafi, 2001). Other hospitals may have no psychiatric resources available to ED staff.

Children with mental health problems represent a real challenge to emergency care providers. Some children present to the ED with highly disruptive behaviors, antagonizing health workers and showing signs of rage. This disruptive behavior can mask the underlying diagnosis of a mental illness (Scheck, 2006). Another major challenge is that specialized psychiatric resources to assess and treat these patients are limited; children in need of psychiatric services often cannot be accommodated immediately. Psychiatric pediatric patients are more likely to require admission than nonpsychiatric pediatric patients (Khan et al., 2002). In many hospitals, however, because of the lack of available psychiatric treatment services, children spend extended lengths of time in the ED or general pediatric inpatient unit waiting for an available psychiatric treatment slot. This situation is particularly problematic in those aged 16–18, who often do not meet the age criteria for adolescent or adult treatment services. In one study, 33 percent of pediatric patients in the ED in need of psychiatric admission were admitted to a pediatric medical floor and waited 1 or more days before being transferred to a psychiatric facility (Mansbach et al., 2003). While assessing the adequacy of mental health resources is beyond the scope of the present study, it is clear that there is a crisis in the mental health system that is having a profound effect on the emergency care system and must be addressed.

Children with Special Health Care Needs

According to the MCHB, children with special health care needs are "those who have or are at increased risk of having chronic physical, developmental, behavioral, or emotional conditions and who also require health and related services of a type or amount beyond that required by children generally" (DHHS et al., 2004). Between 6 and 35 percent of U.S. children meet this definition, depending on which types of disabling conditions are included (AAP, 2002). The number of such children has been growing as medical advances have improved the quality and length of life of children with complex medical conditions. In fact, these children are the most rapidly growing subset of pediatric patients (Sacchetti et al., 2000).

Children with special health care needs have complex, often multiple and lifelong disabilities, and many are dependent upon assistive technological devices and require a specialized approach to assessment, management, and treatment (Spaite et al., 2000; Kastner, 2004). They are also relatively heavy consumers of health care services. Studies of emergency care services for such children in Utah and Los Angeles found that they were more likely than other children to be admitted to the hospital, use EMS for transfer between health care facilities, and receive prehospital treatment such as intravenous therapy (Gausche-Hill, 2000; Suruda et al., 2000). While emergency care providers are increasingly likely to encounter such children (Singh et al., 2003), providers often feel uncertain about their ability to meet these patients' needs (Deschamp and Sneed, 1997), and many EMS agencies do not address these children in their treatment protocols (Singh et al., 2003).

Several efforts have been made by states, communities, and hospitals to develop notification programs for prehospital providers to alert them to children with special health care needs in the area. One of the first was a program called EMS Outreach, developed in 2000 at Children's National Medical Center in Washington, D.C., and supported by the EMS-C program. Under this program, parents and health care providers complete a one-page form with the child's medical information. The form is then faxed to the EMS agency, where the information is entered into the 9-1-1 call center's computers. The EMS stations closes to the child's home also receive the information. The program was expanded to provide all such children with a vinyl index card containing their medical information so that they would have the information with them when away from home. The program also encourages prehospital providers to make home visits so they can become familiar with the children's special needs and establish relationships with both children and parents. In its first year, EMS Outreach enrolled 450 special needs children (Smith et al., 2001).

Similar programs exist in other areas. An EMS-C demonstration grant in New Hampshire was used to develop the Special Needs Identification Project (SNIP). Resources developed through the project are now available online to other states through the EMS-C program's clearinghouse (EMS-C Program, 2003). Certainly as electronic health records advance in the coming years, special needs identification programs are likely to advance as well.

Use of Emergency Care Services by Children

Prehospital Services

Approximately 200 million emergency calls are received by 9-1-1 call centers each year (National Emergency Number Association, 2004); that number includes calls for medical, police, and fire needs. There are no reliable data on the number of pediatric medical calls made to 9-1-1 annually. (The dispatch system is discussed in depth in the committee's companion report, *Emergency Medical Services at the Crossroads*.) However, some data are available on the use of prehospital EMS by children, revealing that in general, their use of such services is relatively low compared with that of adults. The vast majority of pediatric patients under age 15 come to the ED by private vehicle or public transportation and therefore do not receive prehospital emergency care. In 2003, only 3.8 percent of pediatric ED patients under age 15 arrived by ambulance, compared with 11 percent of patients aged 24–44 and 41 percent of those over age 74 (McCaig and Burt, 2005).

Although pediatric patients account for approximately 27 percent of all ED visits, studies suggest that they represent only 5 to 10 percent of all prehospital transports (Seidel et al., 1984; Federiuk et al., 1993). One important source of variation in that percentage is the differing definitions of "child" used by various studies. National data on prehospital calls are not presently collected; therefore, our understanding of pediatric calls is based on studies of individual EMS systems. One of the largest such studies, covering four states, found that most pediatric calls were for boys (56 percent), and most occurred in the evening and daylight hours. Children were transported in 89 percent of the cases, and care was refused by the patient or parents in approximately 8 percent of cases (Joyce et al., 1996). Data from one EMS agency indicate that utilization rates of EMS vary by pediatric age group. In a study of children under age 15 who used the Kansas City, Missouri, EMS system between 1993 and 1995, researchers found that infants under age 1 had the highest rate of use (47.4 children transported per 1,000 persons), followed by those aged 1–4 (26.2), 10–14 (17.5), and 5–9 (17.3) (Murdock et al., 1999).

Approximately half of pediatric prehospital runs are for injury; the rest are for a wide range of medical problems. A 1991 analysis of 10,493 pediatric calls in four California EMS agencies found that 57 percent were for injuries. The most common injuries included head trauma (19 percent of calls), lacerations (16 percent), and contusions (14 percent). Medical calls accounted for the remaining 43 percent, which included knee pain (12 percent), seizures (8.5 percent), neck or back pain (9 percent), ingestions (7 percent), respiratory distress (5 percent), and abdominal pain (5 percent) (Seidel et al., 1991).

However, these statistics mask important differences in prehospital calls across different pediatric age groups. A study of nearly 18,000 transports of children under age 21 in Albuquerque, New Mexico, showed that the most prevalent chief complaints varied by age. Medical complaints predominated in children under 5, while the leading cause of transports among children aged 5–10 was motor vehicle crashes. Assault was a leading cause for transport among patients over age 11 (Sapien et al., 1999).

A number of small studies have investigated the appropriateness of pediatric ambulance transports. Results of these studies generally reveal that the majority of pediatric prehospital runs are not for critical cases (Hamilton et al., 2003) although in general, they are appropriate transports. Foltin and colleagues (1998) developed a tool for evaluating the appropriateness of pediatric ambulance utilization. Applying this tool to patients arriving at two New York City hospitals, they found that the majority of requests for ambulances were appropriate and that dispatchers called for the proper level of care the majority of the time (Foltin et al., 1998).

Still, many pediatric ambulance transports are unnecessary. A study of pediatric transports in Delaware found that they were unnecessary for 28 percent of patients. Of the unnecessary transports, 60 percent were covered by Medicaid. In fact, several studies have shown that children covered by Medicaid have higher rates of EMS transport than other children (Murdock et al., 1999) and higher rates of inappropriate EMS transport (Kost and Arruda, 1999). A study of pediatric ambulance transports in Cleveland that excluded patients needing immediate resuscitation or trauma care found that 82 percent of ambulance transports for children covered by Medicaid were medically unnecessary in the judgment of pediatric emergency physicians. For all medically unnecessary transports, just over half of the caregivers involved cited having no other means of transportation as the reason (Camasso-Richardson et al., 1997). However, determining whether an ambulance transport is medically necessary is much easier retrospectively. Some parents may view ambulance transport as necessary if they lack an alternative means of transportation to an ED (Camasso-Richardson et al., 1997).

Children's Use of the ED

Data from CDC's National Hospital Ambulatory Medical Care Survey (NHAMCS) allow a fairly comprehensive picture of pediatric ED visits. In 2002, there were approximately 29 million pediatric ED visits for children under age 15, representing nearly 27 percent of all ED visits. Data from the National Center for Health Statistics show that the number of pediatric visits to the ED for children under age 15 has been rising since 1997 (see Figure 2-2). In fact, the number of pediatric ED visits increased by nearly 20 percent between 1997 and 2003. The majority of pediatric ED visits (92

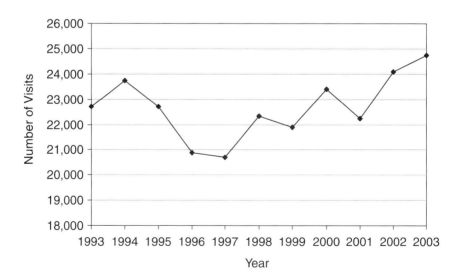

FIGURE 2-2 Number of ED visits for children under age 15 (in thousands).
SOURCE: NHAMCS, ED Summaries for 1993–2003.

percent) are to non-children's hospitals (Gausche-Hill et al., 2004); as noted earlier, however, some general hospitals have specialized pediatric EDs.

Although the majority of pediatric ED visits are for children over age 5, infants (children under age 1) make up a disproportionately large proportion (13 percent) of all pediatric ED visits (see Figure 2-3). In fact, infants have a visit rate of 97.5 visits per 100 persons, much higher than the rate for all children under age 15 (40.8 visits per 100 persons) (McCaig and Burt, 2005). African American children have relatively high rates of ED use—62 visits per 100 children under age 15 compared with 39 visits per 100 for white children. Research on ED utilization for all ages has shown that African Americans had some of the largest increases in ED utilization between 1992 and 1997 (McCaig and Ly, 2002). Hispanic and other non-English-speaking children also use the ED at higher rates.

Nonurgent Use of the ED

Many pediatric visits to the ED are preventable or avoidable. Compared with adults, children make more visits to EDs that can be classified as ambulatory sensitive, meaning that patients do not require care within 12 hours, that immediate care is needed but could be provided in a typical primary care setting, or that immediate care is needed but could have been avoided with timely and effective primary care. Three-quarters of pediatric ED visits that occur overnight and do not result in admission are preventable or avoidable with primary care, suggesting a need for after-hours ambulatory care (Weinick et al., 2003). Perhaps not surprising, parental ED utilization

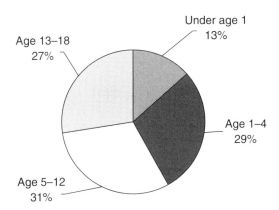

FIGURE 2-3 Percentage of ED visits for children under 18.
SOURCE: 2002 NHAMCS data, calculations by IOM staff.

is significantly associated with increased childhood utilization for both number of visits and number of nonurgent visits (Anderson et al., 2004).

The delivery of nonurgent care in the ED is of concern for three reasons. First, the primary care delivered in the ED may be of lower quality than that in other settings. The ED is designed for rapid, high-intensity responses to acute injuries and illnesses. It is fast-paced and requires intensive concentration of resources for short durations. Such an environment is ill suited to the provision of primary and preventive care (Derlet and Richards, 2000). Physicians in the ED typically do not have a relationship with patients, often lack patients' medical records, face constant interruptions and distractions, and have no means of patient follow-up. Further, because they have low triage priority, nonurgent patients have extremely long wait times—sometimes 6 hours or more. Certainly it would be preferable for children to seek nonurgent care from a medical home.

Second, the literature is unclear as to whether providing nonurgent care in the ED is cost-effective. To some extent, EDs and trauma centers welcome the revenue generated by nonurgent pediatric visits if the hospital would otherwise serve a very low volume of emergent or urgent patients in the ED. Indeed, these revenues can be used to help cover the very large fixed overhead costs associated with maintaining the ED's readiness to provide a full array of services on a round-the-clock basis.

On the other hand, some studies support the notion that costs for nonemergent care in the emergency setting may be substantially higher than those in a primary care setting (Fleming and Jones, 1983; White-Means and Thornton, 1995). Higher costs may be due to the frequent lack of patient records and resultant inability to construct a patient history, which necessitates a high frequency of full workups (Murphy et al., 1996). ED charges for services for minor problems have been estimated to be 2 to 5 times higher than those for a typical office visit (Kusserow, 1992; Baker and Baker, 1994), resulting in $5–7 billion in excess charges in 1993 (Baker and Baker, 1994). While studies probably overestimate the excess cost, it is nevertheless substantial. In contrast, Williams (1996) studied a sample of six hospitals in Michigan and found that average and marginal costs of ED visits were quite low, especially for those classified as nonurgent—perhaps below the cost of a typical physician visit. If hospitals build additional high-cost ED capacity as a result of the increased use of nonurgent care, however, the true cost of treating nonurgent care in the ED will be much higher than the marginal or average cost of treating such patients.

Third, nonurgent utilization may detract from the ED's primary mission of providing emergency and lifesaving care. Regardless of their efficiency on average, EDs do not have unlimited resources. When the ED becomes saturated with patients that could be cared for in a different environment, there are fewer resources—including physicians, nurses, ancillary personnel, equipment, time, and space—available to respond to the population of emergent patients.

Payer Mix

The most common source of payment for ED visits is private insurance, although, as noted above, Medicaid coverage is quite prevalent among pediatric ED users (see Figure 2-4). Indeed, Medicaid represents an important source of health insurance coverage for children; fully 27 percent of all children were covered by the program in 2004 (U.S. Census Bureau, 2005). But looking at insurance status for all pediatric visits masks some important differences by age group. In fact, private coverage becomes more prevalent in higher age groups, while Medicaid coverage declines (see Figure 2-5). Research has shown that Medicaid recipients have disproportionately high rates of ED utilization, and often use the ED for nonurgent care or as their primary source of care (Newacheck, 1992; Gadomski et al., 1995; Liu et al., 1999; Sarver et al., 2002; Irvin et al., 2003). Medicaid patients (of all ages) use the ED at a rate of 81 visits per 100 persons, compared with 41.1 visits per 100 persons with no insurance and 21.5 visits per 100 persons for the privately insured (McCaig and Burt, 2005).

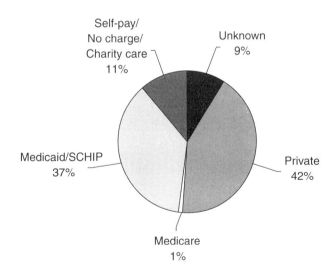

FIGURE 2-4 Pediatric ED visits by payer source.
NOTE: SCHIP = State Children's Health Insurance Program.
SOURCE: 2002 NHAMCS data, calculations by IOM staff.

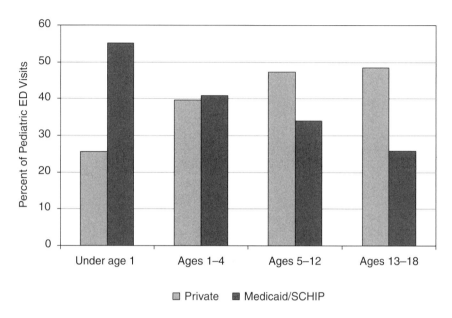

FIGURE 2-5 Percentage of pediatric ED visits covered by private insurance or Medicaid/State Children's Health Insurance Program (SCHIP).
SOURCE: 2002 NHAMCS data, calculations by IOM staff.

There are several reasons why Medicaid enrollees have higher rates of ED utilization. A common assertion is that Medicaid enrollees have poorer access to primary care than other groups, which leads to greater use of the ED (Sharma et al., 2000). This explanation is plausible; because Medicaid reimburses providers at such low rates, it limits access to care, leaving the ED as the only source of care for some individuals. Additionally, Medicaid enrollees may have difficulty seeing primary care providers during regular office hours. According to one study, Medicaid providers who offer evening hours have patients who are less likely to use the ED (Lowe et al., 2005).

On the other hand, a study by Luo and colleagues (2003) suggests that, after controlling for confounding factors, type of insurance coverage is not associated with ED use for nonurgent visits (Luo et al., 2003). Access to primary care (Johnson and Rimsza, 2004) and continuity of care (having a strong relationship with a primary care provider) may be more important deterrents to ED utilization. In a study following 181 children, increased continuity of care with a primary care provider was associated with decreased ED utilization in the first 2 years of life (Brousseau et al., 2004). A larger study that reviewed claims data for more than 46,000 children found that low continuity of care was associated with an increased risk of ED visits and hospitalization (Christakis et al., 2001).

Utilization in Rural Areas

Children in rural areas tend to use the ED more than their urban counterparts. According to data from the National Health Interview Survey (NHIS), 23 percent of rural children versus 20 percent of urban children had made an ED visit within the last year. Higher utilization of the ED in rural areas holds true for adults as well (Center on Aging Society, 2004). Many hypothesize that the shortage of primary care providers is a barrier to physician access for rural populations, where the physician-to-patient ratio is 1 to 3,500, clearly higher than the recommended 1 primary care physician for every 2,000 individuals.

Utilization of Services as a Result of Child Abuse

At least one study has found a link between the number of prior ED visits for injury and subsequent substantiated reports of child maltreatment (Spivey et al., 2005). A focused look at child abuse cases in the ED is needed, however, because national data do not adequately indicate the extent of the prevalence of such cases. Just over 1 percent of all pediatric ED patients are identified as having suffered child abuse; however, it has been estimated that more than 75 percent of all child abuse cases in the ED are missed (Kunen et al., 2003). In one study, researchers retrospectively identified 62 cases of child abuse in the ED. Half of the children had made at least one prior ED visit, and suspicion of abuse had been documented in only 5 cases. Those cases were reported to child protective services, but the children were not placed in protective custody. Of the 62 children identified as child abuse cases, most had made subsequent ED visits, but a history of abuse had not been documented during any of the subsequent visits for trauma (Saade et al., 2002). This study highlights the frequent missed opportunities in the ED to identify cases of abuse and intervene. In fact, abuse is often not recognized until severe injury or death occurs. A review of child abuse fatalities indicates that more than a quarter of the children involved had old fractures consistent with prior abuse and/or recent contact with health care providers (King et al., 2004).

Identification of child abuse varies by hospital type. A recent analysis of infants (children under age 1) admitted to hospitals for treatment for traumatic brain injury or femur fracture (excluding penetrating trauma or motor vehicle injury) shows that children's hospitals diagnosed child abuse more than twice as frequently as did general hospitals (29 and 13 percent, respectively) (Trokel et al., 2006). This is a troubling finding considering that the majority of injured children receive care in general rather than children's hospitals.

The research on this subject indicates two failings. First, identification of child abuse is poor. Although emergency medicine physicians do receive didactic training in child abuse, a survey of residents found that many believed the training was not sufficient (Wagh and Heon, 1999). Results of one study also indicate that prehospital providers lack the knowledge necessary for recognizing, managing, and reporting cases of child abuse (Markenson et al., 2002). Second, high rates of coding errors for pediatric ED visits contribute to underestimates of child abuse. In many cases, child abuse cases identified in the ED are documented using only E-codes. Those cases would be missed in epidemiological studies that select cases using only ICD 995 abuse codes (Kunen et al., 2003).

QUALITY OF CARE

Performance measures specific to emergency care are in the initial stages of development, so formal assessments of the quality of the emergency care system are currently lacking. However, there is reason for concern about the quality of the care delivered. The emergency care system faces a number of challenges that threaten its ability to deliver quality care. Overwhelming demands on the system without the resources necessary to meet those demands contribute to a growing national crisis in emergency care. Under the current system, however, accountability for assuring access to or monitoring the quality of the system is dispersed among many providers. The result is that the system falls short of providing the type of care it should be able to provide.

Growing Pressures on the Emergency Care System

One of the greatest challenges faced by the emergency care system is overwhelming patient loads. The public's dependence on the ED as a source of care is growing; the total number of ED visits rose by 26 percent between 1993 and 2003 (McCaig and Burt, 2005). In some EDs, nonurgent patients must wait 6 to 8 hours before being seen; nationwide, 2 percent of all patients, including pediatric patients, who come to the ED leave before ever being seen (McCaig and Burt, 2005; 2002 NHAMCS data, calculations by IOM staff).

The rising number of patient visits is only part of the problem; EDs are also experiencing great difficulty with moving seriously ill and injured patients from the ED into inpatient beds. In response to cost-cutting measures and lower reimbursement by managed care, Medicaid, and other payers, hospital inpatient bed capacity declined precipitously over the last decade.

To remain viable, some hospitals consolidated and reduced their number of inpatient beds (Brewster and Felland, 2004). Others closed important but unprofitable services, such as trauma, burn, and psychiatric care (IOM, 2003). When no vacant bed is available for an admitted ED patient, most hospitals require ED staff to provide ongoing care to the patient until one becomes available. Many patients are forced to wait hours for an inpatient bed, but some wait days (GAO, 2003). Because most EDs have a limited number of examination rooms and treatment bays, it is not uncommon for admitted patients to be kept on stretchers in ED hallways. This phenomenon, often called "boarding," creates a logjam in the ED because these patients require ongoing attention and care, reducing the resources available to evaluate and treat incoming ED patients. EDs can quickly become overwhelmed by boarders and the crush of patients waiting for care. When patient volume becomes too high for the ED to handle, the hospital may order the ED to go "on diversion," meaning that inbound ambulance traffic is directed to other hospitals. Diversion has become a common occurrence in many areas. In 2003, 45 percent of EDs were on diversion at some point, resulting in the diversion of an estimated 501,000 ambulance runs (Burt et al., 2006).

Diversion has a ripple effect throughout the community, impacting patients, other hospitals, and the community's EMS system. Diversion delays lifesaving care to seriously ill and injured children and adults. By redirecting ambulances to a hospital farther away, it causes valuable time for treating patients to be lost (Neely et al., 1994). For patients who have suffered serious trauma, a heart attack, or a stroke, timely care is essential to prevent death. In these instances, extra minutes spent in transit can have dire, even fatal consequences. For patients with non-life-threatening injuries and illnesses, the extra commute time to an ED bed can cause unnecessary pain and stress. Also, when one hospital goes on EMS diversion, others often follow, either because the inflow of patients becomes too great to handle or because they wish to limit exposure to an influx of uninsured patients to the ED. The result is the health care equivalent of a "rolling blackout" as hospital after hospital closes its doors to ambulance traffic.

When hospitals are on diversion, ambulance transport teams spend more time in transit. The result is not only less accessibility for the community, but also higher levels of stress to providers who are regularly pressured to find an open hospital or care for patients in the ambulance for an extended period of time.

Boarding and ambulance diversion have been prevalent over the past several years. A number of studies have documented the problem, but perhaps most telling is a point-in-time study based on a survey sent to a random sample of hospitals. On Monday, March 12, 2001 (a typical Monday), at 7:00 PM (local time for hospitals), 11 percent of responding hospitals reported being on diversion and 22 percent having patients boarded, awaiting transfer to an inpatient bed (Schneider et al., 2003). However, because most communities and states do not systematically monitor rates of ambulance diversion and the boarding of inpatients in hospital EDs, the extent of these problems and the magnitude of their impact on access to care are largely unknown.

Most studies of boarding and diversion do not specifically address pediatric patients, so the extent to which these problems affect such patients is also unknown. However, a Government Accountability Office (GAO) study found that ED staff have less difficulty transferring patients to pediatric beds than to adult critical care or other adult inpatient beds (GAO, 2003). Some children's hospitals report that they do not go on diversion because there is no alternative source of care for critically injured or ill pediatric patients. However, ED crowding is at least anecdotally an important problem for many children's hospitals. And in hospitals where adults and children are treated in the same ED, the hospital's diversion status will affect pediatric and adult patients equally.

Another challenge to the system is that hospitals are finding it increasingly difficult to identify key specialists, such as neurosurgeons and orthopedists, who are able and willing to take call to treat emergency cases. Surgical specialists typically do not work in the ED full time, but serve in an on-call capacity in case they are needed. Surveys confirm that the availability of on-call specialists, including pediatric specialists, in many areas is rapidly eroding or is already inadequate to meet patients' needs (AAP, 2003; ACEP, 2004; Vanlandingham et al., 2005), and that the problem is worsening (Green et al., 2005; O'Malley et al., 2005).

The role of the emergency care system as a safety net provider also takes a toll. Emergency care providers are the providers of last resort for millions of patients who are uninsured or lack adequate access to care from community providers. Hospitals on the front lines of safety net care encounter patients with intractable social problems, complications resulting from substance abuse or mental illness, and exacerbations of chronic diseases because of inadequate primary care and lack of adherence to medical instructions. Much of the service provided to these difficult patients is compensated poorly or not at all. This care places tremendous financial pressure on safety net hospitals, many of which have closed or are in danger of doing so as a result.

It is within this difficult environment that the emergency care system struggles to meet the unique needs of pediatric patients.

Pediatric Emergency Care and the Six Quality Aims

One way to assess how the current emergency care system is meeting the needs of children is to consider each of the six quality aims for care identified by the IOM in its landmark report *Crossing the Quality Chasm: A New Health System for the 21st Century*: care should be safe, effective, patient-centered, timely, efficient, and equitable. Although evidence often is limited or dated, there is reason to believe that pediatric emergency care is deficient in each of the six aims.

Safe

Patient safety is often compromised in EDs because of overcrowding, the rushed and chaotic environment, frequent provider interruptions, provider fatigue due to long shifts, and limited information on patients' medical histories (Chisholm et al., 2000; Goldberg et al., 2002; Chamberlain et al., 2004). However, it is difficult to determine the safety of emergency care services for children because data on medical errors in emergency care generally are not available. The one exception is evidence suggesting that medication errors in the ED are common for pediatric patients (Selbst et al., 2004; Marcin et al., 2005). Indeed, one study found prescribing errors in the charts of 10 percent of all patients at one pediatric ED (Kozer et al., 2002). Medication errors are especially common for children because doses must be calculated based on the patient's weight; incorrect decimal placement frequently results in 10-fold prescribing errors (Selbst et al., 2004).

Another important threat to the safety of children during emergency care is the lack of knowledge among some providers of how treatment for children differs from that for adults. Without such knowledge, a provider can injure a child while providing care. For example, if a provider does not use special pediatric equipment or exercise proper care when intubating a child, life-threatening errors can be made. Nevertheless, physicians with limited pediatric training or experience are responsible for the majority of patient care in some EDs (Goldmann and Kaushal, 2002). In fact, in many parts of the country, the physicians who staff EDs are not residency trained in emergency medicine or pediatric emergency medicine (Moorhead et al., 2002). Unfortunately, these providers may treat children as they would an adult because of their lack of training and experience (Gausche et al., 1998; Scribano et al., 2000).

Effective

The question of whether commonly practiced emergency care interventions are effective is a surprisingly difficult one to answer for many types of interventions. Particularly in the EMS environment, there is a paucity of evidence to support the treatments that are performed, and few data are collected that could be useful in understanding the effectiveness of interventions (Callaham, 1997). Little or no evidence exists to support basic system design features, such as tiered levels of response, intensity of medical direction, and type of EMS system (e.g., fire department–based, volunteer). The value of deploying paramedics, for example, has been questioned by a recent study (Stiell et al., 2005). A number of clinical practices currently employed, particularly in the prehospital environment (e.g., endotracheal intubation), do not have proven benefits (Gausche et al., 2000; Murray et al., 2000; Wang and Yealy, 2005).

Physician practice patterns for pediatric patients also vary widely, and examples of these variations are numerous. Substantial variations exist among physicians of different specialties—perhaps because of differences in specialty training—in the management of fever (Isaacman et al., 2001), croup (Hampers and Faries, 2002), splenic injury (Davis et al., 2005; Stylianos et al., 2006), diabetic ketoacidosis (Glaser et al., 1997), bronchiolitis (Mansbach et al., 2005), and febrile seizures (Hampers et al., 2000), as well as in resuscitation (Scribano et al., 1997) and use of sedation (Krauss and Zurakowski, 1998). In some of these cases, there are guidelines for treatment (Isaacman et al., 2001); in others, it is unclear which treatment strategy is most beneficial (Glaser et al., 2001; Mansbach et al., 2005), and outcomes are likely to vary based on the treatment provided. This variability in the management of the same conditions suggests that not all children are receiving the most effective care.

Patient-Centered

Patient-centeredness encompasses the qualities of compassion; empathy; and responsiveness to the needs, values, and preferences of patients. In the case of pediatric care, where parents are recognized as the child's primary source of strength and support and play an integral role in the child's health and well-being, the term "family-centered care" is often used instead (Eichner et al., 2003). In the prehospital environment, this means providers should take the time to explain the function of equipment, procedures being performed, and their rationale so family members can be better prepared to make decisions about the child's care. In the ED, family-centered care includes creating a comfortable environment for children and their families, having child life specialists on staff, and enhancing communication between providers and families. In both environments, such care involves giving families the option of being present during procedures and resuscitation as long as doing so does not compromise provider or patient safety.

However, few EDs have written policies or guidelines that allow for the family's presence during invasive procedures (MacLean et al., 2003), and few EMS providers are trained in managing family members or integrating their needs with those of the patient (Loyacono, 2001). Further, many EDs, particularly nonpediatric EDs, can hardly be described as family-friendly, given long wait times to be seen and uncomfortable environments. In some EDs, adults and children wait together and are treated in the same patient care areas, which can frighten children.

Timely

People expect that patients with life-threatening problems will have prompt access to emergency care in the prehospital setting as well as in the ED. But timeliness of care is compromised in overcrowded EDs. The practices of ambulance diversion and patient boarding and their effects in delaying care were discussed above. Likewise, long ED wait times can result in protracted pain and suffering and delays in diagnosis and treatment (Derlet et al., 2001; Derlet, 2002; James et al., 2005). Unfortunately, existing studies on timeliness of care do not include analysis specific to pediatric patients.

Of particular concern are children who leave the ED without being seen. Several studies have investigated which patients leave without being seen and why. Most have concluded that patients do so because the wait was too long (Stock et al., 1994; Quinn et al., 2003), although one Canadian study found that children most often leave because they begin to feel better (Rowe et al., 2003). The majority of patients who leave without being seen have conditions of low acuity (Fernandes et al., 1994), but in some cases such patients are in need of immediate medical attention (Baker et al., 1991; Fernandes et al., 1997). In one study, two-thirds of patients who left without being seen could identify no alternative site of care that would be available to them other than the ED (Baker et al., 1991). Patients who leave without being seen are more likely than those who receive care to report pain or worsening of the seriousness of their problem (Bindman et al., 1991). Many end up returning to the ED at another time, and a small percentage subsequently require hospitalization (Sainsbury, 1990; Bindman et al., 1991).

Specific data on prehospital response times for pediatric patients based on acuity are not currently available. However, seriously ill or injured children pose a real challenge to the system's ability to provide timely care, particularly when pediatric specialists are needed. Ambulances may have to drive to a distant hospital to access providers with pediatric expertise. But more troubling, some EMS agencies authorize ambulances to transport patients only to the nearest hospital, even if that hospital is not appropriate for the patient. In addition, geographic boundaries of an EMS catchment area may limit where ambulances may transport patients.

Timeliness also encompasses the treatment of pain, and there is some evidence indicating that children do not receive pain management in a timely manner. In one study of hospitals in Illinois, only half of children (aged 15 and younger) in severe or moderate pain were offered an analgesic. Older children were more likely to be offered opioids than younger children, particularly those under age 1 (Probst et al., 2005).

Efficient

Efficiency refers to the system's ability to avoid waste, including the waste of equipment, supplies, and energy (IOM, 2001). The considerable patient loads that EDs are required to treat demand efficient care delivery. As discussed earlier, many children who use prehospital and ED services might be treated elsewhere if such care were available. One study found that when Medicaid children are provided enhanced, coordinated access to primary care, utilization of the ED is lower for healthy children, while the total cost of care remains the same (Wang et al., 2005). Whether it is efficient for those patients to receive care in the ED rather than wait for treatment at a later date remains open for debate, however. Although EDs are presumed to have many inefficiencies, the economies of scale resulting from utilization of fixed capital may make it cost-effective to accommodate a certain amount of "after hours" nonurgent care in the hospital ED if doing so enables patients to be treated more quickly and allows parents to work the following day. When the opportunity costs to patients and employers for reduced time loss are factored in, the emergency system may look like a reasonably good alternative. Regardless, for the many patients who use the ED for nonurgent care because they lack access to other sources of care, restricting use of the ED would jeopardize their health.

As noted earlier, under the current system, emergency care providers lack access to patients' medical histories, which can result in the ordering of diagnostic tests that the patient has already received (Cordell et al., 1998). Many emergency care physicians fear the legal consequences of failing to detect rare but dangerous conditions, and compensate by ordering costly diagnostic tests and treatments (Katz et al., 2005). Although some surveys indicate that defensive medicine is not a widespread problem or a major contributor to rising health care costs (Office of Technology Assessment, 1994; Pearson et al., 1995), research suggests that the phenomenon does occur and that physicians who perceive a high risk of a lawsuit are more likely to order tests and procedures that may not be needed (Lawthers et al., 1992). Defensive medicine may be especially likely to occur in emergency settings, where the prevalence of serious illness and injury is high, the public's expectation of diagnostic accuracy is high, and the physician's risk of making an error is increased by the limited time available to make a diagnosis and the lack of an ongoing relationship with the patient and his or her family.

Overall, it would be a considerable stretch to describe the emergency care system as efficient. The practice of boarding patients, long waits in

EDs, ambulance diversion, and long EMS patient off-load times all indicate that the system does not operate smoothly. Yet all of these issues apply to both adult and pediatric patients. There is little information on efficiency specific to pediatric emergency care. An exception is one study that looked at the efficiency of residents in a pediatric ED in terms of number of patients evaluated and treated. The study showed that efficiency varied by residents' subspecialty and years of training (Dowd et al., 2005). Recognizing the paucity of information on the cost-effectiveness of pediatric emergency care, the EMS-C program cited the development of additional economic analyses of pediatric emergency care as an objective in its most recent 5-year plan (MCHB, 2004a).

Equitable

Disparities in health care access and outcomes have long been a problem in the United States (IOM, 2002; AHRQ, 2003). One might assume that because the emergency care system serves all individuals regardless of insurance status, age, race, or income, it is characterized by greater equity relative to the overall health care system. However, of the small number of studies that have looked at equity in emergency care and the still fewer that have examined equity in pediatric emergency care, many indicate that inequities in treatment and access exist.

As discussed above relative to effectiveness, not all patients with the same condition receive the same type of treatment, a fact that indicates a lack of equity in the receipt of care. There is some evidence of variability in treatment based on race and ethnicity for patients of all ages. For example, African Americans and Hispanics are less likely to receive pain medication for certain conditions (Todd et al., 2000), and African American patients are more likely than whites to be denied authorization for ED visits by their primary care provider (Lowe et al., 2001). Such disparities extend to children of different races and ethnicities. Studies indicate that wait times for pediatric patients vary based on race and ethnicity (James et al., 2005), that racial and ethnic disparities exist in the ED care provided to children with mild traumatic brain injury (Bazarian et al., 2003), and that African American children with orthopedic fractures covered by Medicaid are less likely to receive parenteral analgesics and sedatives than other children with similar injuries (Hostetler et al., 2002).

Although only a limited number of studies have looked at racial and ethnic disparities in emergency care, some believe the problem is greater than is currently recognized. Racial and ethnic disparities may occur in the prehospital setting through ambulance destinations, triage assessments, diagnostic testing, and disposition decisions. In the ED, disparate treatment may include the timing and intensity of therapy, patterns of referral or prescription choices, and/or priority for hospital admission or bed decisions (Richardson et al., 2003).

Disparities in care also occur based on age. Prehospital providers are less likely to administer treatment to young children compared with adults (Gausche et al., 1998; Scribano et al., 2000). For example, one study found that paramedics are less likely to perform basic resuscitation procedures for pediatric patients than for equally critical adults (Su et al., 1997). (This issue is discussed further in Chapter 4.) Children are also less likely to receive pain medication than adults, and the youngest children, those under age 2, are less likely to receive such medication than older children (Selbst and Clark, 1990; Petrack et al., 1997; Alexander and Manno, 2003).

Naturally, geography also plays an important role in access to emergency care and pediatric specialists. Issues related to rural pediatric emergency care are explored below.

Not all studies indicate disparities in treatment, however. Two studies found that ED triage and admission decisions were made independently of racial, ethnic, or financial considerations (Kellermann and Haley, 2003; Oster and Bindman, 2003).

Rural Pediatric Emergency Care

In 2000 there were more than 15 million children below age 18 residing in rural areas, constituting 26 percent of the rural population of the United States (U.S. Census Bureau, 2000). While there is no standard definition of a rural area, the basic demographic feature of such a locale is that it is a place of low population density and small aggregate size (IOM, 2005). Children in these areas encounter significant barriers to appropriate emergency care (AAP, 2000). Friedlander and Alessandrini (2004) pointed out that rural children are classically underserved, with conditions of poverty transcending geographic considerations. Rural children are more likely than their nonrural counterparts to be poor, to lack access to primary care and appropriate referral sources, to be covered by a public insurance program, and to utilize an ED.

In 2003, more than 14 percent of people living outside of a metropolitan area lived below the poverty level, compared with 12 percent of their metropolitan counterparts (U.S. Census Bureau, 2004). According to the Kaiser Commission on Medicaid and the Uninsured, 47 percent of rural families have incomes below 200 percent of the poverty level (compared with 27 percent of nonrural families), qualifying a disproportionately large number of rural children for Medicaid benefits and emphasizing their reliance on public insurance. Fewer than half of rural children living in counties not adjacent to a county with a large city have private insurance coverage. Thirty percent of these children are covered by Medicaid or the State Children's Health Insurance Program (SCHIP) (compared with 19 percent of urban/adjacent rural children), and 1 in 5 are uninsured (Kaiser Family Foundation, 2003).

Rural residence has been demonstrated to be predictive of ED use by low-income children (Polivka et al., 2000). Sharma and colleagues (2000) determined that for infants, the highest rate of ED use, 1.8 per person-year, was among rural white infants on Medicaid. The lowest rate, 0.4 visits per person-year, was among urban white infants with commercial insurance (Sharma et al., 2000).

Rural emergency care for pediatric patients is characterized by many of the same issues that affect emergency care in other areas. However, many studies have shown differences in the use of pediatric emergency care between rural and urban areas. In an examination of pediatric coroners' cases in both rural and urban California counties, rural children were found to be less likely to use EMS provider services than their urban counterparts (66 versus 84 percent), and a significantly greater number of rural children died on the street or highway (Gausche et al., 1989). Seidel and colleagues (1991) found that trauma was a more frequent complaint in rural areas of California, responsible for 64 percent of all rural prehospital calls. A study by Svenson and colleagues (1996) found trauma in rural settings of Kentucky to be responsible for nearly 50 percent of EMS calls. Rural trauma centers have also been demonstrated to receive proportionately more victims of motor vehicle crashes (28.5 percent of patients) and "other" categories of injury (28.2 percent), to which bicycle injuries are assigned (Nakayama et al., 1992). Similar injury patterns were noted by Serleth and colleagues (1999) between 1990 and 1993, with more than half of all pediatric trauma admissions being the result of injuries related to falls, recreational activities, and motor vehicle crashes.

Despite the variations in time and setting in the above studies, each found trauma to be a leading cause of EMS activation by rural children. Yet there are deficiencies in the provision of ALS in rural areas. The use of BLS/ALS has been found to be dependent on the patient's age and the level of provider care, with provision of ALS to younger children being less frequent than that to older patients. Failure to provide ALS occurred even though time on scene would not have been prolonged (Svenson et al., 1996). Gausche and colleagues (1989) found that only 66 percent of rural child victims of trauma received ALS interventions, 31 percent fewer than urban children in the same study (Gausche et al., 1989). Thus rural children are more likely to require EMS for traumatic injuries but less likely to obtain EMS services and appropriate life support modalities. Additionally, results of a recent study of admissions in rural EDs indicate higher nonessential admission rates at rural hospitals and by nonpediatric EM physicians, which may reflect a lack of resources, comfort, or expertise among emergency providers for the care of pediatric patients (Derrington et al., 2005).

Rural emergency care providers and provider organizations face a number of operational challenges not encountered by those in urban or suburban areas. In rural areas, the relatively low volume of emergency calls in relation to the high overhead of maintaining a prepared staff results in very high costs per transport. To lower those costs, many rural EMS squads rely on volunteers rather than paid EMS providers, which by nature results in a less stable system. In many rural communities, younger residents are leaving while the remaining population becomes more elderly. As a result, the pool of potential volunteers is dwindling as their average age and the demands on their time increase. The closure or restructuring of many rural hospitals has further increased the demand on rural EMS agencies by creating an environment that requires long-distance, time-consuming, and high-risk interfacility transfers. Another challenge facing some rural areas is that the population can swell—double or triple—during the tourist season. Thus the EMS staffing required throughout the year varies.

Under the Balanced Budget Act of 1997, Congress established the Medicare Rural Hospital Flexibility Program. In additional to providing cost-based reimbursement to certain rural hospitals, the "Flex Program" provides states with grants to support their rural health infrastructure and foster the growth of collaborative rural health care delivery systems. In fiscal year 2003, states received approximately $22 million under the program, with the average state award being approximately $500,000. Development of EMS systems has been a growing focus of state planning efforts under the grants (Flex Monitoring Team, 2004). The committee finds this trend promising and encourages states to focus attention on pediatric needs within rural EMS systems.

REIMBURSEMENT FOR PEDIATRIC EMERGENCY CARE

The costs of providing emergency care services reflect not just the operational costs of responding to each emergency call, but also the costs associated with having personnel available around the clock. Appropriate reimbursement for pediatric emergency care services is of obvious importance. It allows emergency care organizations to increase their readiness by hiring and retaining providers with the right mix of skills and training, to offer continuing pediatric education, and to equip providers with appropriate pediatric supplies. It also allows providers to make investments that can improve the quality of care delivered, from the development of new quality initiatives to the installation of information systems.

Funding for pediatric emergency care differs from that for adult emergency care in that the payer mix is different, which has important implications for reimbursement levels. Emergency care provider organizations are highly dependent on the Medicaid and SCHIP programs for reimbursement for pediatric emergency care services. To the extent that those programs do not adequately cover the cost of services provided to Medicaid and SCHIP enrollees, providers suffer financial losses in caring for those patients. As of this writing, policy makers are facing a dilemma with regard to the Medicaid program's growing expenditures. Among the options being considered are significant cuts in benefits coupled with increases in patient cost sharing. While the committee believes that fair payment for emergency care services under Medicaid is critical, it recognizes the political and economic realities associated with proposing increases in payment at this time. As a result, this section is intended to highlight some of the difficulties related to reimbursement for pediatric emergency care services rather than to suggest immediate changes to payment and policies.

Payer Mix

Although some emergency care providers may receive financial support through public subsidies or private donations, their primary source of income is reimbursement for services. Because reimbursement levels vary based on the insurance status of the patient, payer mix is critical to the financial health of providers.

Data from the March 2004 Current Population Survey (CPS) indicate that in 2003, 61 percent of children were covered by private insurance and 27 percent by Medicaid or other public insurance programs (for example, SCHIP or Medicare), while 12 percent were uninsured (Kaiser Family Foundation, 2004b). If all children used emergency services at the same rate, the payer source for emergency care visits would mirror the data on insurance coverage for children. However, that is not the case. There are important differences in the use of emergency services by insurance status. Table 2-7 displays information on the expected source of payment for ED visits made by children and adults in 2002.

As noted earlier, privately insured children use the ED less than publicly insured or uninsured children. Although 61 percent of children are covered by private insurance, they represent approximately 42 percent of pediatric visits to EDs. Children covered by Medicaid or other public programs tend to use the ED at disproportionately high rates. Only 27 percent of children are covered by Medicaid or other public insurance, but they account for at least 37 percent of all pediatric visits to EDs. Uninsured children tend to use the ED at rates proportionate to their numbers.

The difference in payer mix between nonelderly adult and pediatric ED visits is also of note. Children are more likely to be covered by Medicaid or SCHIP than their adult counterparts, but considerably less likely to be

TABLE 2-7 Payer Mix for ED Visits, Children and Adults, 2002

Source of Payment	Children (<19)	Nonelderly Adults (19–64)
Private Insurance	42%	44%
Medicaid/SCHIP	37	16
Medicare	1	6
Self-Pay	10	20
No Charge	1	2
Workers Compensation	0	3
Unknown	9	10

NOTE: SCHIP = State Children's Health Insurance Program.
SOURCE: 2002 NHAMCS data, calculations by IOM staff.

uninsured. Data on payer mix for prehospital care at the national level are unavailable, but as noted earlier, data from regional ambulance services confirm the heavy reliance of pediatric patients on Medicaid or SCHIP for health insurance coverage. However, these regional data also indicate that a large percentage of pediatric ambulance calls are for uninsured children, and therefore not likely to be reimbursed. Indeed, an examination of EMS transports by the Albuquerque, New Mexico, ambulance service (which provides 99 percent of EMS transports in that city) during 1992–1995 showed that 57 percent of transported patients under age 21 were uninsured. That study also found that payment source varied by patient age, with public insurance being overrepresented among patients younger than age 11, private insurance and lack of insurance being overrepresented among those aged 11–16, and lack of insurance being overrepresented among those aged 17–20 (Sapien et al., 1999).

Medicaid and the State Children's Health Insurance Program

Medicaid is a federal–state health insurance entitlement program that provides coverage for low-income individuals. The program is administered by the states, and the federal government sets guidelines and matches state spending at rates of between 50 and 77 percent, depending on state per capita income (Kaiser Family Foundation, 2004a). Children typically qualify for Medicaid coverage by meeting financial criteria, which vary across states. Federal law mandates coverage of some groups below specified minimum income levels, but also allows states to expand Medicaid eligibility beyond those levels. Medicaid coverage is relatively broad, covering inpatient and outpatient services including emergency services; physician and nurse practitioner services; nursing home and home health care; laboratory and x-ray services; and early and periodic screening, diagnostic, and treatment.

In addition, states commonly cover a wide range of optional Medicaid services, including the costs of prescription drugs, durable medical equipment, and clinic services (Kaiser Family Foundation, 2004a). As of June 2003, more than 42 million individuals were enrolled in Medicaid (CMS, 2003). Children represent approximately 50 percent of Medicaid enrollees (Kaiser Family Foundation, 2004a).

SCHIP is a relatively new public insurance program, introduced in 1997. It is designed to cover "near-poor" children whose family income levels are too high for them to qualify for Medicaid yet too low for them to purchase private coverage. SCHIP operates like the Medicaid program in that it is administered by the states, and funding is matched by the federal government up to a limit. Under the SCHIP program, however, states have greater flexibility in defining eligibility requirements and benefits. Some states design their SCHIP program as essentially an expansion of their Medicaid program; in other states, SCHIP is an entirely separate health insurance program with different benefits and cost-sharing requirements. Unlike Medicaid, SCHIP is not an entitlement program; in fact, some states have a waiting list for enrollment. In the third quarter of 2004, approximately 3.5 million children were enrolled in SCHIP (CMS, 2004).

Children covered under Medicaid and SCHIP are needy in terms of their low family incomes and prevalence of health problems. Compared with privately insured children, those covered by Medicaid or SCHIP are more likely to report only fair or poor health, to have asthma, to have learning disorders, and to have medical conditions that require regular treatment with prescription drugs (Ku and Nimalendran, 2004).

States have considerable freedom to develop their own methods and standards for Medicaid reimbursement. The Omnibus Budget Reconciliation Act of 1989 requires that Medicaid payments to providers be "sufficient to enlist enough providers so that care and services are available under the plan at least to the extent that such care and services are available to the general population in the geographic area." This provision, known as the "equal access" provision, has traditionally not been enforced by the Centers for Medicare and Medicaid Services (CMS). In fact, many states establish physician payment rates without guidance and may not review their rates for several years at a time (AAP, 2002). The result is that Medicaid reimburses care at a lower rate than other payers. Medicaid reimbursement rates are approximately 60 percent of Medicare rates and only 35 to 40 percent of private insurance rates. In a survey conducted by the AAP, more than half of responding pediatricians said that Medicaid payments failed to cover their overhead costs (AAP, 2002).

The low reimbursement rates under Medicaid are evident from the results of a 2001 AAP survey of state Medicaid offices. For three different types of ED visits, the average Medicaid rate was well below the Medicare rate in the vast majority of states. Selected survey results are shown in Table 2-8. These results also reveal the tremendous variation in reimbursement rates across states.

Medicaid rates for emergency services are so low that hospitals tend to collect a greater portion of their charges from the uninsured than from Medicaid patients. Tsai and colleagues (2003) examined payments for ED care using 1998 data from the Medical Expenditure Panel Survey. They found that in 1998, the proportion of charges paid by the uninsured was 58 percent; the proportion paid by Medicaid was only 44 percent. Their analysis included both children and adults.

There are other important problems with Medicaid reimbursement in addition to the low rates. States also have various rules and practices under Medicaid that limit the ability of providers to collect timely payment for services provided. First, some Medicaid programs provide reimbursement for only one service per patient per day. But many children, particularly those with special needs, receive multiple services on the same day. As a result, some services go completely unreimbursed. Second, some states have rules against reimbursing providers if the beneficiary seeks service in another state. This is particularly troubling to providers near a state boarder, such as Washington, D.C., Chicago, and Kansas City. Many patients opt for care outside of their state of residence, particularly if a children's hospital is on the other side of the border. In addition, the Medicaid payment cycle can be twice as long as that of most private insurance payers, so providers do not receive timely reimbursement. Third, some Medicaid programs do not reimburse for a variety of services that are provided to pediatric patients in the ED. An example is sedation and analgesia, which are not reimbursable under the Illinois Medicaid program. Likewise, prevention services provided in the ED are typically not reimbursed even though they have the potential

TABLE 2-8 Medicare and Medicaid Rates for ED Visits, 2001

ED Visit	Medicare Rate	Average Medicaid Rate	Lowest Medicaid Rate	Highest Medicaid Rate	Number of States Where the Medicaid Rate Is Higher Than the Medicare Rate
Low-complexity decision	$30.61	$25.85	$9.00	$50.40	11
Intermediate-complexity decision	$64.66	$41.68	$9.00	$97.00	2
High-complexity decision	$100.62	$61.28	$9.00	$148.91	1

SOURCE: AAP, 2001b.

to reduce future ED visits. Finally, the retrospective nature of Medicaid payment does not account for the diagnostic resources whose use may be necessary during an ED visit. In some states, for example, Medicaid may pay for treatment of a fractured ankle but not a sprained ankle; however, the only way to determine whether the ankle is fractured is with an x-ray. If the x-ray is negative, Medicaid will not pay for it or for the service provided to the patient.

Clearly, there are a number of problems associated with Medicaid payment for pediatric emergency care services. While coverage expansions through SCHIP may aid in offsetting the costs of uncompensated care, the low reimbursement rates and poor payment policies of both programs may not meet the financial needs of operating a pediatric ED.

The impact of Medicaid's poor payment policies is felt most acutely by safety net and children's hospitals because of their sizable dependence on Medicaid as a revenue source. Data from Children's Memorial Hospital in Chicago indicate that a large and growing number of ED patients are covered by Medicaid (see Table 2-9). Because of Medicaid's poor payment rates and policies, the hospital lost $1.2 million in 2004 for treating 28,000 patients covered by Medicaid. If Medicaid paid the same rates paid by Medicare, the hospital would just about break even on those ED patients. While it is true that children's hospitals receive funds from additional sources, such as disproportionate share hospital payments and graduate medical education (GME) funding, those sources still may not cover the hospital's operating expenses. Many children's hospitals pursue philanthropy as a way to cover operating expenses.

Given the low payment rates under Medicaid, it should not be surprising that children—even those with private insurance coverage—have difficulty accessing pediatric specialists in the ED. If specialists expect that one-half of all patients at children's hospital EDs will be covered by Medicaid, they may not be willing to provide care in those settings.

Medicaid payment for prehospital services is no better. Medicaid pays a fixed rate—$25 in some states—for an EMS transport, regardless of the complexity of the case or the resources utilized. Additionally, reimburse-

TABLE 2-9 Growing Dependence on Medicaid at One Children's Hospital

	1999	2000	2001	2002	2003	2004
Total ED Visits	40,556	39,991	43,882	46,841	47,200	49,511
Medicaid ED Visits	20,278	20,395	23,696	26,230	26,902	28,201
Percent Medicaid	50%	51%	54%	56%	57%	57%

SOURCE: Data from Children's Memorial Hospital Emergency Department.

ment is provided only when a patient is transported. This naturally leads to perverse incentives to transport patients to the ED even if they do not require an ED visit.

Other Payment Considerations

While Medicaid concerns are primary, a number of other reimbursement issues specific to pediatric care make it difficult for emergency care providers to collect appropriate revenues for services rendered.

Only a small percentage of children (less than 1 percent) have health insurance coverage under the Medicare program (U.S. Census Bureau, 2005). Medicare is a federal program that provides health care coverage to senior citizens and individuals with disabilities. However, the way Medicare reimburses providers—using the resource based relative value scale (RBRVS)—serves as a model for other payers. The RBRVS is a way of valuating physician services based on the work, associated practice expenses, geographic location, and professional liability expenses. However, the RBRVS does not recognize the considerable effort involved in providing emergency services to children—particularly infants and young children. In fact, there are several reasons why pediatric emergency care requires greater physician time and attention than adult emergency care. First, emergency providers must respond to childrens' fear and anxiety prior to examinations or treatment, which tends to add to the time and stress involved. Providers must also address the needs of parents, which adds an element of complexity. Second, providers must constantly adapt the examination or procedure in response to the patient's level of cooperation or changing behavior. For example, a child may need to be sedated to allow ED staff to perform suturing, whereas suturing an adult is a relatively simple task. Third, pediatric emergencies may require follow-up with a number of different individuals and organizations, including day care facilities, schools, and parents/guardians, which results in increased expenditures of time (Committee on Coding and Nomenclature, 2004). (Certainly similar arguments could be made for other patient groups, such as the elderly, that require extra work likewise not recognized by the RBRVS.)

Like some Medicaid programs, the Medicare program does not provide payment for certain services provided in the ED. Some neonatal and pediatric critical care services, preventive care, some vascular care, immunizations, and sedation/analgesia are not recognized reimbursable pediatric services. Because the Medicare payment system serves as a model for private payers and some Medicaid programs, other payers also exclude reimbursement for those services.

In addition to being an important source of reimbursement for patient services for the elderly, Medicare is the largest source of funding for GME.

In fact, U.S. teaching hospitals receive approximately $7 billion each year to help cover the additional expenses associated with training medical residents (HRSA, 2002). However, because children's hospitals treat children rather than many elderly Medicare recipients, they have largely been excluded from Medicare GME payments (National Association of Children's Hospitals and Related Institutions, 2006). Congress recently addressed this imbalance through special funding for independent teaching children's hospitals. However, children's hospitals are arguably less able than other hospitals to provide financial support for resident training. This situation has resulted in a reluctance on the part of some children's hospitals to have emergency medicine residents train at their facilities because those residents compete with pediatric residents and pediatric specialists for limited training dollars.

Despite the reimbursement problems associated with pediatric emergency care services, a number of hospitals have recently added pediatric EDs. Although this movement appears counterintuitive, hospitals view pediatric EDs as a way of generating revenue for the organization. Parents and caregivers generally prefer to bring their children to a pediatric ED rather than a general ED. In addition, pediatric EDs offer a marketing opportunity by bringing additional family members into contact with the hospital. One study found that an off-site pediatric urgent care clinic helped increase a hospital's market share, enabling it to attract a large number of well-insured patients (Tennyson, 2003). Certainly these new pediatric EDs are not opening in areas where many uninsured and Medicaid children reside, however. In fact, they may be causing additional financial difficulties for children's hospitals if they are drawing privately insured patients away from those hospitals.

REFERENCES

AAP (American Academy of Pediatrics). 1992. AAP task force on infant positioning and SIDS: Positioning and SIDS. *Pediatrics* 89(6 Pt. 1):1120–1126.

AAP. 2000. *Committee on Pediatric Emergency Medicine. History.* [Online]. Available: http://www.aap.org/visit/copemhistory.htm [accessed January 10, 2006].

AAP. 2001a. Care of children in the emergency department: Guidelines for preparedness. *Pediatrics* 107(4):777–781.

AAP. 2001b. Medicaid Reimbursement Survey, 2001. Washington, DC: AAP.

AAP. 2002. *Statement for the Record.* Elk Grove Village, IL: AAP.

AAP. 2003. *Council of Medical Specialty Societies: Workforce Questions.* Washington, DC: AAP.

ACEP (American College of Emergency Physicians). 2004. *Two-Thirds of Emergency Department Directors Report On-Call Specialty Coverage Problems.* [Online]. Available: http://www.acep.org/1,34081,0.html [accessed September 28, 2004].

ACS (American College of Surgeons). 2004. *National Trauma Data Bank Pediatric Report 2004.* Chicago, IL: American College of Surgeons.

Advocates for EMS. 2004. *EMSC Program*. [Online]. Available: http://www.advocatesforems. org/Library/upload/EMSC_Program_Fact_Sheet.pdf [accessed August 2, 2004].

AHRQ (Agency for Healthcare Research and Quality). 2002. *Children's Health Highlights*. Rockville, MD: AHRQ.

AHRQ. 2003. *National Healthcare Disparities Report*. Rockville, MD: DHHS.

Alexander J, Manno M. 2003. Underuse of analgesia in very young pediatric patients with isolated painful injuries. *Annals of Emergency Medicine* 41(5):617–622.

Anderson M, Megan R, Zielinski S. 2004. Decreasing emergency department visits among inner-city children with asthma. *Accident and Emergency Nursing* 2(11):796–797.

Arrowsmith JB, Kennedy DL, Kuritsky JN, Faich GA. 1987. National patterns of aspirin use and Reye syndrome reporting, United States, 1980 to 1985. *Pediatrics* 79(6):858–863.

ATS (American Trauma Society). 2006. *ATS and Trauma*. [Online]. Available: http://www. amtrauma.org/atsandtrauma/atsandtrauma.html [accessed March 12, 2006].

Augustine J, Kellermann A, Koplan J. 2004. America's emergency care system and severe acute respiratory syndrome: Are we ready? *Annals of Emergency Medicine* 43(1):23–26.

Baker DW, Stevens CD, Brook RH. 1991. Patients who leave a public hospital emergency department without being seen by a physician. Causes and consequences. *Journal of the American Medical Association* 266(8):1085–1090.

Baker LC, Baker LS. 1994. Excess cost of emergency department visits for nonurgent care. *Health Affairs* 13(5):164–171.

Bazarian JJ, Pope C, McClung J, Cheng YT, Flesher W. 2003. Ethnic and racial disparities in emergency department care for mild traumatic brain injury. *Academic Emergency Medicine* 10(11):1209–1217.

Beers MH, Berkow R. 2005. *The Merck Manual of Diagnosis and Therapy*. Whitehouse Station, NJ: Merck & Co., Inc.

Belay ED, Bresee JS, Holman RC, Khan AS, Shahriari A, Schonberger LB. 1999. Reye's syndrome in the United States from 1981 through 1997. *New England Journal of Medicine* 340(18):1377–1382.

Bindman AB, Grumbach K, Keane D, Rauch L, Luce JM. 1991. Consequences of queuing for care at a public hospital emergency department. *Journal of the American Medical Association* 266(8):1091–1096.

Bitnun A, Allen U, Heurter H, King SM, Opavsky MA, Ford-Jones EL, Matlow A, Kitai I, Tellier R, Richardson S, Manson D, Babyn P, Read S. 2003. Children hospitalized with severe acute respiratory syndrome-related illness in Toronto. *Pediatrics* 112(4):e261.

Brewster LR, Felland LE. 2004. Emergency department diversions: Hospital and community strategies alleviate the crisis. *Issue Brief (Center for Studying Health System Change)* (78):1–4.

Brousseau DC, Meurer JR, Isenberg ML, Kuhn EM, Gorelick MH. 2004. Association between infant continuity of care and pediatric emergency department utilization. *Pediatrics* 113(4):738–741.

Burt CW, McCaig LF, Valverde RH. 2006. *Analysis of Ambulance Transports and Diversions among U.S. Emergency Departments*. Hyattsville, MD: National Center for Health Statistics.

Callaham M. 1997. Quantifying the scanty science of prehospital emergency care. *Annals of Emergency Medicine* 30(6):785–790.

Camasso-Richardson K, Wilde J, Petrack E. 1997. Medically unnecessary pediatric ambulance transports: A medical taxi service? *Academic Emergency Medicine* 4(12):1137–1141.

CDC (Centers for Disease Control and Prevention). 2004. *Ten Leading Causes of Death*. [Online]. Available: http://www.cdc.gov/ncipc/osp/charts.htm [accessed January 3, 2004].

CDC. 2005. *Child Passenger Safety: Fact Sheet*. [Online]. Available: www.cdc.gov/ncipc/ factsheets/childpas.htm [accessed October 5, 2005].

Center on Aging Society. 2004. *Disease Management Programs: Improving Health While Reducing Costs?* Washington, DC: Center on Aging Society.

Chamberlain J, Slonim A, Joseph J. 2004. Reducing errors and promoting safety in pediatric emergency care. *Ambulatory Pediatrics* 4(1):55–63.

Child Trends Databank. 2004. *Teen Homicide, Suicide, and Firearm Death.* Washington, DC: Child Trends Databank.

Chisholm CD, Collison EK, Nelson DR, Cordell WH. 2000. Emergency department workplace interruptions: Are emergency physicians "interrupt-driven" and "multitasking"? *Academic Emergency Medicine* 7(11):1239–1243.

Christakis DA, Mell L, Koepsell TD, Zimmerman FJ, Connell FA. 2001. Association of lower continuity of care with greater risk of emergency department use and hospitalization in children. *Pediatrics* 107(3):524–529.

Clarke A, Walton WW. 1979. Effect of safety packaging on aspirin ingestion by children. *Pediatrics* 63(5):687–693.

CMS (Centers for Medicare and Medicaid Services). 2003. *Medicaid Managed Care Enrollment as of June 30, 2003.* [Online]. Available: http://www.cms.hhs.gov/medicaid/managedcare/mcsten03.pdf [accessed January 24, 2004].

CMS. 2004. *FY 2004 Third Quarter—Program Enrollment Last Day of Quarter by State—Total SCHIP.* [Online]. Available: http://www.cms.hhs.gov/schip/enrollment/2004pit3qt.pdf [accessed January 24, 2004].

Committee on Coding and Nomenclature. 2004. Application of the resource-based relative value scale system to pediatrics. *Pediatrics* 113(5):1437–1440.

Cooper A. 2006. Organizing the community for pediatric trauma care. In: Wesson D, Cooper A, Scherer III LRT, Stylianos S, Tuggle DW, eds. *Pediatric Trauma. Pathophysiology, Diagnosis, and Treatment.* New York: Taylor & Francis Group.

Cordell WH, Overhage JM, Waeckerle JF. 1998. Strategies for improving information management in emergency medicine to meet clinical, research, and administrative needs. The Information Management Work Group. *Annals of Emergency Medicine* 31(2):172–178.

CPEM (Center for Pediatric Emergency Medicine). 2001. *The Emergency Medical Services for Children Program.* [Online]. Available: http://www.cpem.org/trippals/01EMSC.PDF [accessed December 14, 2004].

Davis DH, Localio AR, Stafford PW, Helfaer MA, Durbin DR. 2005. Trends in operative management of pediatric splenic injury in a regional trauma system. *Pediatrics* 115(1):89–94.

Derlet RW. 2002. Overcrowding in emergency departments: Increased demand and decreased capacity. *Annals of Emergency Medicine* 39(4):430–432.

Derlet RW, Richards J. 2000. Overcrowding in the nation's emergency departments: Complex causes and disturbing effects. *Annals of Emergency Medicine* 35(1):63–68.

Derlet RW, Richards J, Kravitz R. 2001. Frequent overcrowding in U.S. emergency departments. *Academic Emergency Medicine* 8(2):151–155.

Derrington SF, Cole SL, Dean TD, Nasrollahzadeh F, Shontz AM, Marcin JP. 2005. *Increased Nonessential Admissions in Rural Emergency Departments and by Non-Pediatric Emergency Medicine Physicians.* Presented at the Pediatric Academic Societies Meeting, May 2005, Washington, DC.

Deschamp C, Sneed RC. 1997. EMS for children with special healthcare needs. *Emergency Medical Services* 26(11):57–61; quiz 75.

Dey A, Bloom B. 2005. *Summary Health Statistics for U.S. Children: National Health Interview Survey, 2003.* Hyattsville, MD: National Center for Health Statistics.

DHHS (Department of Health and Human Services). 1980. *Promoting Health Preventing Disease: Objectives for the Nation.* Washington, DC: U.S. Government Printing Office.

DHHS. 1990. *Healthy People 2000.* Washington, DC: U.S. Government Printing Office.

DHHS. 1999. *Mental Health: A Report of the Surgeon General.* Rockville, MD: DHHS.

DHHS. 2000. *Healthy People 2010: Understanding and Improving Health* (2nd edition). Washington, DC: U.S. Government Printing Office.

DHHS. 2004. *Emergency Medical Services for Children. Fiscal Year 2003 Program Highlights Report.* [Online]. Available: http://www.ems-c.org/Downloads/PDF/ProgramHighlights/FY03ProgramHighlights.pdf [accessed October 2004].

DHHS, HRSA, MCHB (U.S. Department of Health and Human Services, Health Resources and Services Administration, Maternal and Child Health Bureau). 1995. *Emergency Medical Services for Children Five Year Plan: Emergency Medical Services for Children, 1995-2000.* Washington, DC: EMS-C National Resource Center.

DHHS, HRSA, MCHB. 2000. *Emergency Medical Services for Children Five Year Plan: Midcourse Review.* Washington, DC: EMS-C National Resource Center.

DHHS, HRSA, MCHB. 2001. *Five-Year Plan: Emergency Medical Services for Children, 2001-2005.* Washington, DC: EMS-C National Resource Center.

DHHS, HRSA, MCHB. 2004. *The National Survey of Children with Special Health Care Needs Chartbook 2001.* Washington, DC: US Department of Health and Human Services.

Dowd MD, Tarantino C, Barnett TM, Fitzmaurice L, Knapp JF. 2005. Resident efficiency in a pediatric emergency department. *Academic Emergency Medicine* 12(12):1240–1244.

Eichner JM, Neff JM, Hardy DR, Klein M, Percelay JM, Sigrest T, Stucky ER, Dull S, Perkins MT, Wilson JM, Corden TE, Ostric EJ, Mucha S, Johnson BH, Ahmann E, Crocker E, DiVenere N, MacKean G, Schwab WE. 2003. Family-centered care and the pediatrician's role. *Pediatrics* 112(3):691–696.

EMS-C Program (Emergency Medical Services for Children Program). 2003. *EMSC Product List.* Vienna, VA: Emergency Medical Services for Children Clearinghouse. [Online]. Available: http://www.ems-c.org/Downloads/PDF/Products.pdf [accessed January 2006].

Falsafi N. 2001. Pediatric psychiatric emergencies. *Journal of Child and Adolescent Psychiatric Nursing* 14(2):81–88.

Federiuk CS, O'Brien K, Jui J, Schmidt TA. 1993. Job satisfaction of paramedics: The effects of gender and type of agency of employment. *Annals of Emergency Medicine* 22(4):657–662.

Fernandes CM, Daya MR, Barry S, Palmer N. 1994. Emergency department patients who leave without seeing a physician: The Toronto hospital experience. *Annals of Emergency Medicine* 24(6):1092–1096.

Fernandes CMB, Price A, Christenson JM. 1997. Does reduced length of stay decrease the number of emergency department patients who leave without seeing a physician? *Journal of Emergency Medicine* 15(3):397–399.

Fifield GC, Magnuson C, Carr WP, Deinard AS. 1984. Pediatric emergency care in a metropolitan area. *Journal of Emergency Medicine* 1(6):495–507.

Fildes JJE. 2005. *National Trauma Data Bank Pediatric Report.* Chicago, IL: ACS.

Fleming NS, Jones HC. 1983. The impact of outpatient department and emergency room use on costs in the Texas Medicaid Program. *Medical Care* 21(9):892–910.

Flex Monitoring Team. 2004. *A Synthesis of State Flex Program Plans 2003–2004.* Minneapolis, MN: University of Minnesota, University of North Carolina at Chapel Hill, University of Southern Maine.

Foltin G, Fuchs S. 1991. Advances in pediatric emergency medical service systems. *Emergency Medicine Clinics of North America* 9(3):459–474.

Foltin G, Pon S, Tunik M, Fierman A, Dreyer B, Cooper A, Welborne C, Treiber M. 1998. Pediatric ambulance utilization in a large American city: A systems analysis approach. *Pediatric Emergency Care* 14(4):453–454.

Fong NC, Kwan YW, Hui YW, Yuen LK, Yau EK, Leung CW, Chiu MC. 2004. Adolescent twin sisters with severe acute respiratory syndrome (SARS). *Pediatrics* 113(2):e146–e149.

Fredrickson JM, Bauer W, Arellano D, Davidson M. 1994. Emergency nurses' perceived knowledge and comfort levels regarding pediatric patients. *Journal of Emergency Nursing* 20(1):13–17.

Friedlaender E, Alessandrini E. 2004. Providing optimal emergency care for medically underserved children. *Clinical Pediatric Emergency Medicine* 5:109–119.

Frush K, Hohenhaus S. 2004. *Enhancing Pediatric Patient Safety Grant.* Durham, NC: Duke University Health System.

Gadomski AM, Perkis V, Horton L, Cross S, Stanton B. 1995. Diverting managed care Medicaid patients from pediatric emergency department use. *Pediatrics* 95(2):170–178.

GAO (General Accountability Office). 2003. *Hospital Emergency Departments: Crowded Conditions Vary among Hospitals and Communities.* Report to the Ranking Minority Member, Committee on Finance, U.S. Senate. Washington, DC: GAO.

Gausche M, Seidel JS, Henderson DP, Ness B, Ward PM, Wayland BW. 1989. Violent death in the pediatric age group: Rural and urban differences. *Pediatric Emergency Care* 5(1):64–67.

Gausche M, Rutherford M, Lewis RL. 1995. Emergency department quality assurance/improvement practices for the pediatric patient. *Annals of Emergency Medicine* 25(6):804–808.

Gausche M, Tadeo R, Zane M, Lewis R. 1998. Out-of-hospital intravenous access: Unnecessary procedures and excessive cost. *Academic Emergency Medicine* 5(9):878–882.

Gausche M, Lewis RJ, Stratton SJ, Haynes BE, Gunter CS, Goodrich SM, Poore PD, McCollough MD, Henderson DP, Pratt FD, Seidel JS. 2000. Effect of out-of-hospital pediatric endotracheal intubation on survival and neurological outcome: A controlled clinical trial. *Journal of the American Medical Association* 283(6):783–790.

Gausche-Hill M. 2000. Pediatric continuing education for out-of-hospital providers: Is it time to mandate review of pediatric knowledge and skills? *Annals of Emergency Medicine* 36(1):72–74.

Gausche-Hill M, Lewis R, Gunter C, Henderson D, Haynes B, Stratton S. 2000. Design and implementation of a controlled trial of pediatric endotracheal intubation in the out-of-hospital setting. *Annals of Emergency Medicine* 36(4):356–365.

Gausche-Hill M, Lewis R, Schmitz C. 2004. *Survey of US Emergency Departments for Pediatric Preparedness—Implementation and Evaluation of Care of Children in the Emergency Department: Guidelines for Preparedness. Emergency Medical Services for Children Partnership for Information and Communication Grant #IU93 MC 00184.* Unpublished results.

Glaeser P, Linzer J, Tunik M, Henderson D, Ball J. 2000. Survey of nationally registered emergency medical services providers: Pediatric education. *Annals of Emergency Medicine* 36(1):33–38.

Glaser NS, Kuppermann N, Yee CK, Schwartz DL, Styne DM. 1997. Variation in the management of pediatric diabetic ketoacidosis by specialty training. *Archives of Pediatrics & Adolescent Medicine* 151(11):1125–1132.

Glaser NS, Barnett P, McCaslin I, Nelson D, Trainor J, Louie J, Kaufman F, Quayle K, Roback M, Malley R, Kuppermann N, Pediatric Emergency Medicine Collaborative Research Committee of the American Academy of Pediatrics. 2001. Risk factors for cerebral edema in children with diabetic ketoacidosis. *New England Journal of Medicine* 344:264–269.

Goldberg R, Kuhn G, Andrew L, Thomas H. 2002. Coping with medical mistakes and errors in judgment. *Annals of Emergency Medicine* 39(3):287–292.

Goldmann D, Kaushal R. 2002. Time to tackle the tough issues in patient safety. *Pediatrics* 110(4):823–826.

Graff KJ, Kennedy RM, Jaffe DM. 1996. Conscious sedation for pediatric orthopaedic emergencies. *Pediatric Emergency Care* 12(1):31–35.

Graham CJ, Stuemky J, Lera TA. 1993. Emergency medical services preparedness for pediatric emergencies. *Pediatric Emergency Care* 9(6):329–331.

Green L, Melnick GA, Nawathe A. 2005. *On-Call Physicians at California Emergency Departments: Problems and Potential Solutions.* Oakland, CA: California Healthcare Foundation.

Guidelines for pediatric equipment and supplies for basic and advanced life support ambulances. 1996. Committee on Ambulance Equipment and Supplies, National Emergency Medical Services for Children Resource Alliance. *Annals of Emergency Medicine* 28(6):699–701.

Haddix AC, Mallonee S, Waxweiler R, Douglas MR. 2001. Cost effectiveness analysis of a smoke alarm giveaway program in Oklahoma City, Oklahoma. *Injury Prevention: Journal of the International Society for Child and Adolescent Injury Prevention* 7(4):276–281.

Hamilton S, Adler M, Walker A. 2003. Pediatric calls: Lessons learned from pediatric research. *JEMS: Journal of Emergency Medical Services* 28(7):56–63.

Hampers LC, Faries SG. 2002. Practice variation in the emergency management of croup. *Pediatrics* 109(3):505–508.

Hampers LC, Trainor JL, Listernick R, Eddy JJ, Thompson DA, Sloan EP, Chrisler OP, Gatewood LM, McNulty B, Krug SE. 2000. Setting-based practice variation in the management of simple febrile seizure. *Academic Emergency Medicine* 7(1):21–27.

Harborview Injury Prevention and Research Center. 2006. *Child-Resistant Packaging and the Poison Prevention Packaging Act.* [Online]. Available: http://depts.washington.edu/hiprc/practices/topic/poisoning/packaging.html [accessed February 23, 2006].

Harris BH. 1987. *Progress in Pediatric Trauma.* Presentation at the meeting of the Proceedings of The National Conference on Pediatric Trauma. Boston, MA: The Kiwanis Pediatric Trauma Institute, New England Medical Center.

Hostetler MA, Auinger P, Szilagyi PG. 2002. Parenteral analgesic and sedative use among ED patients in the United States: Combined results from the National Hospital Ambulatory Medical Care Survey (NHAMCS) 1992–1997. *American Journal of Emergency Medicine* 20(3):139–143.

Hoyle J, White L. 2003. Treatment of pediatric and adolescent mental health emergencies in the United States: Current practices, models, barriers, and potential solutions. *Prehospital Emergency Care* 7(1):66–73.

HRSA (Health Resources and Services Administration). 1994. *Emergency Medical Services for Children, Annual Report, FY 1993.* Rockville, MD: HRSA.

HRSA. 2002. *HHS Awards More Than $276 Million to Children's Teaching Hospitals to Ensure Quality Health Care for America's Children (Press Release).* Rockville, MD: DHHS.

IOM (Institute of Medicine). 1993. *Emergency Medical Services for Children.* Washington, DC: National Academy Press.

IOM. 2001. *Crossing the Quality Chasm: A New Health System for the 21st Century.* Washington, DC: National Academy Press.

IOM. 2002. *Unequal Treatment: Confronting Racial and Ethnic Disparities in Health Care.* Washington, DC: National Academy Press.

IOM. 2003. *A Shared Destiny: Community Effects of Uninsurance.* Washington, DC: The National Academies Press.

IOM. 2005. *Quality Through Collaboration: The Future of Rural Health Care.* Washington, DC: The National Academies Press.

Irvin CB, Fox JM, Smude B. 2003. Are there disparities in emergency care for uninsured, Medicaid, and privately insured patients? *Academic Emergency Medicine* 10(11):1271–1277.

Isaacman DJ, Kaminer K, Veligeti H, Jones M, Davis P, Mason JD. 2001. Comparative practice patterns of emergency medicine physicians and pediatric emergency medicine physicians managing fever in young children. *Pediatrics* 108(2):354–358.

James CA, Bourgeois FT, Shannon MW. 2005. Association of race/ethnicity with emergency department wait times. *Pediatrics* 115(3):e310–e315.

Johnson WG, Rimsza ME. 2004. The effects of access to pediatric care and insurance coverage on emergency department utilization. *Pediatrics* 113(3 Pt. 1):483–487.

Joyce S, Brown D, Nelson E. 1996. Epidemiology of pediatric EMS practice: A multistate analysis. *Prehospital Disaster Medicine* 11(3):180–187.

Kaiser Family Foundation. 2003. *Medicaid Benefits.* [Online]. Available: http://www.kff.org/medicaid/benefits/index.cfm [accessed August 20, 2004].

Kaiser Family Foundation. 2004a. *The Medicaid Program at a Glance.* Washington, DC: The Henry J. Kaiser Family Foundation.

Kaiser Family Foundation. 2004b. *Health Coverage for Low-Income Children.* Washington, DC: The Henry J. Kaiser Family Foundation.

Kaplan SL, Mason EO Jr, Wald ER, Schutze GE, Bradley JS, Tan TQ, Hoffman JA, Givner LB, Yogev R, Barson WJ. 2004. Decrease of invasive pneumococcal infections in children among 8 children's hospitals in the United States after the introduction of the 7–valent pneumococcal conjugate vaccine. *Pediatrics* 113(3 Pt. 1):443–449.

Kastner TA. 2004. Managed care and children with special health care needs. *Pediatrics* 114(6):1693–1698.

Katz DA, Williams GC, Brown RL, Aufderheide TP, Bogner M, Rahko PS, Selker HP. 2005. Emergency physicians' fear of malpractice in evaluating patients with possible acute cardiac ischemia. *Annals of Emergency Medicine* 46(6):525–533.

Kellermann AL, Haley LH. 2003. Hospital emergency departments: Where the doctor is always "in." *Medical Care* 41(2):195–197.

Khan ANGA, Carmel M, Rubin DH, Suecoff S. 2002. Pediatric psychiatric illness in the emergency department: An ignored health care issue. *Academic Emergency Medicine* 9(5):390.

King WK, Kiesel EL, Simon HK. 2004. Child abuse fatalities: Are we missing opportunities for intervention? *Academic Emergency Medicine* 11(5):594-a.

Kost S, Arruda J. 1999. Appropriateness of ambulance transportation to a suburban pediatric emergency department. *Prehospital Emergency Care* 3(3):187–190.

Kozer E, Scolnik D, Macpherson A, Keays T, Shi K, Luk T, Koren G. 2002. Variables associated with medication errors in pediatric emergency medicine. *Pediatrics* 110(4):737.

Krauss B, Zurakowski D. 1998. Sedation patterns in pediatric and general community hospital emergency departments. *Pediatric Emergency Care* 14(2):99–103.

Krug S, Kuppermann N. 2005. Twenty years of emergency medical services for children: A cause for celebration and a call for action. *Academic Emergency Medicine* 12(4):345–347.

Ku L, Nimalendran S. 2004. *Improving Children's Health: A Chartbook about the Roles of Medicaid and SCHIP.* Washington, DC: Center on Budget and Policy Priorities.

Kunen S, Hume P, Perret JN, Mandry CV, Patterson TR. 2003. Underdiagnosis of child abuse in emergency departments. *Academic Emergency Medicine* 10(5):546-a.

Kusserow RP. 1992. *Use of Emergency Rooms by Medicaid Recipients.* Washington, DC: DHHS.

Lawthers AG, Localio AR, Laird NM, Lipsitz S, Hebert L, Brennan TA. 1992. Physicians' perceptions of the risk of being sued. *Journal of Health Politics, Policy and Law* 17(3):463–482.

Leung CW, Kwan YW, Ko PW, Chiu SS, Loung PY, Fong NC, Lee LP, Hui YW, Law HK, Wong WH, Chan KH, Peiris JS, Lim WW, Lau YL, Chiu MC. 2004. Severe acute respiratory syndrome among children. *Pediatrics* 113(6):e535–e543.

Liu T, Sayre MR, Carleton SC. 1999. Emergency medical care: Types, trends, and factors related to nonurgent visits. *Academic Emergency Medicine* 6(11):1147–1152.

Lowe RA, Chhaya S, Nasci K, Gavin LJ, Shaw K, Zwanger ML, Zeccardi JA, Dalsey WC, Abbuhl SB, Feldman H, Berlin JA. 2001. Effect of ethnicity on denial of authorization for emergency department care by managed care gatekeepers. *Academic Emergency Medicine* 8(3):259–266.

Lowe RA, Localio AR, Schwarz DF, Williams S, Tuton LW, Maroney S, Nicklin D, Goldfarb N, Vojta DD, Feldman HI. 2005. Association between primary care practice characteristics and emergency department use in a Medicaid managed care organization. *Medical Care* 43(8):792–800.

Loyacono TR. 2001. Family-centered prehospital care. *Emergency Medical Services* 30(6):83.

Luo X, Liu G, Frush K, Hey LA. 2003. Children's health insurance status and emergency department utilization in the United States. *Pediatrics* 112(2):314.

Macias CG. 2005. Pediatric emergency medicine fellowships adopt a new application process. *Pediatric Emergency Care* 21(5):355–356.

MacLean S, Guzzetta C, White C, Fontaine D, Eichhorn D, Meyers T, Desy P. 2003. Family presence during cardiopulmonary resuscitation and invasive procedures: Practices of critical care and emergency nurses. *Journal of Emergency Nursing* 29(3):208–221.

Macpherson AK, MacArthur C. 2002. Bicycle helmet legislation: Evidence for effectiveness. *Pediatric Research* 52(4):472.

Mansbach JM, Wharff E, Austin SB, Ginnis K, Woods ER. 2003. Which psychiatric patients board on the medical service? *Pediatrics* 111(6):e693–e698.

Mansbach JM, Emond JA, Camargo CA Jr. 2005. Bronchiolitis in US emergency departments 1992 to 2000: Epidemiology and practice variation. *Pediatric Emergency Care* 21(4):242–247.

Marcin JP, Seifert L, Cho M, Cole SL, Romano PS. 2005. *Medication Errors among Acutely Ill and Injured Children Presenting to Rural Emergency Departments*. Presentation at the meeting of the Pediatric Academic Societies Meeting, Washington, DC.

Markenson D, Foltin G, Tunik M, Cooper A, Matza-Haughton H, Olson L, Treiber M. 2002. Knowledge and attitude assessment and education of prehospital personnel in child abuse and neglect: Report of a national blue ribbon panel. *Prehospital Emergency Care* 6(3):261–272.

MayoClinic.com. 2005. *Bronchitis*. [Online]. Available: http://www.MayoClinic.com [accessed April 20, 2005].

McCaig LF, Burt CW. 2005. *National Hospital Ambulatory Medical Care Survey: 2003 Emergency Department Summary*. Hyattsville, MD: National Center for Health Statistics.

McCaig LF, Ly N. 2002. National Hospital Ambulatory Medical Care Survey: 2000 Emergency Department Summary. *Advance Data from Vital and Health Statistics; No. 326*. Hyattsville, MD: National Center Health Statistics.

MCHB (Maternal and Child Health Bureau). 2004a. *Emergency Medical Services for Children. Five Year Plan 2001–2005: Midcourse Review*. Washington, DC: EMS-C National Resource Center.

MCHB. 2004b. *Tube Tools: Rapid Sequence Intubation and Related Pediatric Airway Techniques, Version 1.0*. Rockville, MD: DHHS.

MCHB. 2005a. *Emergency Medical Services for Children*. [Online]. Available: http://www.mchb.hrsa.gov/programs/emsc/ [accessed October 4, 2005].

MCHB. 2005b. *EMSC Program*. Rockville, MD: HRSA.

Melese-d'Hospital IA, Olson LM, Cook L, Skokan EG, Dean JM. 2002. Children presenting to emergency departments with mental health problems. *Academic Emergency Medicine* 9(5):528-a.

Middleton KR. 2005. *National Center for Health Statistics Survey, "Emergency Pediatric Services and Equipment Supplement" to the National Hospital Ambulatory Medical Care Survey*. Presentation at the meeting of the 2005 EMSC Annual Grantee Meeting, Washington, DC.

Middleton KR, Burt CW. 2006. *Availability of Pediatric Services and Equipment in Emergency Departments: United States, 2002–03*. Hyattsville, MD: National Center for Health Statistics.

Mittelstaedt EA, Simon SR. 2004. Developing a child safety seat program. *Military Medicine* 169(1):30–33.

Moorhead JC, Gallery ME, Hirshkorn C, Barnaby DP, Barsan WG, Conrad LC, Dalsey WC, Fried M, Herman SH, Hogan P, Mannle TE, Packard DC, Perina DG, Pollack CV Jr, Rapp MT, Rorrie CC Jr, Schafermeyer RW. 2002. A study of the workforce in emergency medicine: 1999. *Annals of Emergency Medicine* 40(1):3–15.

Moreland JE, Sanddal ND, Sanddal TL, Pickert CB. 1998. Pediatric equipment in ambulances. *Pediatric Emergency Care* 14(1):84.

Murdock TC, Knapp JF, Dowd MD, Campbell JP. 1999. Bridging the emergency medical services for children information gap. *Archives of Pediatrics & Adolescent Medicine* 153(3):281–285.

Murphy AW, Bury G, Plunkett PK, Gibney D, Smith M, Mullan E, Johnson Z. 1996. Randomised controlled trial of general practitioner versus usual medical care in an urban accident and emergency department: Process, outcome, and comparative cost. *British Medical Journal* 312(7039):1135–1142.

Murray JA, Demetriades D, Berne TV, Stratton SJ, Cryer HG, Bongard F, Fleming A. 2000. Prehospital intubation in patients with severe head injury. *Journal of Trauma* 49(6):1065–1070.

Nakayama DK, Copes WS, Sacco W. 1992. Differences in trauma care among pediatric and nonpediatric trauma centers. *Journal of Pediatric Surgery* 27(4):427–431.

NAS, NRC (National Academy of Sciences, National Research Council). 1966. *Accidental Death and Disability: The Neglected Disease of Modern Society*. Washington, DC: National Academy of Sciences.

NASEMSD (National Association of State EMS Directors). 2004. *Pediatric Disaster and Terrorism Preparedness*. Falls Church, VA: NASEMSD.

National Association of Children's Hospitals and Related Institutions. 2006. *Education*. [Online]. Available: http://www.childrenshospitals.net/Template.cfm?Section=Home&CONTENTID=3703&TEMPLATE=/ContentManagement/ContentDisplay.cfm [accessed January 25, 2006].

National Cancer Institute. 2005. *Digital vs. Film Mammography in the Digital Mammographic Imaging Screening Trial (DMIST)*. [Online]. Available: http://www.cancer.gov/newscenter/pressreleases/DMISTQandA/ [accessed January 10, 2006].

National Center for Complementary and Alternative Medicine. 2002. *NIH Launches Large Clinical Trial on EDTA Chelation Therapy for Coronary Artery Disease*. [Online]. Available: http://nccam.nih.gov/news/2002/chelation/pressrelease.htm [accessed January 10, 2006].

National Center for Health Statistics. 2004. Deaths: Final data for 2002. *National Vital Statistics Reports* 53(5). Hyattsville, MD: National Center for Health Statistics.

National Center for Injury Prevention and Control. 2001. *Injury Fact Book 2001–2002*. Atlanta, GA: CDC.

National Clearinghouse on Child Abuse and Neglect Information. 2004. *Child Abuse and Neglect Fatalities: Statistics and Interventions*. Washington, DC: DHHS.

National Emergency Number Association. 2004. *9-1-1 Fast Facts*. Arlington, VA: National Emergency Number Association.

National Institute of Neurological Disorders and Stroke. 2006. *NINDS Reye's Syndrome Information Page*. [Online]. Available: http://www.ninds.nih.gov/disorders/reyes_syndrome/reyes_syndrome.htm [accessed February 24, 2006].

National Institute on Deafness and Other Communication Disorders. 2002. *Ear Infections: Facts for Parents About Otitis Media*. [Online]. Available: http://www.nidcd.nih.gov/health/hearing/otitismedia.asp [accessed December 7, 2006].

National Safe Kids Campaign. 2004. *Trends in Unintentional Injury Fact Sheet*. Washington, DC: National Safe Kids Campaign.

Neely KW, Norton RL, Young GP. 1994. The effect of hospital resource unavailability and ambulance diversions on the EMS system. *Prehospital Disaster Medicine* 9(3):172–176; discussion 177.

Newacheck PW. 1992. Characteristics of children with high and low usage of physician services. *Medical Care* 30(1):30–42.

Newacheck PW, Hughes DC, Hung YY, Wong S, Stoddard JJ. 2000. The unmet health needs of America's children. *Pediatrics* 105(4 Pt. 2):989–997.

O'Malley AS, Gerland AM, Pham HH, Berenson RA. 2005. *Rising Pressure: Hospital Emergency Departments: Barometers of the Health Care System*. Washington, DC: The Center for Studying Health System Change.

Office of Technology Assessment. 1989. *Rural Emergency Medical Services—Special Report*. Washington, DC: Office of Technology Assessment.

Office of Technology Assessment. 1994. *Defensive Medicine and Medical Malpractice*. Washington, DC: U.S. Government Printing Office.

Oster A, Bindman AB. 2003. Emergency department visits for ambulatory care sensitive conditions: Insights into preventable hospitalizations. *Medical Care* 41(2):198–207.

Pantridge JF, Geddes JS. 1967. A mobile intensive-care unit in the management of myocardial infarction. *Lancet* 2(7510):271–273.

Pearson SD, Goldman L, Orav EJ, Guadagnoli E, Garcia TB, Johnson PA, Lee TH. 1995. Triage decisions for emergency department patients with chest pain: Do physicians' risk attitudes make the difference? *Journal of General Internal Medicine* 10(10):557–564.

PECARN (Pediatric Emergency Care Applied Research Network). 2004. *About PECARN*. [Online]. Available: http://www.pecarn.org/about_pecarn.htm [accessed August 2, 2004].

Peddle N, Wang C-T. 2002. *Current Trends in Child Abuse Prevention, Reporting, and Fatalities*. Chicago, IL: Prevent Child Abuse America.

Pena ME, Snyder BL. 1995. Pediatric emergency medicine. The history of a growing discipline. *Emergency Medicine Clinics of North America* 13(2):235–253.

Perez K. 1998. *Emergency Medical Services for Children*. Washington, DC: National Council of State Legislatures.

Petrack EM, Christopher NC, Kriwinsky J. 1997. Pain management in the emergency department: Patterns of analgesic utilization. *Pediatrics* 99(5):711.

Piacentini J, Rotheram-Borus MJ, Gillis JR, Graae F, Trautman P, Cantwell C, Garcia-Leeds C, Shaffer D. 1995. Demographic predictors of treatment attendance among adolescent suicide attempters. *Journal of Consulting & Clinical Psychology* 63(3):469–473.

Polivka BJ, Nickel JT, Salsberry PJ, Kuthy R, Shapiro N, Slack C. 2000. Hospital and emergency department use by young low-income children. *Nursing Research* 49(5):253–261.

Porter SC, Fein JA, Ginsburg KR. 1997. Depression screening in adolescents with somatic complaints presenting to the emergency department. *Annals of Emergency Medicine* 29(1):141–145.

Probst BD, Lyons E, Leonard D, Esposito TJ. 2005. Factors affecting emergency department assessment and management of pain in children. *Pediatric Emergency Care* 21(5):298–305.

Quinn JV, Polevoi SK, Kramer NR, Callaham ML. 2003. Factors associated with patients who leave without being seen. *Academic Emergency Medicine* 10(5):523-b, 524.

Ramenofsky ML. 2006. Organizing the hospital for pediatric trauma care. In: Wesson D, Cooper A, Scherer III LRT, Stylianos S, Tuggle DW, eds. *Pediatric Trauma. Pathophysiology, Diagnosis, and Treatment*. New York: Taylor & Francis Group.

Ramenofsky ML, Luterman A, Quindlen E, Riddick L, Curreri PW. 1984. Maximum survival in pediatric trauma: The ideal system. *The Journal of Trauma* 24(9):818–823.

Richardson LD, Babcock Irvin C, Tamayo-Sarver JH. 2003. Racial and ethnic disparities in the clinical practice of emergency medicine. *Academic Emergency Medicine* 10(11):1184–1188.

Rivara FP, Grossman DC, Cummings P. 1997. Injury prevention. Second of two parts. *New England Journal of Medicine* 337(9):613–618.

Rosen P. 1995. *History of Emergency Medicine.* New York: Josiah Macy, Jr. Foundation. Pp. 59–79.

Rosenblatt R, Law S, Rosenbaum S. 2001. *Law and the American Health Care System.* New York: Foundation Press.

Rowe BH, Channan P, Bullard M, Alibha A, Saunders D. 2003. Reasons why patients leave without being seen from the emergency department. *Academic Emergency Medicine* 10(5):513.

Saade DN, Simon HK, Greenwald M. 2002. Abused children: Missed opportunities for recognition in the ED. *Academic Emergency Medicine* 9(5):524.

Sacchetti A, Sacchetti C, Carraccio C, Gerardi M. 2000. The potential for errors in children with special health care needs. *Academic Emergency Medicine* 7(11):1330–1333.

Sainsbury S. 1990. Emergency patients who leave without being seen. *Military Medicine* 155(10):460–464.

Santucci KA, Sather J, Douglas M. 2000. Psychiatry-related visits to the pediatric emergency department: A growing epidemic (abstract). *Pediatric Research* 47(4):117A.

Santucci KA, Sather J, Baker MD. 2003. Emergency medicine training programs' educational requirements in the management of psychiatric emergencies: Current perspective. *Pediatric Emergency Care* 19(3):154–156.

Sapien RE, Fullerton L, Olson LM, Broxterman KJ, Sklar DP. 1999. Disturbing trends: The epidemiology of pediatric emergency medical services use. *Academic Emergency Medicine* 6(3):232–238.

Sarver JH, Cydulka RK, Baker DW. 2002. Usual source of care and nonurgent emergency department use. *Academic Emergency Medicine* 9(9):916–923.

Scheck A. 2006, January. Children with psychiatric disorders now younger and more common in EDs. *Emergency Medicine News.* P. 1.

Schneider SM, Gallery ME, Schafermeyer R, Zwemer FL. 2003. Emergency department crowding: A point in time. *Annals of Emergency Medicine* 42(2):167–172.

Scribano PV, Baker MD, Ludwig S. 1997. Factors influencing termination of resuscitative efforts in children: A comparison of pediatric emergency medicine and adult emergency medicine physicians. *Pediatric Emergency Care* 13(5):320–324.

Scribano PV, Baker MD, Holmes J, Shaw KN. 2000. Use of out-of-hospital interventions for the pediatric patient in an urban emergency medical services system. *Academic Emergency Medicine* 7(7):745–750.

Seidel JS. 1986a. A needs assessment of advanced life support and emergency medical services in the pediatric patient: State of the art. *Circulation* 74(6 Pt. 2):IV129–IV133.

Seidel JS. 1986b. Emergency medical services and the pediatric patient: Are the needs being met? II. Training and equipping emergency medical services providers for pediatric emergencies. *Pediatrics* 78(5):808.

Seidel JS, Hornbein M, Yoshiyama K, Kuznets D, Finklestein JZ, St Geme JW Jr. 1984. Emergency medical services and the pediatric patient: Are the needs being met? *Pediatrics* 73(6):769–772.

Seidel JS, Henderson DP, Ward P, Wayland BW, Ness B. 1991. Pediatric prehospital care in urban and rural areas. *Pediatrics* 88(4):681.

Selbst SM, Clark M. 1990. Analgesic use in the emergency department. *Annals of Emergency Medicine* 19(9):1010–1013.

Selbst SM, Levine S, Mull C, Bradford K, Friedman M. 2004. Preventing medical errors in pediatric emergency medicine. *Pediatric Emergency Care* 20(10):702–709.

Serleth HJ, Cogbill TH, Perri C, Lambert PJ, Ross AJ III, Thompson JE. 1999. Pediatric trauma management in a rural Wisconsin trauma center. *Pediatric Emergency Care* 15(6):393–398.

Sharma V, Simon SD, Bakewell JM, Ellerbeck EF, Fox MH, Wallace DD. 2000. Factors influencing infant visits to emergency departments. *Pediatrics* 106(5):1031–1039.

Shults R. 2004. Child passenger deaths involving drinking drivers—United States, 1997–2002. *Morbidity and Mortality Weekly Report* 53(4):77–79.

Sills MR, Bland SD. 2002. Summary statistics for pediatric psychiatric visits to US emergency departments, 1993–1999. *Pediatrics* 110(4):e40.

Singh T, Wright J, Adirim T. 2003. Children with special health care needs: A template for prehospital protocol development. *Prehospital Emergency Care* 7(3):336–351.

Smith E, Singh T, Adirim T. 2001. Outstanding outreach: A prehospital notification system makes a difference for special needs children. *JEMS: Journal of Emergency Medical Services* 26(5):48–55.

Spaite D, Karriker K, Seng M, Conroy C, Battaglia N, Tibbitts M, Salik R. 2000. Training paramedics: Emergency care for children with special health care needs. *Prehospital Emergency Care* 4(2):178–185.

Spivey M, Schnitzer P, Slusher P, Kruse R, Jaffe D. 2005. *Emergency Department Injury Visits for Infants and Children. Evaluation of Frequency as an Indicator for Child Maltreatment.* Presentation at the meeting of the Pediatric Academic Societies Annual Meeting, Washington, DC.

Starko KM, Ray CG, Dominguez LB, Stromberg WL, Woodall DF. 1980. Reye's syndrome and salicylate use. *Pediatrics* 66(6):859–864.

Stenklyft P. 1999, March. Pediatric emergency medicine: Past, present, and future. *Jacksonville Medicine Magazine.* [Online]. Available: http://www.dcmsonline.org/jax-medicine/1999journals/march99/pediatricer.htm [accessed January 31, 2007].

Stiell IG, Nesbitt LP, Osmond MH, Campbell S, Gerein R, Munkley DP, Luinstra LG, Maloney JP, Wells GA, for the OPALS Study Group. 2005. OPALS Pediatric Study: What is the impact of advanced life support on out-of-hospital cardiac arrest? *Academic Emergency Medicine* 12(5 Suppl. 1):17-b, 18.

Stock LM, Bradley GE, Lewis RJ, Baker DW, Sipsey J, Stevens CD. 1994. Patients who leave emergency departments without being seen by a physician: Magnitude of the problem in Los Angeles County. *Annals of Emergency Medicine* 23(2):294–298.

Stylianos S, Egorova N, Guice KS, Arons RR, Oldham KT. 2006. Variation in treatment of pediatric spleen injury at trauma centers versus nontrauma centers: A call for dissemination of American pediatric surgical association benchmarks and guidelines. *Journal of the American College of Surgeons* 202(2):247–251.

Su E, Mann NC, McCall M, Hedges JR. 1997. Use of resuscitation skills by paramedics caring for critically injured children in Oregon. *Prehospital Emergency Care* 1(3):123–127.

Subedar N, Rathore MH. 1995. Changing epidemiology of childhood meningitis. *Journal of the Florida Medical Association* 82(7):467–469.

Sullivan AM, Rivera J. 2000. Profile of a comprehensive psychiatric emergency program in a New York City municipal hospital. *The Psychiatric Quarterly* 71(2):123–138.

Suruda A, Vernon D, Diller E, Dean J. 2000. Usage of emergency medical services by children with special health care needs. *Prehospital Emergency Care* 4(2):131–135.

Svenson JE, Nypaver M, Calhoun R. 1996. Pediatric prehospital care: Epidemiology of use in a predominantly rural state. *Pediatric Emergency Care* 12(3):173–179.

Tennyson DH. 2003. Hospital-affiliated pediatric urgent care clinics: A necessary extension for emergency departments? *Health Care Management* 22(3):190–202.

Todd KH, Lee T, Hoffman JR. 1994. The effect of ethnicity on physician estimates of pain severity in patients with isolated extremity trauma. *Journal of the American Medical Association* 271(12):925–928.

Todd KH, Deaton C, D'Adamo A, Goe L. 2000. Ethnicity and analgesic practice. *Annals of Emergency Medicine* 35(1):11–16.

Traffic Safety Center. 2002. The "forgotten child" is getting some attention at last. *Traffic Safety Center Online Newsletter* 1(2).

Trokel M, Wadimmba A, Griffith J, Sege R. 2006. Variation in the diagnosis of child abuse in severely injured infants. *Pediatrics* 117(3):722–728.

Tsai AC, Tamayo-Sarver JH, Cydulka RK, Baker DW. 2003. Declining payments for emergency department care, 1996–1998. *Annals of Emergency Medicine* 41(3):299–308.

United Nations Children's Fund. 2001. *A League Table of Child Deaths by Injury in Rich Nations.* Florence, Italy: UNICEF Innocenti Research Center.

U.S. Census Bureau. 2000. *Census 2000.* [Online]. Available: http://www.census.gov [accessed October 2004].

U.S. Census Bureau. 2004. *Current Population Survey, 2003 and 2004 Annual Social and Economic Supplements.* Washington, DC: U.S. Census Bureau.

U.S. Census Bureau. 2005. *Current Population Survey, 2005 Annual Social and Economic Supplement.* Washington, DC: U.S. Census Bureau.

U.S. Consumer Product Safety Commission. 1997. *Hospital-Based Pediatric Emergency Resources Survey.* Bethesda, MD: Division of Hazard and Injury Data Systems.

U.S. Department of State. 2006. *Avian Influenza Frequently Asked Questions.* [Online]. Available: http://travel.state.gov/travel/tips/health/health_2747.html [accessed April 5, 2006].

Vanlandingham BD, Powe NR, Diener-West M, Marone B, Rubin H. 2005. *Patient Insurance Status and Specialist On-Call Coverage in U.S. Hospital Emergency Departments: A National Study.* Presented at AcademyHealth in Boston, MA.

Wagh A, Heon D. 1999. Self assessment of emergency medicine residents' training and confidence in evaluating pediatric physical and sexual abuse. *Academic Emergency Medicine* 6(5):465.

Wang C, Villar ME, Mulligan DA, Hansen T. 2005. Cost and utilization analysis of a pediatric emergency department diversion project. *Pediatrics* 116(5):1075–1079.

Wang HE, Yealy DM. 2005. Out-of-hospital endotracheal intubation: It's time to stop pretending that problems don't exist. *Academic Emergency Medicine* 12(12):1245.

Watson W, Litovitz T, Klein-Schwartz W, Rodgers G, Youniss J, Reid N, Rouse W, Rembert R, Borys D. 2003. *2003 Annual Report of the American Association of Poison Control Centers Toxic Exposure Surveillance System.* Washington, DC: American Association of Poison Control Centers.

Weinick RM, Billings J, Thorpe JM. 2003. Ambulatory care sensitive emergency department visits: A national perspective. *Academic Emergency Medicine* 10(5):525-b, 526.

White-Means SI, Thornton MC. 1995. What cost savings could be realized by shifting patterns of use from hospital emergency rooms to primary care sites? *American Economic Review* 85(2):138–142.

Williams RM. 1996. The costs of visits to emergency departments. *New England Journal of Medicine* 334(10):642–646.

Willinger M. 1995. SIDS prevention. *Pediatric Annals* 24(7):358–364.

3

Building a 21st-Century Emergency and Trauma Care System

The committee's vision for the emergency and trauma care system is rather simple. The committee envisions a system in which patients of all ages and in all communities receive well-planned and -coordinated emergency care services. Consideration of pediatric concerns during the planning stages will ensure that the system meets the needs of children. Dispatch, emergency medical services (EMS), emergency department (ED) providers, trauma care, public safety, and public health will be fully interconnected and united in an effort to ensure that each patient receives the most appropriate care, at the optimal location, with the minimum delay. From the standpoint of pediatric patients and their parents or guardians, delivery of emergency care services will be seamless. All service delivery will be evidence-based, and innovations will be rapidly adopted and adapted to each community's needs. The performance of the system will be completely transparent, so that emergency medical technicians (EMTs) and parents will know which hospitals are best able to deliver care to critically ill or injured children (see Box 3-1).

The committee recognizes that improved care for children cannot be accomplished without addressing some of the failings in the larger emergency care system. The committee's vision centers on three goals: coordination, regionalization, and accountability. While this vision may appear innovative, many of its elements have been advocated for decades. However, early progress toward achieving these elements was derailed as a result of deeply entrenched political interests and cultural attitudes, as well as funding cutbacks and practical impediments to change. These obstacles remain today, and represent the chief challenges to realizing the committee's vision. Con-

---

BOX 3-1
A Vision of Pediatric Emergency Care in 2010

In a rural area, a car slides off the road and crashes 30 minutes from the nearest town. An automated crash notification system provides an emergency response center with detailed information about the location and characteristics of the crash. Passenger weights indicate that an adult and child, both properly restrained, are in the car. A dashboard displays information about the crash to air and ground response teams, emergency departments, and trauma facilities throughout the region. Because of the large impact of the crash, the automated triage system launches two advanced life support (ALS) response teams. An air medical response team is placed on standby.

Once the EMS teams are on the scene, patients' complete medical histories and alerts, obtained through a regional information system, are instantly available. Using an evidence-based triage protocol, one of the EMS teams determines that the child, an 8-year-old boy, is suffering from serious injuries. In accordance with regional transport protocols, the first responders call for air transport to bring the boy to the nearest trauma center. The paramedics stabilize the boy using age- and size-scaled equipment and drugs, and begin transmission of telemetry and on-board diagnostic scans to the trauma center. The other EMS team assesses the child's father and determines that although he requires a lower level of care, he should be transported to the trauma center to accompany his son.

An air transport team arrives at the scene and transports the child and father to a level I trauma center with the resources and medical experts needed to handle high-level pediatric and adult trauma cases. Care continues to be

---

certed, cooperative efforts at multiple levels of government and the private sector are necessary to finally break through and achieve these goals.

This chapter is dedicated to describing the three goals of the committee's vision for the emergency care system of the future, with a special focus on pediatric emergency care. In some areas of the country, states and regions are already developing coordinated, regionalized systems that incorporate elements of accountability; some of these efforts are described as well.

GOAL 1: COORDINATION

The current emergency care system faces a number of problems, but among the most long-standing of these is that emergency services are fragmented, resulting in poor communication and delayed services. EMS,

delivered en route in accordance with evidence-based treatment guidelines. The pediatric trauma specialist—alerted to the emergency when the air medical team was dispatched—performs emergency surgery when the child arrives at the hospital, and a pediatric intensivist is available for consult. The child receives the highest level of care based on the available clinical evidence. His medications, all approved for use in children, are delivered according to dosage guidelines for his age and size. The child's pediatrician and father's primary care provider are notified of the event.

The child's mother, who was not in the vehicle, is contacted immediately and apprised of the status of her husband and son. While understandably upset at the news, she takes some comfort in knowing that her husband and son are at a trauma center that has earned high marks for quality care delivery. When the mother arrives at the hospital, she is met by a social worker and nurse and given a clear explanation of the surgery being performed on her son. Hospital staff remain available to answer all of her questions. After surgery, the child is admitted to the hospital, where he spends a couple of days in recovery. When the child is eventually released from the hospital, the parents are given clear instructions for his continued care.

A record of the event is automatically collected by the region's emergency care information system, capturing information from the ground and flight paramedics as well as the hospital. A copy of that information is sent to both the state trauma registry and the National Trauma Data Bank. Additionally, the automatic crash notification system identifies that the crash occurred in an area where crashes are common and sends a notification to the public health department.

hospitals, trauma centers, and public health have traditionally worked in silos, a situation that largely persists today (NHTSA, 1996). For example, public safety and EMS agencies often lack common communications frequencies and protocols for communicating with each other during disasters. Similarly, emergency care providers do not have access to patient medical histories that could be useful in decision making. Even within those silos, coordination may be limited. For example, only about half of hospitals with EDs have pediatric interfacililty transfer agreements (MCHB, 2004), which are necessary in case a hospital receives a critically ill or injured child but lacks the resources to properly manage his or her care. Jurisdictional borders also contribute to fragmentation under the current system. For example, one county in Michigan has 18 different EMS systems with different service models and protocols. Medicaid and other payer policies contribute to geographic fragmentation when reimbursement does not follow patients seamlessly across state lines.

The problem is exacerbated in some regions by turf wars between fire-fighters and EMS personnel that were documented in a series of articles for *USA Today* (Davis, 2003). Even within EDs, there may be friction between emergency staff trying to admit patients and personnel on understaffed in-patient units who have no incentive for speeding up the admissions process. Lack of coordination between EMS and hospitals can result in delays that compromise care, and EDs may clash with on-call specialists over delays in response.

Also contributing to fragmentation is that pediatric concerns often are not included in the initial planning stages of the emergency care system. Either pediatric concerns are overlooked entirely, or planning for adult and pediatric care occurs independently. This is particularly true of disaster and trauma planning. A 2003 National Association of State EMS Directors (NASEMSD) survey found that only 14 states involved pediatric experts in state, regional, and local disaster planning. It is not surprising, then, that the majority of state disaster plans fail to address pediatric equipment and medications at hospitals (NASEMSD, 2004). Only about half of states report having designated pediatric trauma centers and trauma registries, indicating another important gap in planning (MCHB, 2004).

Importance of Linkages with Public Health

The ED has a special relationship with the community and state and local public health departments because it serves as a community barometer of both illness and injury trends (Malone, 1995). In her analysis of heavy users of ED services, Malone argued that "emergency departments remain today a 'window' on wider social issues critical to health care reforms" (p. 469). A commonly cited example is the use of seat belts. We now know that increased utilization of seat belts reduces the number of seriously injured car crash victims in the ED—the ED served as a proving ground for documenting the results of seat belt enforcement initiatives. Although prevention activities have been limited in the emergency care setting, that setting represents an important teaching opportunity. To take advantage of this opportunity, emergency care providers would benefit from the resources and experiences of public health agencies and experts in the implementation of injury prevention measures.

Perhaps now more than ever, with the threat of bioterrorism and outbreaks of such diseases as avian influenza and severe acute respiratory syndrome (SARS), it is essential that EMS, EDs, trauma centers, and state and local public health agencies partner to conduct surveillance for disease prevalence and outbreaks and other health risks. Hospital EDs can recognize the diagnostic clues that may indicate an unusual infectious disease outbreak so that public health authorities can respond quickly (GAO, 2003). However, a solid partnership must first be in place—one that allows for easy communication of information between emergency providers and public health officials.

Importance of Linkages with Other Medical Care Providers

According to the American College of Emergency Physicians (ACEP), EDs "define their mission in terms of unlimited access regardless of citizenship, insurance status, ability to pay, day of week, or time of day . . . it is the only source of care available for certain populations" (O'Brien, 1999, p.19). Indeed, EDs fill many existing gaps within the health care network, serving as key safety net providers in many communities (Lewin and Altman, 2000). Studies have shown that a significant number of patients use the ED for nonurgent purposes because of financial barriers, lack of access to clinics after hours, transportation barriers, convenience, and lack of a usual source of care (Grumbach et al., 1993; Young et al., 1996; Peterson et al., 1998; Koziol-McLain et al., 2000; Cunningham and May, 2003). There is also evidence that clinics and physicians are increasingly using EDs as an adjunct to their practice, referring patients to the ED for a variety of reasons, such as their own convenience after regular hours, reluctance to take on a complicated case, the need for diagnostic tests they cannot perform in the office, and liability concerns (Berenson et al., 2003; Studdert et al., 2005). Unfortunately, in many communities there is little interaction between emergency care services and community safety net providers—this even though they share a common base of patients, and their actions may affect one another substantially. The absence of coordination represents missed opportunities for enhanced access; improved diagnosis, patient follow-up, and compliance; and enhanced quality of care and patient satisfaction.

Previous Calls for Improved Coordination

The value of integrating and coordinating emergency care has long been recognized. The 1966 National Academy of Sciences/National Research Council (NAS/NRC) report *Accidental Death and Disability: The Neglected Disease of Modern Society* called for better coordination of emergency care through Community Councils on Emergency Medical Services, which would bring together physicians, medical facilities, EMS, public health, and others "to procure equipment, construct facilities and ensure optimal emergency care on a day to day basis as well as in disaster or national emergency" (NAS and NRC, 1966, p.7). In 1972, the NAS/NRC report *Roles and Responsibilities of Federal Agencies in Support of Comprehensive Emergency Medical Services* promoted an integrated, systems approach to planning at the state, regional, and local levels and called for the Department of Health, Education, and Welfare (DHEW) to take an administrative and leadership role in federal EMS activities. The Emergency Medical Services Systems Act of 1973 (P.L. 93-154) created a new grant program in the Division of EMS within DHEW to foster the development of regional EMS systems. The Robert Wood Johnson Foundation added support by funding the development of 44 regional EMS systems. Although the drive toward system development waned after the demise of the DHEW program and the block granting of EMS funds in 1981, the goal of system planning and co-ordination has remained paramount within the emergency care community. In 1996, the National Highway Traffic Safety Administration's (NHTSA) *Emergency Medical Services Agenda for the Future* also emphasized the goal of system coordination:

> EMS of the future will be community-based health management that is fully integrated with the overall health care system. It will have the ability to identify and modify illness and injury risks, provide acute illness and injury care and follow-up, and contribute to treatment of chronic conditions and community health monitoring. . . . [P]atients are assured that their care is considered part of a complete health care program, connected to sources for continuous and/or follow-up care, and linked to potentially beneficial health resources. . . . EMS maintains liaisons, including systems for communication with other community resources, such as other public safety agencies, departments of public health, social service agencies, departments of public health, social service agencies and organizations, health care provider networks, community health educators, and others. . . . EMS is a community resource, able to initiate important follow-up care for patients, whether or not they are transported to a health care facility. (NHTSA, 1996, pp. 7, 10)

Successes Achieved

While progress toward a highly integrated emergency care system has been slow, there have been some important successes in the coordination of emergency care services, which point the way toward solutions to the fragmentation that dominates the system today. For example, the trauma system in Maryland, described in more detail later in this chapter, provides a comprehensive and coordinated approach to the care of injured children. Children's hospitals have also been successful at accomplishing regional co-ordination to ensure the transport and appropriate care of children needing specialized services. The pediatric intensive care system is a leading example of regional coordination among hospitals, community physicians, and EMTs (Gausche-Hill and Wiebe, 2001). These are but a few examples demonstrating the possibilities for enhancing coordination of the system as a whole.

One promising public health surveillance effort is Insight, a computer-based clinical information system at the Washington Hospital Center (WHC) in Washington, D.C., designed to record and track patient data, including geographic and demographic information. The software proved useful during the 2001 anthrax attacks, when it enabled WHC to transmit complete, real-time data to the Centers for Disease Control and Prevention (CDC) while other hospitals were sending limited information with a lag time of one or more days. The success of Insight attracted considerable grant funding for the system's expansion; WHC earmarked $7 million for Insight to link it to federal and regional agencies and to integrate it with other hospital systems (Kanter and Heskett, 2002).

Many communities have established primary care networks that integrate hospital EDs into their planning and coordination efforts. A rapidly growing number of communities, such as San Francisco and Boston, have developed regional health information organizations that coordinate the development of information systems to facilitate patient referrals and track the sharing of medical information between providers to optimize a patient's care across settings. The San Francisco Community Clinic Consortium brings together primary and specialty care providers and EDs in a planning and communications network that closely coordinates the care of safety net patients throughout the city.

The Importance of Communications

Communications are a critical factor in establishing systemwide coordination. An effective communications system is the glue that can hold together effective, integrated emergency care services. It provides the key link between 9-1-1/dispatch and EMS responders and is necessary to ensure that on-line medical direction is available when needed. It enables ambulance dispatchers to tell callers what to do until help arrives and to track a patient's progress following the arrival of EMS responders. An effective communications system also enables ambulance dispatchers to assist EMS personnel in directing patients to the most appropriate facility based on the nature of their illness or injury and the capacity of receiving facilities. It links the emergency medical system with other public safety providers—such as police and fire departments, emergency management services, and public health agencies—and facilitates coordination between the medical response system and incident command in both routine and disaster situations. It helps hospitals communicate with each other to organize interfacility transfers and arrange for mutual aid. And it facilitates medical and operational oversight and quality control within the system.

GOAL 2: REGIONALIZATION

The goal of regionalization is to improve patient outcomes by directing patients to facilities with the optimal capabilities and best outcomes for any given type of illness or injury. A regionalized system ensures access to care at a level appropriate to patient needs while maintaining efficient use of available resources (Wright and Klein, 2001). Because not all hospitals within a community have the personnel and resources to support high-level pediatric emergency care delivery, critically ill and injured children should not be directed simply to the closest facility, but to the nearest facility with the pediatric expertise and resources needed to deliver high-level care.

Regionalization of emergency care is not a new concept. The Institute of Medicine (IOM) report *Emergency Medical Services for Children* noted that "categorization and regionalization are essential for full and effective operation of [pediatric emergency care] systems" (IOM, 1993, p. 171). Steps to regionalize certain pediatric services were supported by the American College of Critical Care Medicine and the Society of Critical Care Medicine in their 2000 *Consensus Report for Regionalization of Services for Critically Ill or Injured Children* (Committee on Pediatric Emergency Medicine Pediatric Section and Task Force on Regionalization of Pediatric Critical Care, 2000). Because of higher volume, regional providers gain experience in treating severely injured children, which in turn results in higher-quality care. Two recent studies found that child trauma patients have better outcomes at specialized pediatric centers (Stylianos, 2005; Densmore et al., 2006). Mortality among pediatric patients with respiratory failure or head injury is lower in hospitals that provide tertiary-level pediatric intensive care than in those that do not (Pollack et al., 1991; Tilford et al., 2005).

There is substantial evidence that regionalization of services to designated hospitals with greater experience improves outcomes and reduces costs across a range of high-risk conditions and procedures for adult patients, including cardiac arrest and stroke (Grumbach et al., 1995; Imperato et al., 1996; Nallamothu et al., 2001; Chang and Klitzner, 2002; Bardach et al., 2004). The literature also shows improved outcomes and lower costs associated with the regionalization of care for severely injured patients (Mullins and Mann, 1999; Jurkovich and Mock, 1999; Mann et al., 1999; Nathens et al., 2001; Chiara and Cimbanassi, 2003; Bravata et al., 2004), although the evidence in this regard is not uniformly positive (Glance et al., 2004). Regionalization benefits triage, medical care, outbreak investigations, security management, and emergency management. It may also be a cost-effective strategy for developing and training teams of response personnel (Bravata et al., 2004).

An example of a pediatric regionalization effort is the regionalization of neonatal care. The use of neonatal intensive care services in the 1960s and 1970s proved to decrease neonatal mortality (Williams and Chen, 1982), but not all hospitals could purchase and support the sophisticated equipment and specialized staff needed to care for the small number of infants requiring such care (Holloway, 2001). In the interest of using resources efficiently and ensuring access to neonatal care, in 1976 a Committee on Perinatal Health organized by the March of Dimes recommended the development of a regionalized system of neonatal intensive care (Cifuentes et al., 2002). Under the system, premature or very ill newborns were to be transferred to the nearest designated center to receive the level of care they required (Jones, 2004). While it is difficult to draw a definitive conclusion, studies suggest that regionalization has contributed to lower neonatal mortality rates (Bode et al., 2001; Holloway, 2001; Cifuentes et al., 2002).

Another example is organized trauma systems, which have been shown to improve outcomes of trauma care and to reduce mortality from traumatic injury through regionalization (Mullins et al., 1994; Jurkovich and Mock, 1999; MacKenzie, 1999; Mullins and Mann, 1999; Nathens et al., 2000; MacKenzie et al., 2006). While the literature has long reported benefits of such systems for adult patients, there is less evidence for children (Wright and Klein, 2001); however, the limited available research indicates benefits from regionalized pediatric trauma care. The initiation of a regionalized trauma system in Oregon resulted in a reduction in the risk of death from serious pediatric injuries (Hulka et al., 1997; Hulka, 1999). In New York, the triage of moderately to severely injured children to centers within regionalized systems reduced the risk of death compared with nonregionalized systems operating in other parts of the state (Cooper et al., 1993; Hulka, 1999).

Many states and/or communities have taken steps toward regionalizing pediatric emergency care by designating hospitals that meet certain requirements as "stand-by emergency departments approved for pediatrics" (SEDPs), "emergency departments approved for or accepting pediatrics" (EDAPs), and/or "emergency pediatric centers" (EPCs) (Gausche-Hill and Wiebe, 2001). In some areas, only EDAP or EPC hospitals are allowed to accept pediatric patients who have been transported by advanced life support (ALS) EMS providers. However, a state-by-state analysis shows that many states have still not formally regionalized pediatric intensive care or trauma (Adomako and Melese-d'Hospital, 2004). Most pediatric trauma patients are not brought to pediatric trauma centers, and they receive less-than-optimal care as a result (Densmore et al., 2006).

Simply designating hospitals as SEDPs, EDAPs, or EPCs and formalizing pediatric EMS transport protocols to reflect those designations is not sufficient, however. As noted in Chapter 2, the vast majority of children do not access EMS before arriving at an ED (McCaig and Burt, 2005), and in part for this reason, most children are seen in general EDs (Gausche-Hill et al., 2004). In all likelihood, many of these EDs are not designated as SEDPs, EDAPs, or EPCs; this is certainly so if the state lacks a designation process. It is natural for many parents simply to bring their children to the closest ED. Therefore, all hospitals, especially those not recognized as having the ability to care for critically ill or injured pediatric patients, must be linked to a broader regional system. There must be clear protocols for transferring such patients from an ED without specialized pediatric capabilities to a better-equipped facility. Regionalization of emergency care helps ensure that pediatric patients receive definitive care as soon as possible, even in rural or remote areas.

Concerns About Regionalization

One concern about the regionalization of pediatric emergency and trauma care is that moving too many children to regional centers would further dilute the pediatric experience of community hospitals. But all hospitals must have some baseline of pediatric readiness. As noted above, they must have the capability to stabilize pediatric patients and must have formal transfer agreements in place with regional pediatric centers.

Another concern is that regionalizing services could adversely impact the overall availability of other services in a community. For example, loss of certain type of patients could result in the closure of a hospital unit or an entire hospital, particularly a small, rural hospital. The survival of small, rural facilities may require identification and treatment of those illnesses and injuries that do not require the capacities and capabilities of larger facilities, as well as repatriation to the local facility after stabilization at the tertiary center for long-term care and follow-up. A systems approach to regionalization considers the full effects of regionalizing services on a community. Determining the appropriate metrics for this type of analysis and defining the process for applying them within each region are significant research and practical issues. Nonetheless, in the absence of rigorous evidence to guide the process, planning authorities should take these factors into account in developing regionalized systems of emergency care.

Configuration of Services

The design of the emergency care system envisioned by the committee bears similarities to the inclusive trauma system concept that was espoused by the American College of Surgeons (ACS) and has been widely adopted throughout the United States. Under the ACS approach, every hospital in the community can play a role in the trauma system by undergoing verification and designation as a level I to level IV/V trauma center, based on its capabilities. Trauma care is optimized in the region through protocols and transfer agreements that are designed to direct trauma patients to the most appropriate level of care available given the type of injury and the relative travel times to each center. As discussed earlier, the advantages of such a system are evident from studies demonstrating improved outcomes when patients receive care at designated facilities with specialized resources. These benefits accrue to pediatric patients as well as adults (Stylianos, 2005; Densmore et al., 2006).

The committee's vision expands this concept beyond trauma to encompass all illnesses and injuries, and beyond hospitals to encompass the entire continuum of emergency care—including 9-1-1 and dispatch and prehospital EMS, as well as clinics and urgent care providers that may play a role in emergency care. In this model, every provider organization can play a role in providing emergency care in the community according to its capabilities. All hospitals are categorized in a manner similar to the way some states and communities have designated SEDPs, EDAPs, and EPCs. Initially, this categorization may simply be based on the existence of a dedicated pediatric ED; recommended pediatric equipment; and specialized pediatric services, such as pediatric neurosurgery. Over time, the categorization process may evolve to include detailed information, such as the times specific emergency procedures are available; arrangements for on-call pediatric specialty care; service-specific outcomes; or general emergency service indicators, such as time to treatment, frequency of diversion, and ED boarding. Prehospital EMS services may be similarly categorized according to pediatric capabilities. The result is a complete inventory of emergency care assets and capabilities within a community.

A standard national approach to the categorization of emergency care providers that reflects both adult and pediatric capabilities is needed. Categories should reflect meaningful differences in the types of emergency care available, yet be simple enough to be understood easily by the provider community and the public. The use of national definitions will ensure that the categories are understood by providers and by the public across states or regions of the country, and will also promote benchmarking of performance.

The committee concludes that a standard national approach to the categorization of emergency care is essential for the optimal allocation of resources and provision of critical information to an informed public. Therefore, the committee recommends that **the Department of Health and Human Services and the National Highway Traffic Safety Administration, in part-**

nership with professional organizations, convene a panel of individuals with multidisciplinary expertise to develop evidence-based categorization systems for emergency medical services, emergency departments, and trauma centers **based on adult and pediatric service capabilities (3.1).** The categorization systems should be developed within 18 months of the release of this report. The two federal agencies should fund the process and convene the panel of emergency care experts and medical professionals to review the literature and develop the categorization systems. The multidisciplinary nature of the process should help ensure that the categories reflect the viewpoints of the various stakeholders and facilitate familiarity with the categories, as well as their adoption. The results of this process should be a complete inventory of emergency care assets for each community, which should be updated regularly to reflect the rapid changes in delivery systems nationwide.

Treatment, Triage, and Transport

The information generated by the implementation of recommendation 3.1 could be used to develop protocols that would guide EMTs in the transport of patients. But more research and discussion are needed to develop transport protocols. For example, it is unclear whether pediatric dispatch cards, which vary across jurisdictions, are appropriate. More research and discussion are needed to determine under what circumstances patients should be brought to the closest hospital for stabilization and transfer as opposed to being transported directly to the highest level of care, even if that facility is farther away. A debate remains over whether EMS providers should perform ALS procedures in the field or whether rapid transport to definitive care is best (Wright and Klein, 2001). The answer to this question likely depends, at least in part, on the type of emergency condition. It is evident, for example, that whether a patient will survive out-of-hospital cardiac arrest depends almost entirely on actions taken at the scene, including rapid defibrillation, provision of cardiopulmonary resuscitation (CPR), and perhaps other ALS interventions. Delaying these actions until the unit reaches a hospital results in dismal rates of survival and poor neurological outcomes. Conversely, there is little that prehospital personnel can do to stop internal bleeding from major trauma. In this instance, rapid transport to definitive care in an operating room offers the victim the best odds of survival. For example, a recent study showed that bypassing a level II trauma center in favor of a more distant level I trauma center may be optimal for head trauma patients (McConnell et al., 2005).

EMS responders who provide stabilization before the patient arrives at a critical care unit are sometimes subject to criticism because of a strongly held bias among some physicians that out-of-hospital stabilization only delays definitive treatment without adding value; however there is little evidence that the prevailing "scoop and run" paradigm of EMS is always optimal (Orr et al., 2006). Decisions regarding the appropriate steps to take should be resolved using the best available evidence. The committee concludes that there should be a national approach to the development of prehospital protocols. Therefore, the committee recommends that **the National Highway Traffic Safety Administration, in partnership with professional organizations, convene a panel of individuals with multidisciplinary expertise to develop evidence-based model prehospital care protocols for the treatment, triage, and transport of patients, including children (3.2).** These protocols should be developed within 18 months of the release of this report. NHTSA should fund the process and convene the panel of emergency care experts and medical professionals to review the literature and develop the protocols. In addition, the process of updating these protocols will be important because it will determine how rapidly patients receive the current standard of care. This effort need not start from scratch. The Model Pediatric Protocols developed by the National Association of EMS Physicians and supported by the Emergency Medical Services for Children (ESM-C) program, which cover the treatment of pediatric patients in the prehospital environment, can serve as a starting point for the initiative as it relates to pediatric patients.

Treatments may require modification to reflect local resources, capabilities, and transport times; however, the basic pathophysiology of human illness is the same in all areas of the country. Once in place, the national protocols could be tailored to local assets and needs. Regional protocols should reflect the state of readiness of given facilities within a region at a given point in time. Real-time, concurrent information on the availability of hospital resources and specialties should be made available to EMS providers to inform transport decisions. Figure 3-1 shows an example of the service configuration in a regionalized system.

In addition to the use of the EMS system to direct patients to the optimum location for emergency care, hospital emergency care designations should be posted prominently. Particularly for pediatric patients, who are generally transported to the ED by their parents or caregivers rather than by EMS, public information about an ED's pediatric capabilities is essential.

Again, the concept of categorization of hospitals based on capabilities is not new. It was recommended not only in the 1993 IOM Report *Emergency Medical Services for Children*, but also in the 1966 NAS/NRC report *Accidental Death and Disability* (NAS and NRC, 1966). According to that report:

> Hospital emergency departments should be surveyed . . . to determine the numbers and types of emergency facilities necessary to provide optimal emergency treatment for the occupants of each region. . . . Once the required numbers and types of treatment facilities have been determined, it may be necessary to lessen the requirements at some institutions, increase them in others, and even

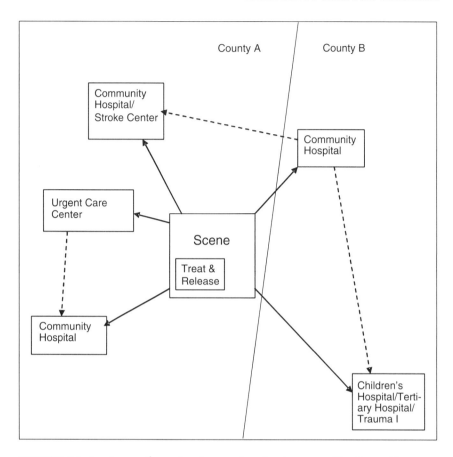

FIGURE 3-1 Service configuration in a regionalized system. The figure illustrates some potential transport options within a regionalized system. The basic structure of current EMS systems is not altered, but protocols are refined to ensure that patients go to the optimal facility given their type of illness or injury, the travel time involved, and facility status (e.g., ED and intensive care unit bed availability). For example, instead of taking a pediatric trauma victim to the closest general community hospital within the county, EMTs could cross county lines and transport the patient to a nearby pediatric center. Over time, based on evidence on the effectiveness of alternative delivery models, some pediatric patients may be transported to a nearby urgent care center for stabilization or treated and released at the scene. Whichever pathway the patient follows, communications are enhanced, data collected, and the performance of the system evaluated and reported so that future improvements can be made.

redistribute resources to support space, equipment, and personnel in the major emergency facilities. Until patient, ambulance driver, and hospital staff are in accord as to what the patient might reasonably expect and what the staff of an emergency facility can logically be expected to administer, and until effective transportation and adequate communication are provided to deliver casualties to proper facilities, our present levels of knowledge cannot be applied to optimal care and little reduction in mortality and/or lasting disability can be expected. (p. 20)

GOAL 3: ACCOUNTABILITY

Accountability is perhaps the most important of the three goals envisioned by the committee because it is necessary to achieving the other two. Lack of accountability has contributed to the failure of the emergency care system to adopt these changes in the past. Without accountability, participants in the system need not accept responsibility for failures and can avoid making changes necessary to improve the delivery of care.

Accountability is difficult to establish in emergency care because responsibility is dispersed across many different components of the system; thus it is difficult even for policy makers to determine where system breakdowns occur and how they can subsequently be addressed. When hospitals lack transfer agreements, when providers receive no continuing pediatric education, and when pediatric specialists and on-call specialists are not available, no one party is to blame—it is a system failure. Ambulance diversion is another good example. When a city recognizes it has an unacceptably high frequency of diversion, whom should it hold accountable? EMS can blame the hospitals for crowding and excessively long off-loading times; hospitals can blame the on-call specialists or the discharge sites that are unwilling to take additional referrals; and both can blame the state public health department for inadequate funding of community-based alternatives or community physicians for excessive referrals of their patients to the ED.

The unpredictable and infrequent nature of emergency care contributes to the lack of accountability. Most people have limited exposure to the emergency care system—an ambulance call or a visit to the ED is a rare event. Therefore, the performance of the system is generally not in the forefront of public awareness. Further, public awareness is hindered by the lack of nationally defined indicators of system performance. Few localities can answer basic questions about their emergency care services, such as how well 9-1-1, dispatch, prehospital EMS, hospital emergency and trauma care, and other components of the system perform and how their performance compares with that in other regions and the rest of the nation. Consequently, few understand the present crisis facing the system. By and large, the public assumes that the system functions better than it actually does (Harris Interactive, 2004).

Building Accountability

The committee believes three steps are required to bring accountability into the emergency care system: development of national performance indicators, measurement of performance within communities, and public dissemination of information on system performance.

Development of National Performance Indicators

There is currently no shortage of standards-setting efforts. ED performance measures have been developed by Qualis Health and Lindsay (Lindsay et al., 2002). The Data Elements for Emergency Department Systems (DEEDS) project and Health Level Seven (HL7) are working to develop uniform specifications for ED performance data (Pollock et al., 1998; National Center for Injury Prevention and Control, 2004; Health Level 7, 2005; Personal communication, R.W. Sattin, November 30, 2005). And the ACS and several partners have developed surgical process and outcome measures under the National Surgical Care Improvement Project.

The EMS Performance Measures Project is coordinated by the National Association of State EMS Officials in partnership with the National Association of EMS Physicians, and is supported by NHTSA and the Health Resources and Services Administration (HRSA). The project is working to develop consensus measures of EMS system performance that will assist in demonstrating the system's value and defining an adequate level of EMS service and preparedness for a given community (EMS Performance Measures Project, 2005). The consensus process of the project has sought to unify disparate efforts to measure performance previously undertaken nationwide that have lacked consistency in definitions, indicators, and data sources. Work undertaken under the project in 2004 resulted in the development of 138 indicators of EMS performance. This list was pared down to 25 indicators in 2005. The list included system measures such as "What are the time intervals in a call?" and "What percentage of transports is conducted with red lights and sirens?" and clinical measures such as "How well was my pain relieved?" The questions were defined using data elements from the National EMS Information System (NEMSIS) dataset so that results could be compared across EMS systems.

In addition, statewide trauma and EMS systems are evaluated by the ACS, HRSA's Division of Trauma and EMS, and NHTSA's Office of EMS. There are also various components of the system with independent accrediting bodies. Hospitals, for example, are accredited by the Joint Commission on Accreditation of Healthcare Organizations, ambulance services are accredited by the Commission on Accreditation of Ambulance Services, and air medical services are voluntarily accredited by the Commission on

Accreditation of Medical Transport Systems. Each of these organizations collects performance information.

However, many performance measurement efforts have two major shortcomings. First, many such efforts do not specifically address pediatric performance measures. As discussed in Chapter 5, it is critical that information systems incorporate specific attributes of pediatric illness and injury. Second, the measures developed cannot be used to assess the performance of the full emergency care system within each community and benchmark that performance against statewide and national performance metrics. A credible entity to develop such measures would not be strongly tied to any one component of the emergency care continuum. One approach would be to form a collaborative entity that would include representation from all of the system components—hospitals, trauma centers, EMS agencies, physicians, nurses, and others. Certainly individuals with pediatric expertise must be involved as well.

Another approach would be to work with an existing organization, such as the National Quality Forum (NQF), to develop a set of emergency care–specific measures. NQF grew out of the President's Advisory Commission on Consumer Protection and Quality in the Health Care Industry in 1998. It operates as a not-for-profit membership organization made up of national, state, regional, and local groups representing consumers, public and private purchasers, employers, health care professionals, provider organizations, health plans, accrediting bodies, labor unions, supporting industries, and organizations involved in health care research or quality improvement. NQF has reviewed and endorsed measure sets applicable to several health care settings and clinical areas and services, including hospital care, home health care, nursing-sensitive care, nursing home care, cardiac surgery, and diabetes care (NQF, 2002, 2003, 2004a,b, 2005).

The committee concludes that a standard national approach to the development of performance indicators is essential and recommends that **the Department of Health and Human Services convene a panel of individuals with emergency and trauma care expertise to develop evidence-based indicators of emergency and trauma care system performance, including the performance of pediatric emergency care (3.3).** The federal government must play a lead role in this effort because of the need for an independent, national process involving the broad participation of every component of emergency care. The Department of Health and Human Services (DHHS) should fund the process and convene the panel of individuals with emergency and trauma care expertise to review the research and develop performance indicators. The committee intends this to be a discrete project to be conducted within a brief timeframe. The set of performance indicators should be selected within 18 months of the release of this report.

The measures developed should include structure and process measures, but evolve toward outcome measures over time. They should be nationally standardized so that statewide and national comparisons can be made. Measures should evaluate the performance of individual provider organizations within the system, as well as that of the system as a whole. Measures should also be sensitive to the interdependence among the components of the system; for example, EMS response times may be related to EDs going on diversion. Naturally, measures should also be appropriate for assessing the performance of pediatric emergency care. To this end, it may be necessary to include additional, pediatric-specific measures in data collection efforts.

Furthermore, because an episode of emergency care can span multiple settings, each of which can have a significant impact on the final outcome, it is important that patient-level data from each setting be captured and combined. Currently it is difficult to piece together an episode of emergency care. To address this need, states should develop guidelines for the sharing of patient-level data from dispatch through post–hospital release. The federal government should support such efforts by sponsoring the development of model procedures that can be adopted by states to minimize their administrative costs and liability exposure as a result of sharing these data.

Measurement of Performance

Using measures developed through a national consensus process, performance data should be collected on a regular basis from all of the emergency care providers in a community. The data should be tabulated in ways that can be used to measure, report on, and benchmark system performance. For example, emergency care systems across the country might be tasked with providing data on time-critical pediatric conditions, such as respiratory arrest. Data from the various system components would allow researchers to measure how well the system ensures the appropriate performance of each link in the chain of survival for the care of children (9-1-1, first response, EMS, ED, trauma), and would be useful for ongoing feedback and process improvement. Using their regulatory authority over health care services, states should play a lead role in collecting and analyzing these performance data. Careful attention by the states will be required to ensure that the reporting of performance measures by provider organizations results in real improvements in care processes and outcomes, as opposed to being simply cosmetic paper exercises that demonstrate compliance.

While a full-blown data collection and reporting system for performance measurement is the desired ultimate outcome, the committee believes a handful of key indicators of regional system performance should be collected and promulgated as soon as possible. These could include, for example, indicators of diversion, boarding, and EMS times to arrival. It is essential that pediatric indicators be included in initial data collection and performance assessment efforts. Examples include time to administration of antibiotics for treatment of meningitis or time to first nebulization for treatment of asthma. Indicators should also aim to be outcome-based. For example, systems could collect data on pediatric respiratory arrest or respiratory failure—time-sensitive sentinel conditions that are amenable to an outcome assessment.

Public Dissemination of Information on System Performance

Public dissemination of performance data is crucial to drive the needed changes in the delivery of emergency care services. Dissemination can take various forms, including public report cards, annual reports, and state public health reports. Public dissemination of health care information is still in a state of development despite the proliferation of such initiatives over the past two decades. Problems include the costs associated with data collection, the sensitivity of individual provider information, concerns about the interpretation of data by the public, and a lack of public interest. There are many examples from which to learn: the Health Plan Employer Data and Information Set (HEDIS), which reports on managed care plans to purchasers and consumers; the Centers for Medicare and Medicaid Services' (CMS) reports on home health and nursing home care—the *Home Health Compare* and *Nursing Home Compare* websites, respectively (CMS, 2005e); and *Hospital Compare* from the Hospital Quality Alliance, which reports comparative quality data on hospitals (CMS, 2005d). A number of states and regional business coalitions have also developed report cards on managed care plans and hospitals (State of California Office of the Patient Advocate, 2005). Because of the unique status of the emergency care system as an essential public service and the public's limited awareness of the significant problems facing the system, the public is likely to take an active interest in this information. The committee believes dissemination of these data will have an important impact on public awareness and the development of integrated regional systems.

Public reporting can be at a detailed or aggregate level. Because of the potential sensitivity of performance data, they should initially be reported in the aggregate, at the national, state, and regional levels, rather than at the level of the individual provider. Prematurely reporting provider performance data may inhibit participation and divert providers' resources to public relations rather than corrective efforts. At the same time, however, movement toward public reporting should begin as swiftly as possible. Moreover, individual providers should have full access to their own data so they can understand and improve their individual performance, as well as their contribution to the overall system. Over time, information on individual provider organizations should become an important part of the public information on the system. Eventually, the data may be used to drive performance-based payment for emergency care.

CURRENT APPROACHES

A number of current efforts to establish emergency care systems achieve some or all of the committee's goals of coordination, regionalization, and accountability. Some are purely voluntary, while others have the force of state regulation. Some are local and regional in scope, while others are statewide or national. This section highlights several such efforts that provide insights for future initiatives.

The Maryland EMS and Trauma System

Maryland has a unique statewide system that coordinates all EMS and trauma activity throughout the state. The Maryland Institute for EMS Systems (MIEMSS) is an independent state agency governed by an 11-member board that is appointed by the governor. The system provides training and certification, has established statewide EMS protocols, coordinates care through a central communications center, and operates the air medical system in coordination with the Maryland State Police. The system is funded in part through a surcharge on state driver's license fees.

Coordination

MIEMSS has an EMS for children program that oversees grants from the federal EMS-C program and provides a focal point for statewide resources and networking on emergency care for children and their families. The Maryland EMS for children program develops state guidelines and resources for care, reviews pediatric emergency care and facility regulations, and coordinates pediatric education programs. Additionally, the program works with organizations, including the Safe Kids Coalition, the National Study Center for Trauma and Emergency Medical Systems, the Maryland Highway Safety Office, and the American Trauma Society, to foster and support education and injury prevention programs.

A statewide communications center coordinates all communications between EMS and other components of the system. The system links ambulances, helicopters, and hospitals and enables direct communications between components at any time. For example, a paramedic in western Maryland can talk directly with a local ED physician or obtain on-line consultation with a specialty hospital in Baltimore. While the local 9-1-1 centers initiate dispatch, they are usually too busy to follow patients through the continuum of care. The statewide communications center provides support by maintaining communications links, providing medical direction, and maintaining continuity of care. The center has direct links to incident command to facilitate management of EMS resources as an event unfolds.

The state also is developing a new wireless digital capability that will connect EMS with other public safety entities (police, fire, emergency management, public health) throughout the state. In addition, the state has developed a County Hospital Alert Tracking System (CHATS) to monitor the status of hospitals and EMS assets so ambulances can be directed to less crowded facilities. This capability can also be applied to individual services—for example, patients with acute coronary syndrome can be directed to facilities based on the current availability of reperfusion suites. The Facility Resource Emergency Database system was designed to gather detailed information electronically from hospitals on bed availability, staffing, medications, and other critical capacity issues during disasters, but is also used to monitor and report on system capacity issues on a regular basis.

The state ensures coordination and compliance with protocols through its statewide training, provider designation, and licensure functions. In addition to providing EMS training and certification, the system offers statewide disaster preparedness training for members of the National Disaster Medical System.

Regionalization

While EMS and 9-1-1 are operated locally, they utilize statewide protocols that promote regionalization of pediatric services to two designated centers. Regionalization is also used to direct adult patients to trauma, stroke, burn, eye, perinatal, and hand referral centers. The control of air medical services by the state facilitates the regionalization of care through the active operation of dispatch.

Accountability

The state monitors performance at the provider and system levels through a provider review panel that regularly evaluates the operation of the system. As a state agency, the system reports on its performance goals and improvements. Also, CHATS enables participating hospitals and the public to view the status of hospitals at all times through its website, including data on availability of cardiac monitor beds, ED beds, and trauma beds. Paper ambulance run sheets are being replaced with an electronic system so that data can be collected and analyzed quickly to facilitate real-time performance improvement.

While Maryland is relatively advanced in achieving the goals of coordination, regionalization, and accountability, it is not clear how easily its system could be replicated in other states. The system has benefited from strong and stable leadership in the state office, adequate funding, a high concentration of resources, and limited geography—features that many states do not currently enjoy.

Austin/Travis County, Texas

Austin/Travis County and four surrounding counties agreed to form a single EMS and trauma system to provide seamless care to emergency and trauma patients throughout the region. The initiative, 10 years in the making, started with a fragmented delivery system consisting of the Austin EMS system, 13 separate fire departments, and a 9-1-1 service run through the sheriff's office that lacked unified protocols. These different entities agreed to come together to form a unified system that would coordinate all emergency care within the region. The system operates through a Combined Clinical Council that includes representatives of the different agencies and providers within the geographic area, including fire departments, 9-1-1, EMS, air medical services, and corporate employers. This is a "third service" system—it is separate from fire and other public safety entities.

Coordination

Coordination of care is achieved through several means. A unified set of clinical guidelines was developed and is maintained by the system in accordance with current clinical evidence. These guidelines provide a common framework for the care and transport of patients throughout the system. Any changes to the guidelines must be evaluated and approved by the Combined Clinical Council.

All providers in the region have a common set of credentials and are given badges that identify them as certified providers within the system, substantially reducing the multijurisdictional fragmentation that is common across metropolitan areas. In addition, there is no distinction within the system between volunteer and career providers. The integrated structure facilitates both incident command and disaster planning.

Regionalization

The unified system supports the regional emergency and trauma care system through clinical operating guidelines that determine the care and transport of all emergency and trauma patients. But the system is focused more on coordination and medical direction of EMS than on regionalization of care.

Accountability

A Healthcare Quality Committee is charged with reviewing the performance of the system and recommending specific actions to improve quality.

San Diego County, California

San Diego County has a regionalized trauma system that is characterized by a strong public–private partnership between the county and its five adult and one children's trauma centers. Public health, assessment, policy development, and quality assurance are core components of the system, which operates under the auspices of the state EMS Authority.

Coordination

A countywide electronic system (QA Net) provides the real-time status of every trauma center and ED in the county, including the reason for diversion status, intensive care unit (ICU) bed availability, and trauma resuscitation capacity. The system has been in place for over 10 years and is a critical part of the coordination of emergency and trauma care in the county.

A regional communications system serves as the backbone of the emergency and trauma care system for both day-to-day operations and disasters. It includes an enhanced 9-1-1 system and a countywide network that allows all ambulance providers and hospitals to communicate. The network is used to coordinate decisions on EMS destinations and bypass information, and allows each hospital and EMS provider to know the status of every other hospital and provider on a real-time basis. Because the system's authority comes from the state to the local level, all prehospital and emergency hospital services are coordinated through one lead agency. This arrangement provides continuity of services, standardized triage, treatment and transport protocols, and an opportunity to improve the system as issues are identified.

Regionalization

The county is divided into five service areas, each of which has at least a level II trauma center. Adult trauma patients are triaged and transported to the appropriate trauma center, while the children's hospital provides trauma care to all seriously injured children below the age of 14. Serious burn cases are taken to the University of California-San Diego Burn Center. The county is considering regionalization for other conditions, such as stroke and heart attack, based on the trauma model. The system includes the designation of regional trauma centers, designation of base hospitals to provide medical direction to EMS personnel, establishment of regional medical policies and procedures, and licensure of EMS services.

Accountability

Accountability is driven by a quality improvement program in which a medical audit committee meets monthly to review systemwide patient deaths and complications. The committee includes trauma directors; trauma nurse managers; the county medical examiner; the chief of EMS; and representatives of key specialty organizations, including orthopedic surgeons and neurosurgeons, as well as a representative for nondesignated facilities. A separate prehospital audit committee that includes ED physicians and prehospital providers also meets monthly and discusses any relevant prehospital issues.

Palm Beach County, Florida

An initiative currently under way in Palm Beach County, Florida, is more limited in scope than the systems highlighted above and is in the initial stages of development. The goal of the initiative is to find regional solutions to the limited availability of physician specialists who provide on-call emergency care services. In spring 2004, physician leaders, hospital executives, and public health officials formed the Emergency Department Management Group to address this problem. One approach being explored is to attack the rising cost of malpractice insurance for emergency care providers, which discourages specialists from serving on on-call panels. The organization is developing a group captive insurance company to offer liability coverage for physicians providing care in county EDs.

Coordination

The Emergency Department Management Group is developing a web-based, electronic ED call schedule so the EMS system can track which specialists are available at all hospitals throughout the county. This will enable the system to direct transport to the most appropriate facility based on a patient's type of injury or illness.

Regionalization

The Emergency Department Management Group is exploring the regionalization of certain high-demand specialties, such as hand surgery and neurosurgery, so that the costs of maintaining full on-call coverage can be concentrated in those few hospitals where the volume of cases makes it feasible to maintain such coverage. Hospitals throughout the county would pay a "subscription fee" to support the cost of on-call coverage at designated hospitals. The fee would be set at a level below what it would cost to have hospitals manage their on-call coverage individually.

Accountability

The initiative includes the development of a countywide quality assurance program under which all hospitals would submit certain data elements for assessment. It is unclear at this time how far this system would go toward public disclosure of system performance.

NEED FOR A DEMONSTRATION PROGRAM

States and regions face a variety of situations, and no one approach to building emergency care systems will achieve the goals discussed in this chapter. There is, for example, substantial variation across states and regions in the level of development of trauma systems; the effectiveness of state EMS offices and regional EMS councils; and the degree of coordination and integration among fire departments, EMS, hospitals, trauma centers, and emergency management. The baseline conditions and needs also vary. For example, rural areas face very different problems from those of urban areas, and an approach that works for one may be counterproductive for the other.

In addition to these varying needs and conditions, the problems involved are too complex for the committee to prescribe an a priori solution. A number of different avenues should be explored and evaluated to determine what does and does not work. Over time and over a number of controlled initiatives, such a process should yield important insights about what works and under what conditions. These insights can provide best-practice models that can be widely adopted to advance the nation toward the committee's vision.

The process described here is one that can be supported effectively through federal demonstration projects. Such an approach can provide funding critical to project success; guidance for design and implementation; waivers from federal laws that might otherwise impede the process; and standardized, independent evaluations of projects and overall national assessment of the program. At the same time, the demonstration approach allows for significant variations according to state and regional needs and conditions within a set of clearly defined parameters. The IOM report *Fostering Rapid Advances in Health Care: Learning from System Demonstrations* articulated the benefits of the demonstration approach: "There is no accepted blueprint for redesigning the health care sector, although there is widespread recognition that fundamental changes are needed. . . . For many important issues, we have little experience with alternatives to the status quo. . . . [T]he committee sees the launching of a carefully crafted set of demonstrations as a way to initiate a 'building block' approach" (IOM, 2002).

The committee therefore recommends that **Congress establish a demonstration program, administered by the Health Resources and Services Administration, to promote coordinated, regionalized, and accountable emergency care systems throughout the country, and appropriate $88 million over 5 years to this program (3.4).** The demonstration projects should aim to optimize emergency services for both adults and children. The essential features of the proposed program are described below.

Recipients

Grants would be targeted at states, which could develop projects at the state, regional, or local level; cross-state collaborative proposals would be encouraged. Grantees would be selected through a competitive process based on the quality of proposals and assessment of the likelihood of success in achieving the stated goal(s). Grantees could propose approaches addressing one, two, or all three of the goals of coordination, regionalization, and accountability. Proposals would not have to address more than one goal, but should address the implications of the proposed project for both pediatric and adult patients.

Purpose of the Grants

Each proposal would be required to describe the proposed approach in detail, explain how it would achieve the stated goal(s), identify who would carry out the responsibilities associated with the initiative, identify the costs associated with its implementation, and describe how success would be measured. Proposals should describe the state's current stage of development and sophistication with regard to the stated goal(s) and explain how the grant would be used to enhance system performance in that regard.

Grants could be used in a number of different ways. Grant funds could be used to enhance communications so as to improve coordination of services; of particular interest would be the development of centralized communications centers at the regional or state level. Grants could be used to establish convening and planning functions, such as the creation of a regional or state advisory group of stakeholders for the purposes of building collaboration and designing and executing plans to improve coordination. Grant funds could be used to hire consultants and staff to manage the planning and coordination functions, as well as to pay for data collection, analysis, and public reporting. In very limited circumstances, they could also be used to implement information systems for the purpose of improving coordination of services. Grant funds should not, however, be used for routine functions that would be performed in the absence of the demonstration project, such as the hiring or training of pediatric specialists or the purchase of pediatric equipment. Funds could also be used to enhance linkages between rural and urban emergency services within broadly defined regions so as to improve rural emergency care through communications, telemedicine, training, and coordination activities.

Funding Levels

The committee proposes a two-phase program. In phase I, the program would fund up to 10 projects at up to $6 million over 3 years. The committee recommends support for 10 projects for two reasons. First, the committee hopes that the publication of its recommendations in this report will stimulate a desire among states and communities to undertake efforts to achieve the committee's vision. Resources should be available to encourage and support these efforts. Second, there is likely to be considerable variation in the types of projects proposed. A good number of projects will be needed to generate appropriate lessons learned.

Based on successful results that appeared to be replicable and sustainable in other states, the program would launch phase II, in which smaller, 2-year demonstration grants—up to $2 million each—would be made available to up to 10 additional states. This phase of the program would also include a technical assistance program designed to disseminate results and practical guidance to all states. Program administration would encompass evaluation of the program throughout its 5 years, including reports and public comments at 2.5 and 5 years after program initiation. The committee estimates funding for the program as follows:

- Phase I grants: $60 million (over 3 years)
- Phase II grants: $20 million (over 2 years)
- Phase II technical assistance: $4 million (over 2 years)
- Overall program administration: $4 million (over 5 years)
- Total program funding: $88 million (over 5 years)

Granting Agency

No single agency has responsibility for the multiple components of the nation's emergency care system. This responsibility is currently shared among multiple agencies—principally NHTSA, HRSA, CDC, and the Department of Homeland Security (DHS). If, as recommended below, a lead agency is established to consolidate funding and provide leadership for these multiple activities, it would be the appropriate agency to lead this proposed effort. Until that consolidation occurs, however, the committee believes this demonstration program should be placed within HRSA. HRSA currently directs the EMS-C program and sponsored the Trauma-EMS Systems Program, both of which share many of the broad goals of the proposed demonstration program. HRSA has already shown a willingness and ability to collaborate effectively with other relevant federal agencies and should be encouraged to consider them as partners in this enterprise. The agency or agencies that oversee the program should be sure that grantees address pediatric concerns within their demonstration projects.

REDUCING BARRIERS TO IMPLEMENTATION

If the process of redesigning the emergency care system to achieve the goals outlined by the committee is to be successful, it must be supported. As stated in *Fostering Rapid Advances in Health Care*, ". . . we must both plant the seeds of innovation and create an environment that will allow success to proliferate. Steps must be taken to remove barriers to innovation and to put in place incentives that will encourage redesign and sustain improvements" (IOM, 2002). The process used to redesign the system must include payment policies that reward successful strategies. It must recognize the interdependencies within emergency care and address systemic problems. It must balance the interests of many different stakeholders. And it must involve leadership at many levels taking responsibility for creating change. A number of institutional barriers to the adoption of coordinated, regionalized, accountable emergency care systems currently exist. These include payment systems, the legal framework that defines much of the structure of emergency care delivery, and the level of coordination of emergency care at the federal level.

Aligning Payment with Incentives

No major change in health care can take place without strong financial incentives. The way emergency care services are reimbursed reinforces certain modes of delivery that are inefficient and are a barrier to achieving the committee's vision of emergency care. Under Medicare and Medicaid, for example, prehospital providers are not paid unless they transport a patient to the hospital. This makes it difficult for regional systems to introduce innovations such as "treat and release" or other nontransport approaches that could result in better care for patients and more efficient system design. CMS and all other payers should eliminate this requirement and develop a payment system for prehospital care that reflects the costs of providing those services.

Similarly, many hospitals do not have a strong economic motivation to address the problems of ED crowding, boarding, and ambulance diversion; indeed, they may even benefit from these practices. Several payment approaches could eliminate this perverse incentive. One is to eliminate or compensate for the differential in payment between scheduled and ED admissions that relates to differences in both payer mix and severity of illness. Another approach is to provide hospitals with direct financial rewards or penalties based on their management of patient throughput. CMS, through its purchaser and regulatory power, has the ability to drive hospitals to address and manage patient flow and ensure timely access to quality care for its clients. All payers, including Medicare, Medicaid, and private insurers, could also develop contracts that would penalize hospitals for chronic delays in treatment, crowding, and diversion. CMS should lead the way in the development of innovative payment approaches that would accomplish these objectives. All payers should be encouraged to do the same.

Adapting the Legal and Regulatory Framework

The way hospitals and EMS agencies deliver emergency care is shaped largely by federal laws, including the Emergency Medical Treatment and Active Labor Act (EMTALA) and the Health Insurance Portability and Accountability Act (HIPAA). The application of these laws to the actual provision of care is guided by regulatory rules and advisories, enforcement decisions, and court decisions, as well as by providers' understanding of these.

EMTALA was passed in 1986 to prevent hospitals from refusing to serve uninsured patients and "dumping" them on other hospitals. The act established a mandate for hospitals and physicians who provide emergency and trauma care to provide a medical screening exam to all patients and properly stabilize patients or transfer them to an appropriate facility if an emergency medical condition exists (GAO, 2001). This requirement applies regardless of patients' ability to pay.

EMTALA also has implications for the regional coordination of care. The act was written to provide individual patient protections—it focuses on the obligations of an individual hospital to an individual patient (Rosenbaum and Kamoie, 2003). The statute is not clearly adaptable to a highly integrated regional emergency care system in which the optimal care of patients may diverge from conventional patterns of emergency treatment and transport.

Until recently, EMTALA appeared to hinder the regional coordination of services in several ways—for example, requiring a hospital-owned ambulance to transport a patient to the parent hospital even if it was not the optimal destination for that patient, requiring a hospital to interrupt the transfer to administer a medical screening exam for a patient being transferred from ground transport to helicopter if the hospital's helipad was used, and limiting the ability of hospitals to direct nonemergent patients who entered the ED to an appropriate and readily available ambulatory care setting. Interim guidance published by CMS in 2003 appeared to mitigate these problems (CMS, 2003). It established, for example, that a patient visiting an off-campus hospital site that does not normally provide emergency care does not create an EMTALA obligation, that a hospital-owned ambulance need not return the patient to the parent hospital if it is operating under the authority of a communitywide EMS protocol, and that hospitals are not obligated to provide treatment for clearly nonemergency situations as determined by qualified medical personnel. Further, hospitals involved in disasters need not adhere strictly to EMTALA if operating under a community disaster plan. Despite these changes, however, uncertainty surrounding the interpretation and enforcement of EMTALA remains a damper on the development of coordinated, integrated emergency care systems.

In 2005, CMS convened a technical advisory group to study EMTALA and address additional needed changes (CMS 2005a,b,c). To date, the advisory group has focused on incremental modifications to the act. While the recent CMS guidance and deliberations of the EMTALA advisory group are positive steps, the committee envisions a more fundamental rethinking of EMTALA that would support and facilitate the development of regionalized emergency systems, rather than simply addressing each obstacle on a piecemeal basis. The new EMTALA would continue to protect patients from discrimination in treatment while enabling and encouraging communities to test innovations in the design of emergency care systems, such as direct transport of patients to non–acute care facilities—dialysis centers and ambulatory care clinics, for example—when appropriate.

HIPAA was enacted to facilitate electronic transmission of data between providers and payers while protecting the privacy of patient health information. In protecting patient confidentiality, HIPAA can present certain challenges for providers, such as making it more complicated for a physician to send information about a patient to another physician for a consultation. Regional coordination is based on the seamless delivery of care across multiple provider settings. Patient-level information must flow freely between these settings—from dispatch to emergency response to hospital care—to ensure that appropriate information will be available for clinical decision making and coordination of services. Current interpretations of HIPAA would make it difficult to achieve the required degree of information fluidity. Additionally, HIPAA can be a barrier to family-centered care by limiting access to information to parents or legally identified caregivers of children.

Both EMTALA and HIPAA protect patients from potential abuses and serve invaluable purposes. As they are written and interpreted, however, compliance with these statutes can be difficult and costly for providers. More important, the acts are likely to impede the development of regional systems. The committee believes appropriate modifications could be made to both acts that would preserve their original purpose while reducing their adverse impact on the development of regional systems. The committee recommends that **the Department of Health and Human Services adopt rule changes to the Emergency Medical Treatment and Active Labor Act and the Health Insurance Portability and Accountability Act so that the original goals of the laws are preserved, but integrated systems may further develop (3.5).**

Coordinating Federal Leadership in Emergency Care

The committee's vision of a coordinated, regionalized, and accountable emergency and trauma care system for adults and children is impeded by the structure of federal programs that currently support emergency and trauma care. To function effectively, the components of the emergency and trauma care system must be highly integrated. Operationally, this means that all of the key players in a given region—hospital emergency and trauma departments, EMS dispatchers, state public health officials, trauma surgeons, EMS agencies, ED nurses, hospital administrators, firefighters, police, community safety net providers, and others—must work together to make decisions, deploy resources, and monitor and adjust system operations based on performance feedback.

As documented in this report, however, fragmentation, silos, and entrenched interests prevail throughout emergency and trauma care. The organization of federal government programs that support and regulate emergency and trauma care services largely reflects the fragmentation of emergency and trauma care services at the local level. Responsibility for emergency and trauma care is widely dispersed among multiple federal agencies within DHHS, the U.S. Department of Transportation (DOT), and DHS. This situation reflects the history and inherent nature of emergency and trauma care—essential public services that operate at the intersection of medical care, public health, and public safety (police, fire departments, and emergency management agencies).

In the 1960s, the mounting toll of highway deaths led NHTSA to become the first government home for EMS, where it has remained. Thus although EMS is primarily a medical discipline, federal responsibility for EMS rests with DOT. This responsibility was recently reinforced by the elevation of NHTSA's EMS program to the status of the Office of EMS within the agency. Today, NHTSA sponsors a number of workforce and research initiatives and the development of the National EMS Information System, and it recently received funding for a major nationwide initiative to promote the development of next-generation 9-1-1 service.

DHHS has played an important supporting role in the development of EMS and has taken the lead role with respect to hospital-based emergency and trauma care. It housed the Division of Emergency Medical Services and the Division of Trauma and EMS for many years, and most recently the Trauma-EMS Systems Program. All of these programs have been eliminated; the latter was recently zeroed out of the federal budget for fiscal year 2006. DHHS continues to support CDC's National Center for Injury Prevention and Control, the EMS-C program, and the National Bioterrorism Hospital Preparedness program. These programs have made important contributions to emergency and trauma care despite inconsistent funding and the frequent threat of elimination. The Agency for Healthcare Research and Quality (AHRQ), another DHHS agency, has historically been the principal federal agency funding research in emergency care delivery, including much of the early research on management of out-of-hospital cardiac arrest. Recently, AHRQ has funded important studies of ED crowding, operations management, and patient safety issues. It is active as well in funding research on preparedness, bioterrorism planning, and response.

DHS also plays an important role in emergency and trauma care. The Federal Emergency Management Agency (FEMA), once an independent cabinet-level agency now housed in DHS, provides limited amounts of grant funding to local EMS agencies through the U.S. Fire Administration. DHS also houses the Metropolitan Medical Response System (MMRS), a grant program designed to enhance emergency and trauma preparedness in major population centers. This program was migrated from DHHS to DHS in 2003. In addition, DHS houses the Disaster Medical Assistance Team (DMAT) program, through which health professionals volunteer and train as locally organized units so they can be deployed rapidly, under federal direction, in response to disasters nationwide. However, this program will migrate to DHHS in January 2007.

Efforts have been made to improve interagency collaboration at the federal level, especially in recent years. Over the last decade, federal agencies have worked collaboratively to provide leadership in the emergency and trauma care field, to minimize gaps and overlaps across programs, and to pool resources to jointly fund promising research and demonstration programs. For example, NHTSA and HRSA jointly supported the development of the *Emergency Medical Services Agenda for the Future*, which was published in 1996. This degree of collaboration has not been universal, however, and has been evident in some agencies more than others. Furthermore, collaborative efforts are limited by the constraints of agency authorization and funding. At some point, agencies must pursue their own programmatic goals at the expense of joint initiatives. Furthermore, to the degree that successful collaboration has occurred, it has generally depended on the good will of key individuals in positions of leadership, limiting the sustainability of these efforts when personnel changes occur.

In an effort to enhance the sustainability of collaborative initiatives, a number of agencies have participated in informal planning groups. For example, the Interagency Committee on Emergency Medical Services for Children Research (ICER), which is sponsored by HRSA, brings together representatives from a number of federal programs for the purposes of sharing information and improving research in emergency and trauma care for children.

A broader initiative is the Federal Interagency Committee on EMS (FICEMS), a planning group designed to coordinate the efforts of the various federal agencies involved in emergency and trauma care. FICEMS was established in the late 1970s. After a subsequent period of dormancy, it was reconstituted in the mid-1980s. The organization had no statutory authority until 2005, when it was given formal status by the Safe, Accountable, Flexible, Efficient Transportation Equity Act: A Legacy for Users (SAFETEA-LU), DOT's reauthorization legislation. While the focus of FICEMS is EMS, the group has in practice reached beyond the strict boundaries of prehospital care to facilitate coordination and collaboration with agencies involved in other aspects of hospital-based emergency and trauma care (see Box 3-2). NHTSA is charged with providing administrative support for FICEMS, which must submit a report to Congress annually. The central aims of the group are as follows:

• To ensure coordination among the federal agencies involved with state, local, or regional EMS and 9-1-1 systems.
• To identify state, local, or regional needs in EMS and 9-1-1 services.
• To recommend new or expanded programs, including grant programs, for improving state, local, or regional EMS and implementing improved EMS communications technologies, including wireless 9-1-1.
• To identify ways of streamlining the process through which federal agencies support state, local, or regional EMS.
• To assist state, local, or regional EMS in setting priorities based on identified needs.
• To advise, consult, and make recommendations on matters relating to the implementation of coordinated state EMS programs.

Problems with the Current Structure

Despite recent efforts at improved federal collaboration, there is widespread agreement that the various components of emergency care (EMS for

BOX 3-2
FICEMS Membership

The 2005 Safe, Accountable, Flexible, Efficient Transportation Equity Act: A Legacy for Users designated the following agencies as members of FICEMS. Each year, members elect a representative from one of these member organizations as the FICEMS chairperson.

- National Highway Traffic Safety Administration (DOT)
- Preparedness Division, Directorate of Emergency Preparedness and Response (DHS)
- Health Resources and Services Administration (DHHS)
- Centers for Disease Control and Prevention (DHHS)
- U.S. Fire Administration, Directorate of Emergency Preparedness and Response (DHS)
- Centers for Medicare and Medicaid Services (DHHS)
- Under Secretary of Defense for Personnel and Readiness (Department of Defense [DoD])
- Indian Health Service (DHHS)
- Wireless Telecommunications Bureau, Federal Communications Commission
- A representative of any other federal agency appointed by the Secretary of Transportation or the Secretary of Homeland Security through the Under Secretary for Emergency Preparedness and Response, in consultation with the Secretary of Health and Human Services, as having a significant role in relation to the purposes of the interagency committee
- A state EMS director appointed by the Secretary

adults and children, trauma care, hospital-based care) individually have not received sufficient attention, stature, and funding within the federal government. The scattered nature of federal responsibility for emergency care limits the visibility necessary to secure and maintain federal funding. The result has been marked fluctuations in budgetary support and the constant risk that key programs will be dramatically downsized or eliminated. The lack of a clear point of contact for the public and for stakeholders makes it difficult to build a unified constituent base that can advocate effectively for funding and provide feedback to the government on system performance. The lack of a unified budget has created overlaps, gaps, and idiosyncratic funding of various programs (for example, separate hospital surge capacity initiatives are currently taking place in AHRQ, CDC, HRSA, and DHS).

Finally, the lack of unified accountability disperses responsibility for system failures and perpetuates divisions between public safety and medical-based emergency and trauma care professionals. The degree to which the scattered responsibility for emergency and trauma care at the federal level has contributed to this disappointing performance is unclear. Regardless, the committee believes a new approach is warranted.

Alternative Approaches

Strong federal leadership for emergency and trauma care is at the heart of the committee's vision for the future, and continued fragmentation of responsibility at the federal level is unacceptable. The committee considered two options for remedying the situation: (1) maintain the status quo, giving the FICEMS approach time to strengthen and mature, or (2) designate or create a new lead agency within the federal government for emergency and trauma care. Some of the key differences between these two approaches are summarized in Table 3-1.

Option 1: Maintain the status quo and allow FICEMS to strengthen The committee considered the ramifications of maintaining the status quo. The problems associated with fragmented federal leadership of emergency care, documented above, include variable funding, periodic program cuts, programmatic duplication, and critical program gaps. With the recent enactment of a statutory framework for FICEMS, however, the committee considered the possibility that the need for a lead federal agency has diminished. The committee carefully examined the rationale for delaying the move toward a lead federal agency and allowing FICEMS time to gain strength. The central argument in support of this strategy is that there have been a number of recent improvements in collaboration at the federal level, and these efforts should be given a chance to work before an unproven and politically risky approach is pursued. Several recent developments support this view: the enactment of a statutory framework for FICEMS; the increasing level of collaboration among some federal agencies; the substantial new NHTSA funding for a next-generation 9-1-1 initiative; and the elevation of the NHTSA EMS program to the Office of EMS, which has the potential to improve visibility and funding for EMS, and perhaps other aspects of emergency and trauma care, within the federal government.

While the committee applauds these positive developments, setbacks have occurred as well. As noted above, DHHS's Division of Emergency Medical Services, its Division of Trauma and EMS, and most recently its Trauma-EMS Systems Program were recently zeroed out of the federal budget. Federal funding for AHRQ, nonbioterrorism programs at CDC, and other federal programs related to emergency and trauma care at the

TABLE 3-1 Comparison of the Current FICEMS Approach and the Committee's Lead Agency Proposal

	Maintain the Status Quo, Allowing FICEMS to Gain Strength	Designate or Create a New Lead Agency
Description	• Current agencies retain autonomy, but the FICEMS process fosters collaboration in planning.	• Combines emergency care functions from several agencies into a new lead agency.
Authority	• FICEMS has the authority to convene meetings, but no authority to enforce planning, evaluation, and coordination of programs and funding.	• Lead agency would have planning and budgetary authority over the majority of emergency care activities at the federal level.
Funding	• No guarantee of coordinated program funding. • Distributed responsibility for federal functions means that if programs are cut, others remain, reducing the risk of losing all federal support for emergency and trauma care.	• Consolidates visibility and political representation of emergency care, enhancing federal funding opportunities. • Emergency care funding is fully coordinated. • Risk of losing significant funding for emergency care in a hostile budget environment.
Collaboration	• Brings together the key emergency and trauma care agencies. • FICEMS cannot enforce coordination or collaboration.	• Unified agency would drive collaboration among all components of emergency and trauma care to achieve systemwide performance goals.
Public Identity	• Still lacks a unified point of authority from the public's perspective. • FICEMS facilitates response to the public.	• Provides for a unified federal emergency and trauma care presence for interaction with the public and stakeholder groups.
Professional Identity	• Fragmented federal representation makes it difficult to break down silos in the field.	• Provides a home for emergency and trauma care, which can project and enhance the professional identity of emergency and trauma care providers over time. • Lead agency could consolidate constituencies and engender stronger political representation.

TABLE 3-1 Continued

	Maintain the Status Quo, Allowing FICEMS to Gain Strength	Designate or Create a New Lead Agency
Efficiency	• May reduce redundancy through enhanced collaboration. • Very low administrative overhead costs.	• Eliminates redundant administrative structure, reducing administrative overhead costs. • Consolidated funding would allow for better allocation of federal dollars across the various emergency care needs (e.g., would eliminate overlapping programs).
Transition	• FICEMS is established in law, and implementation is under way. • Given FICEMS' limited powers, risks to individual programs and constituencies are minimal.	• Substantial startup costs associated with the transition to a single agency. • Potential for changes in program and funding emphasis during the transition, which could create winners and losers. • Potential dissension among emergency care agencies and constituencies could impact the organization's effectiveness.

federal level have been cut. These developments suggest that a fragmented organizational structure at the federal level would significantly hinder the creation of a coordinated, regionalized, accountable emergency and trauma care system. FICEMS can be a valuable body, but it is a poor substitute for formal agency consolidation. FICEMS is expressly focused on EMS, and ultimately has limited power over even this sphere. It is not a federal agency and therefore cannot regulate, spend, or withhold funding. It cannot even hold its own member agencies accountable for their actions—or lack of action.

Option 2: Designate or create a new federal lead agency   The possibility of a lead agency for emergency and trauma care has been discussed for years and was highlighted in the 1996 report *Emergency Medical Services Agenda for the Future.* While the concept of a lead agency promoted in that report was focused on prehospital EMS, the committee believes a lead agency should encompass all components involved in the provision of emergency and trauma care. This federal lead agency would unify federal policy development related to emergency and trauma care, provide a central point of contact for the various constituencies in the field, serve as a federal advocate for emergency and trauma care within the government, and coordinate grants so that federal dollars would be allocated efficiently and effectively.

A lead federal agency could better move the emergency and trauma care system toward improved integration; unify funding and other decisions; and represent all emergency and trauma care patients, providers, and settings, including prehospital EMS (both ground and air), hospital-based emergency and trauma care, pediatric emergency and trauma care, rural emergency and trauma care, and medical disaster preparedness. Specifically, a federal lead agency could:

• Provide federal leadership on important policy issues that cut cross agency boundaries.
• Create unified accountability for the performance of the emergency and trauma care system.
• Rationalize funding across the various aspects of emergency and trauma care to optimize the allocation of resources in achieving system outcomes.
• Coordinate programs to eliminate overlaps and gaps in current and future funding.
• Create a large combined federal presence, increasing the visibility of emergency and trauma care within the government and among the public.
• Provide a recognizable entity that would serve as a single point of contact for stakeholders and the public, resulting in consolidated and efficient data collection and dissemination and coordinated program information.
• Enhance the professional identity and stature of emergency and trauma care practitioners.
• Bring together multiple professional groups and cultures, creating cross-cultural and interdisciplinary interaction and collaboration that would model and reinforce the integration of services envisioned by the committee.

Although creating a lead agency could yield many benefits, such a move would also involve significant challenges. Numerous questions must be addressed regarding the location of such an agency in the federal government, its structure and functions, and the possible risk of weakening or losing current programs. HRSA's rural EMS and EMS-Trauma System programs have already been defunded, and the EMS-C program is under the constant threat of elimination. There is real concern that proposing an expensive and uncertain agency consolidation could jeopardize programs already at risk, such as EMS-C, as well as cripple new programs just getting started, such as NHTSA's enhanced 9-1-1 program. This is particularly likely if there is resistance to the consolidation from within the current agency homes for these programs.

A related concern is that the priority currently given to certain programs could shift, resulting in less support for existing programs. EMS advocates have expressed concern that hospital-based emergency and trauma care issues would dominate the agenda of a new unified agency. The pediatric community is worried about getting lost in a new agency, and has fought hard to establish and maintain strong categorical programs supported by historically steady funding streams. There is concern that under the proposed structure, the current focus of the EMS-C program could get lost or diminished or simply lose visibility in the multitude of programs addressed by the new agency.

There is also the potential for administrative and funding disruptions. Combining similar agencies, particularly those that reside within the same department, may be straightforward. But combining agencies with different missions across departments with different cultures may prove highly difficult. The problems experienced during the consolidation of programs in DHS increase anxiety about this proposal.

Another concern is that removing medical-related functions from DHS and DOT could exacerbate rather than reduce fragmentation. Operationally, nearly half of EMS services are fire department–based. Thus, there is concern that separating EMS and fire responsibilities at the federal level could splinter rather than strengthen relationships.

The Committee's Recommendation

Despite the concerns outlined above, the committee believes the potential benefits of consolidation outweigh the potential risks. A lead federal agency is required to fully realize the committee's vision of a coordinated, regionalized, and accountable emergency and trauma care system. The committee recognizes that a number of challenges are associated with the establishment of a new lead agency, though it believes these concerns can be mitigated through appropriate planning. The committee therefore recommends that **Congress establish a lead agency for emergency and trauma care within 2 years of the release of this report. The lead agency should be housed in the Department of Health and Human Services, and should have primary programmatic responsibility for the full continuum of emergency medical services and emergency and trauma care for adults and children, including medical 9-1-1 and emergency medical dispatch, prehospital emergency medical services (both ground and air), hospital-based emergency and trauma care, and medical-related disaster preparedness. Congress should establish a working group to make recommendations regarding the structure, funding, and responsibilities of the new agency, and develop and monitor the transition. The working group should have representation from federal and state agencies and professional disciplines involved in emergency care (3.6).**

Objectives of the lead agency   The lead agency's mission would be to enhance the performance of the emergency and trauma care system as a whole, as well as to improve the performance of the various components of the system, such as prehospital EMS, hospital-based emergency care, trauma systems, pediatric emergency and trauma care, prevention, rural emergency and trauma care, and disaster preparedness. The lead agency would set the overall direction for emergency and trauma care planning and funding; would be the primary collector and repository of data in the field; and would be the key source of information about emergency and trauma care for the public, the federal government, and practitioners themselves. It would be responsible for allocating federal resources across all of emergency and trauma care to achieve systemwide goals, and should be held accountable for the performance of the system and its components.

Location of the lead agency   The lead agency would be housed within DHHS. The committee considered many factors in selecting DHHS over DOT and DHS. The factor that drove this decision above all others was the need to unify emergency and trauma care within a medical care/public health framework. Emergency and trauma care is by its very nature involved in multiple arenas—medical care, public safety, public health, and emergency management. The multiple identities that result from this multifaceted involvement reinforce the fragmentation that is endemic to the emergency and trauma care system. For too long, the gulf between EMS and hospital care has hindered efforts at communication, continuity of care, patient safety and quality of care, data collection and sharing, collaborative research, performance measurement, and accountability. It will be difficult for emergency and trauma care to achieve seamless and high-quality performance across the system until the entire system is organized within a medical care/public health framework while also retaining its operational linkages with public safety and emergency management.

Only DHHS, as the department responsible for medical care and public health in the United States, can encompass all of these functions effectively. Although DOT has played an important role in both EMS and acute trauma care and has collaborated effectively with other agencies, its EMS and highway safety focus is too narrow to represent all of emergency and trauma care. DHS houses the Fire Service, which is closely allied with EMS, particularly at the field operations level. But the focus of DHS on disaster preparedness and bioterrorism is also too narrow to encompass the broad scope of emergency and trauma care.

Because emergency and trauma care functions would be consolidated in a department oriented toward medical care and public health, there is a risk that public safety and emergency management components could receive less attention, stature, or funding. Therefore, it is imperative that the mission of the new agency be understood and clearly established by statute so that the public safety and emergency management aspects of emergency and trauma care will not be neglected.

Programs included in the lead agency The committee envisions that the lead agency would have primary programmatic responsibility for the full continuum of EMS; emergency and trauma care for adults and children, including medical 9-1-1 and emergency medical dispatch; prehospital EMS (both ground and air); hospital-based emergency and trauma care; and medical-related disaster preparedness. The agency's focus would be on program development and strategic funding to improve the delivery of emergency and trauma care nationwide. It would not be primarily a research funding agency, with the exception of a few of the existing grant programs mentioned above. Funding for basic, clinical, and health services research in emergency and trauma care would remain the primary responsibility of existing research agencies, including the National Institutes of Health (NIH), AHRQ, and CDC. Because of the limited research focus of the lead agency, it would be imperative for existing research agencies, NIH in particular, to work closely with the new agency and strengthen their commitment to emergency and trauma care research. On the other hand, it may be appropriate to keep certain clinical and health services research initiatives with the programs in which they are housed, and therefore bring them into the new agency. For example, responsibility for funding the infrastructure for the Pediatric Emergency Care Applied Research Network (PECARN) would be moved into the new agency along with the rest of the EMS-C program.

In addition to existing functions, the lead agency would become the home for future programs related to emergency and trauma care, including new programs that would be dedicated to the development of inclusive systems of emergency and trauma care.

Working group While the committee envisions consolidation of most of the emergency care–related functions currently residing in other agencies and departments, it recognizes that many complex issues are involved in determining which programs should be combined and which left in their current agency homes. A deliberate process should be established to determine the exact composition of the new agency and to coordinate an effective transition. For these reasons, the committee is recommending the establishment of an independent working group to make recommendations regarding the structure, funding, and responsibilities of the new agency, and to coordinate and monitor the transition process. The working group should include representatives from federal and state agencies and professional disciplines involved in emergency care. The committee considered whether FICEMS would be an appropriate entity to assume this advisory and oversight role and concluded that, as currently constituted, it lacks the scope and independence to carry out this role effectively.

Role of FICEMS FICEMS is a highly promising entity that is complementary to the proposed new lead agency. FICEMS would play a vital role during the proposed interim 2-year period by continuing to enhance coordination and collaboration among agencies and providing a forum for public input. In addition, it could play an important advisory role to the independent working group. Once the lead agency had been established, FICEMS would continue to coordinate work between the lead agency and other agencies, such as NIH, CMS, and DoD, that would remain closely involved in various emergency and trauma care issues.

Structure of the lead agency While the principle of integration across the multiple components of emergency and trauma care should drive the structure, operation, and funding of the new lead agency, the committee envisions distinct program offices to provide focused attention and programmatic funding for key areas, such as the following:

- Prehospital EMS, including 9-1-1, dispatch, and both ground and air medical services
  - Hospital-based emergency and trauma care
  - Trauma systems
  - Pediatric emergency and trauma care
  - Rural emergency and trauma care
  - Disaster preparedness

To ensure that current programs would not lose visibility and stature within the new agency, it would be critical for each program office to have equal status and reporting relationships within the agency's organizational structure. The committee lacks the expertise to specify the organizational structure in further detail. Rather, it envisions a national dialogue over the coming year—coordinated by the proposed independent working group, aided by input from FICEMS, and with the involvement of the Office of Management and Budget and congressional committees with jurisdiction—to implement the committee's recommendation.

Funding for the lead agency Existing programs transferring to the new agency would bring with them their full current and projected funding. Congress should also establish additional funding to cover the costs associated with the transition to and the new administrative overhead associated with the lead agency. In addition, Congress should add new funding for the offices of hospital-based emergency and trauma care, rural emergency and trauma care, and trauma systems. In light of the pressing challenges confronting emergency care providers and the American public, this would be money well spent. While the committee is not qualified to estimate the costs associated with establishing a unified lead agency, it recognizes that these costs would be substantial. At the same time, however, the committee believes that substantial cost savings would result from reduced duplication and lower overhead. New funding that flowed into the agency would result in new programming, rather than an increase in existing overhead.

Mitigation of concerns regarding the establishment of a lead federal agency The committee recognizes that transitioning to a single lead agency would be a difficult challenge under any circumstances, but would be especially difficult for an emergency and trauma care system that is already under duress from funding cutbacks, elimination of programs, growing public demand on the system, and pressure to enhance disaster preparedness. During this critical period, it is imperative that support for emergency and trauma care programs already in place in the various federal agencies be sustained. In particular, the Office of EMS within NHTSA has ongoing programs that are critical to the EMS system. Similarly, existing emergency care–related federal programs, such as those in HRSA's EMS-C program and Office of Rural Health Policy and at CDC, should be supported during the transition period. If the committee's proposal is to be successful, the constituencies associated with established programs must not perceive that they are being politically weakened during the transition.

The committee believes the proposed consolidation of agencies would enhance support for emergency and trauma care across the board, benefiting all current programs. But it also believes avoiding disruptions that could adversely affect established programs is critically important. Therefore, the committee considers it imperative for legislation creating the new agency to protect current levels of funding and visibility for existing programs. The new agency should balance its funding priorities by adding to current funding levels, not by diverting funds away from existing programs.

The committee acknowledges the concern that removing medical-related emergency and trauma functions from DHS and DOT would create additional fragmentation. The committee believes the public safety aspects of emergency and trauma care must continue to be addressed as a core element of the emergency and trauma care system. But the primary focus of the system must be medical care and public health if the recognition, stature, and outcomes that are critical to the system's success are to be achieved.

THE EMERGENCY MEDICAL SERVICES
FOR CHILDREN PROGRAM

It is the committee's hope and expectation that in the future, existing deficiencies in pediatric emergency care will be eliminated, and providers will be equally prepared for the care of both children and adults. However, the work of the EMS-C program today remains relevant and vital.

In the chapters that follow, the committee outlines a number of recommendations for improving pediatric emergency care. Implementing these recommendations will require the leadership of a well-recognized, well-respected entity not just within pediatrics, but within the broader emergency care system. The EMS-C program, with its long history of working with federal partners, state policy makers, researchers, providers, and professional organizations across the spectrum of emergency care, is in the best position to assume this leadership role. The committee recommends that **Congress appropriate $37.5 million per year for the next 5 years to the Emergency Medical Services for Children program (3.7)**.

The committee is not suggesting that the EMS-C program should assume full responsibility for funding the implementation of the recommendations presented in this report; rather, the program should serve as a facilitator to initiate the implementation process. For example, the EMS-C program could convene national conferences involving individuals with multidisciplinary expertise to address how the committee's various recommendations should be implemented. However, additional funding will be needed to ensure that the program has the capacity to initiate these efforts. An additional $500,000 should be allocated to the program's budget to sponsor four to five national conferences per year.

The program's budget should also be expanded to accommodate an increase in the award size for the State Partnership Grants. In fiscal year 2005, EMS agencies (or a designated alternative) in 54 U.S. states and territories received grant support from the program to institutionalize pediatric EMS improvements. In many states, however, the award from the EMS-C program ($100,000 to $115,000) represents the state's largest or only investment in pediatric emergency care. After covering salary and overhead for a staff person, the current size of the grant leaves little to be spent on programmatic initiatives. An additional $8 million per year is needed to increase the annual award amount to $250,000 per state/territory. This additional funding would better enable a state representative to initiate improvements, which could include organizing pediatric disaster drills, increasing the level of available pediatric emergency care training, participating in and organizing statewide pediatric emergency care planning, and meeting with provider organizations to encourage and facilitate improvements in pediatric preparedness.

The EMS-C program also provides financial support for the infrastructure of PECARN through its network demonstration cooperative agreements. The importance of PECARN cannot be overstated. While it remains small in size, it is perhaps the best resource for conducting multicenter randomized trials in pediatric emergency care. As the network is currently organized, however, its linkages to prehospital providers are limited, thereby constraining the ability of researchers to conduct analyses across the continuum of care. Additional funding is needed to build a sustainable link between the four research nodes of PECARN and the prehospital providers in those nodes. EMS-C program funding should be increased to provide each research node $1 million per year to establish data linkages with local prehospital providers, for a total cost of $4 million per year. Looking to the future of PECARN, its administrators should also explore the possibility of integrating more general hospitals into the network and expanding research nodes in the south and southeast to improve the network's geographic reach.

Finally, the program is in need of additional funding that could be directed toward special initiatives or one-time projects addressing important needs. For example, the program is currently funding two projects for the development of clinical practice guidelines ($250,000 per year for 3 years for each project). Justification for expanding this initiative is provided in Chapter 4, where the committee calls for the development, evaluation, and updating of pediatric clinical practice guidelines. An additional $5 million per year would allow the EMS-C program to support approximately 18 similar large projects. Examples of other types of special projects that could be supported with this funding are the development of pediatric dosing guidelines for certain medications and the development of labeling techniques to reduce medication errors.

The 5-year timeframe is suggested so that the program will have the capacity to address the deficiencies in the pediatric emergency care system quickly. The program should focus on creating sustainable activities and strive to integrate pediatrics into emergency care planning at the federal, state, and local levels. The proposed 5-year period is not intended as a limit on federal funding dedicated to improving pediatric emergency care; indeed, there will always be a need to monitor and study emergency care for children. However, the committee's expectation is that the various elements of emergency care leadership at the federal level will be better integrated and consolidated in the future (as discussed above). Support for pediatric emergency care will always remain a vital aspect of that federal leadership, but it may not be in the form of a separate program. After 5 years, it will be necessary to reexamine how best to identify and fund pediatric emergency care objectives at the federal level, as well as to reevaluate future funding levels for the EMS-C program.

SUMMARY OF RECOMMENDATIONS

3.1 The Department of Health and Human Services and the National Highway Traffic Safety Administration, in partnership with professional organizations, should convene a panel of individuals with multidisciplinary expertise to develop evidence-based categorization systems for emergency medical services, emergency departments, and trauma centers based on adult and pediatric service capabilities.

3.2 The National Highway Traffic Safety Administration, in partnership with professional organizations, should convene a panel of individuals with multidisciplinary expertise to develop evidence-based model prehospital care protocols for the treatment, triage, and transport of patients, including children.

3.3 The Department of Health and Human Services should convene a panel of individuals with emergency and trauma care expertise to develop evidence-based indicators of emergency and trauma care system performance, including the performance of pediatric emergency care.

3.4 Congress should establish a demonstration program, administered by the Health Resources and Services Administration, to promote coordinated, regionalized, and accountable emergency care systems throughout the country, and appropriate $88 million over 5 years to this program.

3.5 The Department of Health and Human Services should adopt rule changes to the Emergency Medical Treatment and Active Labor Act and the Health Insurance Portability and Accountability Act so that the original goals of the laws are preserved, but integrated systems may further develop.

3.6 Congress should establish a lead agency for emergency and trauma care within 2 years of the release of this report. The lead agency should be housed in the Department of Health and Human Services, and should have primary programmatic responsibility for the full continuum of emergency medical services and emergency and trauma care for adults and children, including medical 9-1-1 and emergency medical dispatch, prehospital emergency medical services (both ground and air), hospital-based emergency and trauma care, and medical-related disaster preparedness. Congress should establish a working group to make recommendations regarding the structure, funding, and responsibilities of the new agency, and develop and monitor the transition. The working group should have representation from federal and state agencies and professional disciplines involved in emergency and trauma care.

3.7 Congress should appropriate $37.5 million per year for the next 5 years to the Emergency Medical Services for Children program.

REFERENCES

Adomako SA, Melese-d'Hospital I. 2004. *State-by-State Profiles: The Integration of Pediatric Care Components into the EMS System.* Rockville, MD: MCHB, NHTSA, HRSA.

Bardach NS, Olson SJ, Elkins JS, Smith WS, Lawton MT, Johnston SC. 2004. Regionalization of treatment for subarachnoid hemorrhage: A cost-utility analysis. *Circulation* 109(18):2207–2212.

Berenson RA, Kuo S, May JH. 2003. Medical malpractice liability crisis meets markets: Stress in unexpected places. *Issue Brief (Center for Studying Health System Change)* 68:1–7.

Bode MM, O'Shea TM, Metzguer KR, Stiles AD. 2001. Perinatal regionalization and neonatal mortality in North Carolina, 1968–1994. *American Journal of Obstetrics and Gynecology* 184(6):1302–1307.

Bravata D, McKonald K, Owens D, Wilhelm ER, Brandeau ML, Zaric GS, Holty JC, Sundaram V. 2004. *Regionalization of Bioterrorism Preparedness and Response.* Rockville, MD: AHRQ.

Chang RK, Klitzner TS. 2002. Can regionalization decrease the number of deaths for children who undergo cardiac surgery? A theoretical analysis. *Pediatrics* 109(2):173–181.

Chiara O, Cimbanassi S. 2003. Organized trauma care: Does volume matter and do trauma centers save lives? *Current Opinion in Critical Care* 9(6):510–514.

Cifuentes J, Bronstein J, Phibbs CS, Phibbs RH, Schmitt SK, Carlo WA. 2002. Mortality in low birth weight infants according to level of neonatal care at hospital of birth. *Pediatrics* 109(5):745–751.

CMS (Centers for Medicare and Medicaid Services). 2003. Emergency Medical Treatment and Active Labor Act (EMTALA) Interim Guidance. Letter to State Survey Agency Directors. Ref: S&C-04-10.

CMS. 2005a. *Report Number One to the Secretary, U.S. Department of Health and Human Services, from the Inaugural Meeting of the Emergency Medical Treatment and Labor Act Technical Advisory Group.* Washington, DC: CMS.

CMS. 2005b. *Report Number Two to the Secretary, U.S. Department of Health and Human Services, from the Emergency Medical Treatment and Labor Act Technical Advisory Group.* Washington, DC: CMS.

CMS. 2005c. *Report Number Three to the Secretary, U.S. Department of Health and Human Services, from the Emergency Medical Treatment and Labor Act Technical Advisory Group.* Washington, DC: CMS.

CMS. 2005d. *Hospital Compare.* [Online]. Available: http://www.hospitalcompare.hhs.gov/hospital/home2.asp [accessed November 23, 2005].

CMS. 2005e. *Medicare Spotlights.* [Online]. Available: http://www.medicare.gov [accessed November 22, 2005].

Committee on Pediatric Emergency Medicine Pediatric Section and Task Force on Regionalization of Pediatric Critical Care. 2000. Consensus report for regionalization of services for critically ill or injured children. *Pediatrics* 105(1):152–155.

Cooper A, Barlow B, DiScala C, String D, Ray K, Mottley L. 1993. Efficacy of pediatric trauma care: Results of a population-based study. *Journal of Pediatric Surgery* 28(3):299–303; discussion 304–305.

Cunningham P, May J. 2003. Insured Americans drive surge in emergency department visits. *Issue Brief (Center for Studying Health System Change)* 70:1–6.

Davis R. 2003, July. The method: Measure how many victims leave the hospital alive. *USA Today.* P. A1.

Densmore JC, Lim HJ, Oldham KT, Guice KS. 2006. Outcomes and delivery of care in pediatric injury. *Journal of Pediatric Surgery* 41(1):92–98; discussion 92–98.

EMS Performance Measures Project. 2005. *Performance Measures in EMS.* [Online]. Available: http://www.measureems.org/performancemeasures2.htm [accessed January 5, 2006].

GAO (General Accounting Office). 2001. *Emergency Care. EMTALA Implementation and Enforcement Issues.* Washington, DC: GAO.

GAO. 2003. *Infectious Diseases: Gaps Remain in Surveillance Capabilities of State and Local Agencies.* Washington, DC: GAO.

Gausche-Hill M, Wiebe R. 2001. Guidelines for preparedness of emergency departments that care for children: A call to action. *Pediatrics* 107(4):773–774.

Gausche-Hill M, Lewis R, Schmitz C. 2004. *Survey of US Emergency Departments for Pediatric Preparedness: Implementation and Evaluation of Care of Children in the Emergency Department: Guidelines for Preparedness.* Unpublished results.

Glance LG, Osler TM, Dick A, Mukamel D. 2004. The relation between trauma center outcome and volume in the national trauma databank. *Journal of Trauma-Injury Infection & Critical Care* 56(3):682–690.

Grumbach K, Keane D, Bindman A. 1993. Primary care and public emergency department overcrowding. *American Journal of Public Health* 83(3):372–378.

Grumbach K, Anderson GM, Luft HS, Roos LL, Brook R. 1995. Regionalization of cardiac surgery in the United States and Canada. Geographic access, choice, and outcomes. *Journal of the American Medical Association* 274(16):1282–1288.

Harris Interactive. 2004. *Trauma Care: Public's Knowledge and Perception of Importance.* Rochester, NY: The Coalition for American Trauma Care.

Health Level 7. 2005. *Emergency Care Special Interest Group.* [Online]. Available: http://www.hl7.org/Special/committees/emergencycare/index.cfm [accessed November 30, 2005].

Holloway MY. 2001. *The Regionalized Perinatal Care Program.* Princeton, NJ: The Robert Wood Johnson Foundation.

Hulka F. 1999. Pediatric trauma systems: Critical distinctions. *The Journal of Trauma* 47(Suppl. 3):S85–S89.

Hulka F, Mullins RJ, Mann NC, Hedges JR, Rowland D, Worrall WH, Sandoval RD, Zechnich A, Trunkey DD. 1997. Influence of a statewide trauma system on pediatric hospitalization and outcome. *The Journal of Trauma* 42(3):514–519.

Imperato PJ, Nenner RP, Starr HA, Will TO, Rosenberg CR, Dearie MB. 1996. The effects of regionalization on clinical outcomes for a high risk surgical procedure: A study of the whipple procedure in New York state. *American Journal of Medical Quality* 11(4):193–197.

IOM (Institute of Medicine). 1993. *Emergency Medical Services for Children.* Washington, DC: National Academy Press.

IOM. 2002. *Fostering Rapid Advances in Health Care: Learning from System Demonstrations.* Washington, DC: National Academy Press.

Jones J. 2004. Neonatal nursing: The first six weeks. *Critical Care Nursing* (Suppl.):6–8.

Jurkovich GJ, Mock C. 1999. Systematic review of trauma system effectiveness based on registry comparisons. *Journal of Trauma-Injury Infection & Critical Care* 47(Suppl. 3): S46–S55.

Kanter RM, Heskett M. 2002. *Washington Hospital Center (B): The Power of Insight.* Watertown, MA: Harvard Business School Publishing.

Koziol-McLain J, Price DW, Weiss B, Quinn AA, Honigman B. 2000. Seeking care for nonurgent medical conditions in the emergency department: Through the eyes of the patient. *Journal of Emergency Nursing* 26(6):554–563.

Lewin ME, Altman S. 2000. *America's Health Care Safety Net.* Washington DC: National Academy Press.

Lindsay P, Schull M, Bronskill S, Anderson G. 2002. The development of indicators to measure the quality of clinical care in emergency departments following a modified-delphi approach. *Academic Emergency Medicine* 9(11):1131–1139.

MacKenzie EJ. 1999. Review of evidence regarding trauma system effectiveness resulting from panel studies. *Journal of Trauma-Injury Infection & Critical Care* 47(Suppl. 3): S34–S41.

MacKenzie EJ, Rivara FP, Jurkovich GJ, Nathens AB, Frey KP, Egleston BL, Salkever DS, Scharfstein DO. 2006. A national evaluation of the effect of trauma-center care on mortality. *New England Journal of Medicine* 354(4):366–378.

Malone RE. 1995. Heavy users of emergency services: Social construction of a policy problem. *Social Science Medicine* 40(4):469–477.

Mann NC, Mullins RJ, MacKenzie EJ, Jurkovich GJ, Mock CN. 1999. Systematic review of published evidence regarding trauma system effectiveness. *Journal of Trauma-Injury Infection & Critical Care* 47(Suppl. 3):S25–S33.

McCaig LF, Burt CW. 2005. *National Hospital Ambulatory Medical Care Survey: 2003 Emergency Department Summary.* Hyattsville, MD: National Center for Health Statistics.

McConnell KJ, Newgard CD, Mullins RJ, Arthur M, Hedges JR. 2005. Mortality benefit of transfer to level I versus level II trauma centers for head-injured patients. *Health Services Research* 40(2):435–457.

MCHB (Maternal and Child Health Bureau). 2004. *Emergency Medical Services for Children. Five Year Plan 2001–2005: Midcourse Review.* Washington, DC: EMS-C National Resource Center.

Mullins RJ, Mann NC. 1999. Population-based research assessing the effectiveness of trauma systems. *Journal of Trauma-Injury Infection & Critical Care* 47(Suppl. 3):S59–S66.

Mullins RJ, Veum-Stone J, Helfand M, Zimmer-Gembeck M, Hedges JR, Southard PA, Trunkey DD. 1994. Outcome of hospitalized injured patients after institution of a trauma system in an urban area. *Journal of the American Medical Association* 271(24):1919–1924.

Nallamothu BK, Saint S, Kolias TJ, Eagle KA. 2001. Clinical problem-solving of nicks and time. *New England Journal of Medicine* 345(5):359–363.

NAS, NRC (National Academy of Sciences, National Research Council). 1966. *Accidental Death and Disability: The Neglected Disease of Modern Society.* Washington, DC: National Academy of Sciences.

NASEMSD (National Association of State EMS Directors). 2004. *Pediatric Disaster and Terrorism Preparedness.* Falls Church, VA: NASEMSD.

Nathens AB, Jurkovich GJ, Rivara FP, Maier RV. 2000. Effectiveness of state trauma systems in reducing injury-related mortality: A national evaluation. *The Journal of Trauma* 48(1):25–30; discussion 30–31.

Nathens AB, Jurkovich GJ, Maier RV, Grossman DC, MacKenzie EJ, Moore M, Rivara FP. 2001. Relationship between trauma center volume and outcomes. *Journal of the American Medical Association* 285(9):1164–1171.

National Center for Injury Prevention and Control. 2004. *DEEDS—Data Elements for Emergency Department Systems.* [Online]. Available: http://www.cdc.gov/ncipc/pub–res/deedspage.htm [accessed November 25, 2005].

NHTSA (National Highway Traffic Safety Administration). 1996. *Emergency Medical Services Agenda for the Future.* Washington, DC: U.S. DOT.

NQF (National Quality Forum). 2002. *National Voluntary Consensus Standards for Adult Diabetes Care.* [Online]. Available: http://www.qualityforum.org/txdiabetes–public.pdf [accessed November 23, 2005].

NQF. 2003. *National Voluntary Consensus Standards for Hospital Care: An Initial Performance Measure Set.* [Online]. Available: http://www.qualityforum.org/txhospmeasBEACHpublicnew.pdf [accessed November 23, 2005].

NQF. 2004a. *National Voluntary Consensus Standards for Nursing Home Care.* [Online]. Available: http://www.qualityforum.org/txNursingHomesReportFINALPUBLIC.pdf [accessed November 23, 2005].

NQF. 2004b. *National Voluntary Consensus Standards for Nursing-Sensitive Care: An Initial Performance Measure Set.* [Online]. Available: http://www.qualityforum.org/txNCFINALpublic.pdf [accessed November 23, 2005].

NQF. 2005. *National Voluntary Consensus Standards for Home Health Care.* [Online]. Available: http://www.qualityforum.org/webHHpublic09-23-05.pdf_ [accessed November 23, 2005].

O'Brien PM. 1999. The emergency department as a public safety net. In: Fields W, ed. *Defending America's Safety Net.* Dallas, TX: American College of Emergency Physicians.

Orr RA, Han YY, Roth K. 2006. Pediatric transport: Shifting the paradigm to improve patient outcome. In: Fuhrman B, Zimmerman J, eds. *Pediatric Critical Care* (3rd edition). Mosby, Elsevier Science Health. Pp. 141–150.

Peterson LA, Burstin HR, O'Neil AC. 1998. Non-urgent emergency department visits: The effect of having a regular doctor. *Medical Care* 36:1249–1255.

Pollack MM, Alexander SR, Clarke N, Ruttimann UE, Tesselaar HM, Bachulis AC. 1991. Improved outcomes from tertiary center pediatric intensive care: A statewide comparison of tertiary and nontertiary care facilities. *Critical Care Medicine* 19(2):150–159.

Pollock DA, Adams DL, Bernardo LM, Bradley V, Brandt MD, Davis TE, Garrison HG, Iseke RM, Johnson S, Kaufmann CR, Kidd P, Leon-Chisen N, MacLean S, Manton A, McClain PW, Michelson EA, Pickett D, Rosen RA, Schwartz RJ, Smith M, Snyder JA, Wright JL. 1998. Data elements for emergency department systems, release 1.0 (deeds): A summary report. Deeds Writing Committee. *Journal of Emergency Nursing* 24(1):35–44.

Rosenbaum S, Kamoie B. 2003. Finding a way through the hospital door: The role of EMTALA in public health emergencies. *Journal of Law, Medicine & Ethics* 31(4):590–601.

State of California Office of the Patient Advocate. 2005. *2005 HMO Report Card.* [Online]. Available: http://www.opa.ca.gov/report_card/ [accessed January 12, 2006].

Studdert DM, Mello MM, Sage WM, DesRoches CM, Peugh J, Zapert K, Brennan TA. 2005. Defensive medicine among high-risk specialist physicians in a volatile malpractice environment. *Journal of the American Medical Association* 293(21):2609–2617.

Stylianos S. 2005. Outcomes from pediatric solid organ injury: Role of standardized care guidelines. *Current Opinion in Pediatrics* 17(3):402–406.

Tilford JM, Aitken ME, Anand KJS, Green JW, Goodman AC, Parker JG, Killingsworth JB, Fiser DH, Adelson PD. 2005. Hospitalizations for critically ill children with traumatic brain injuries: A longitudinal analysis. *Critical Care Medicine* 33(9):2140–2141.

Williams RL, Chen PM. 1982. Identifying the sources of the recent decline in perinatal mortality rates in California. *New England Journal of Medicine* 306(4):207–214.

Wright JL, Klein BL. 2001. Regionalized pediatric trauma systems. *Clinical Pediatric Emergency Medicine* 2:3–12.

Young GP, Wagner MB, Kellermann AL, Ellis J, Bouley D. 1996. Ambulatory visits to hospital emergency departments. Patterns and reasons for use. 24 hours in the ED Study Group. *Journal of the American Medical Association* 276(6):460–465.

4

Arming the Emergency Care Workforce with Pediatric Knowledge and Skills

This chapter provides an overview of the emergency care workforce. The review focuses on the level of pediatric education and training that providers receive and evidence of their ability to treat children appropriately. What becomes clear from the discussion is that pediatric care represents a relatively limited component of educational requirements for many emergency care providers; moreover, many emergency care providers treat critically ill or injured pediatric patients infrequently and therefore may be unable to maintain the requisite level of skill. The result is that some emergency care providers are ill prepared to address the broad spectrum of ailments that children encounter, from common to critical injuries and illnesses. This is a long-standing problem that has improved somewhat over time, but naturally has led to continued concerns about the ability of the emergency care workforce to care properly for pediatric patients. To reduce the consequences of illness and injury, the workforce must have the knowledge and skills necessary to deliver appropriate pediatric emergency care. The committee offers several recommendations for enhancing and supporting providers' ability to deliver quality care to children.

PREHOSPITAL EMERGENCY CARE

The term "first responder" is often used to identify the first care provider on the scene. In the mid-1990s, the term was used by the National Highway Traffic Safety Administration (NHTSA) in its formal classification of emergency medical services (EMS) responders. First responders represent the most basic level of EMS response and are trained to provide basic emergency medical care. They have more training than first aid, but less than an emergency medical technician (EMT). A certification exists for first responders, and many firefighters, police officers, and other emergency workers have first responder training, which is useful since they may arrive on the scene before an EMT. First responders use a limited amount of equipment to perform initial assessment and intervention and are trained to assist EMTs once the EMTs arrive on the scene (NHTSA and MCHB, 1995; Bureau of Labor Statistics and U.S. Department of Labor, 2004).

EMTs are the backbone of prehospital emergency care in the United States as they are usually the first providers of direct medical care to patients needing emergency treatment. There are generally three levels of EMT: EMT-B (Basic), EMT-I (Intermediate), and EMT-P (Paramedic).

EMT-Bs are those trained to provide basic, noninvasive prehospital care, although their scope of practice varies by state and may include certain invasive procedures in some states. EMT-Bs provide care to patients at the scene of a medical emergency (e.g., car crash) and during transport to the hospital. They perform the following tasks:

- Examine victims to determine the nature and scope of their injury or illness.
- Administer basic life support (BLS), including providing oxygen or performing cardiopulmonary resuscitation (CPR).
- Use automated or semiautomated defibrillators to administer life-saving shocks to a stopped heart.
- Upon arrival at the hospital or medical center, help the staff provide preadmittance treatment and obtain patient medical histories (Bureau of Labor Statistics, 2002; State of California Employment Development Department Labor Market Information Division, 1995).

EMT-Ps are the most highly skilled EMTs, and they provide the most extensive care. Paramedics are trained in all phases of emergency prehospital care, including advanced life support (ALS) treatment. In addition to the tasks performed by EMT-Bs, they may also:

- Administer drugs (usually intravenously).
- Administer intravenous fluids.
- Use manual defibrillators to administer lifesaving shocks to a stopped heart.
- Use advanced airway techniques and equipment to assist those patients experiencing a respiratory emergency.
- Perform endotracheal intubations and perhaps other invasive airway maneuvers.
- Interpret the results of heart-monitoring equipment (Bureau of Labor

Statistics, 2002; State of California Employment Development Department Labor Market Information Division, 1995).

Most states recognize a level of practice between that of EMT-Bs and EMT-Ps. Sometimes known as EMT-I, this level encompasses all the tasks of an EMT-B, but also may include some of the tasks of a paramedic. The scope of practice of these EMT-Is varies by state, but is always broader than that of an EMT-B in the same state and narrower than that of an EMT-P.

The EMT profession is different from most medical occupations in that a substantial number of workers serve in a volunteer capacity. According to data gathered from a sample of members of the National Registry of Emergency Medicine Technicians (NREMT), 36.5 percent of registered EMTs are volunteers. The vast majority of volunteer EMTs are EMT-Bs (89.5 percent), while paid EMTs are much more likely to be registered as EMT-Ps (46.3 percent) (NREMT, 2003). Volunteer personnel have traditionally been the lifeblood of rural EMS agencies. Since the development of EMS systems began in the 1960s, millions of hours of time and effort have been donated by rural EMTs to the care of their neighbors, friends, and complete strangers.

Staffing Challenges

Working conditions for EMTs tend to be very challenging, leading to high rates of turnover. EMTs may experience burnout, or even post-traumatic stress disorder, as a result of the emotional and psychological stressors of their job. Many EMTs work irregular hours, and some are not well compensated in salary or retirement benefits. The work of EMTs is also occasionally dangerous, as they must respond to unpredictable and uncontrolled situations and may be exposed to the threat of violence or infectious disease (Franks et al., 2004). Moreover, there is no well-defined career ladder for EMTs, and those in fire department–based services sometimes must leave EMS work for other duties to advance within their organization. Many individuals work as an EMT as a step toward becoming a physician assistant, registered nurse (RN), or physician.

Recruitment and retention are a constant problem for EMS agencies; at a recent EMS conference, administrators ranked recruitment and retention as a top priority (EMS Insider, 2005). Anecdotal reports indicate that many regions are facing shortages of prehospital personnel. Some reports indicate a critical shortage of EMTs in rural areas, but even some urban areas struggle. For example, the District of Columbia Fire and EMS Service Department reported a shortage of EMS personnel that had driven staffing levels below half of what is needed to staff the city's fleet of ambulances. In 2005, 57 of the 166 paramedic positions in the District of Columbia were vacant. As a result, the city is staffing ALS ambulances with a paramedic and a lesser-trained EMT rather than two paramedics (Wilber, 2005). Reports indicate that staffing shortfalls appear to be most pronounced at the paramedic level. This is likely due to the increased education required for this level of EMT and attrition of personnel to fire services (Personal communication, M. Williams, March 27, 2006).

Demand for EMTs will continue to be strong in rural and smaller metropolitan areas (Bureau of Labor Statistics, 2002). Volunteer staffing has become increasingly more difficult to maintain in rural areas for a variety of reasons. Decades ago it was common for volunteers to be on call virtually 24 hours a day. Today, increased time demands due to the need for two-income family support and vying interests create an environment in which volunteers may donate just one specific weeknight or a few hours on a weekend. Rural EMS agencies face particular volunteer staffing shortages during the weekday work hours.

Pediatric Training

Although there are National Standard Curricula for all levels of EMT training, those curricula are not mandatory, so training requirements for certification vary across states. A written exam is required in most states, and some require an additional practical exam to obtain certification. Generally, the national standards for BLS are a minimum of 110 hours of instructional training with additional field training requirements that vary by state. For ALS, training at the paramedic level entails 1,000–1,200 hours of didactic training beyond the EMT-B level (DOT, 1998), with additional practicum time. Certification in all states needs to be renewed (every 2 years for most states). Renewal usually requires completion of continuing education, verification of skills by a medical director, and current affiliation with an EMS agency.

Pediatric care has traditionally been a small component of EMT training. In a mid-1980s survey of EMT training programs nationwide, Seidel (1986) found that 41 percent of such programs offered 10 hours or less of didactic training in pediatrics; 5 percent of programs offered none. All EMTs received on average 8 hours of didactic training in pediatrics; paramedics received 15 hours. Seidel also identified wide variation in the pediatric topics covered in the curriculum. Most training programs covered epiglottitis (98 percent of agencies), croup (98 percent), respiratory distress (98 percent), asthma (97 percent), and seizures (95 percent). However, half of programs did not offer pediatric field simulation, half did not cover pediatric dysrhythmias, 36 percent did not cover hypotension, 26 percent did not cover drowning, 22 percent did not cover pediatric ALS, and 16 percent did not cover neonatal resuscitation.

Since the early 1990s, a number of efforts have been made to improve pediatric training opportunities for EMTs. Among the earliest courses designed specifically for EMTs was the Prehospital Trauma Life Support course, developed in 1990 by the National Association of EMTs in cooperation with the American College of Surgeons' (ACS) Committee on Trauma. This continuing education course incorporates material on prehospital pediatric assessment and stabilization. It is an intensive 16- to 20-hour course attended by all levels of EMTs.

In 1992, the first national consensus curriculum on prehospital pediatrics was published by the California Pediatric Emergency and Critical Care Coalition, the California Emergency Medical Services for Children (EMS-C) Project, and the American College of Emergency Physicians (ACEP). The initiative grew, and in 1995 a task force produced the Pediatric Education for Paramedics (PEP) course, which built on the work of several state projects funded by the federal EMS-C program (AAP, 2005a). That course was eventually expanded by a steering committee assembled by the American Academy of Pediatrics (AAP) to serve both BLS and ALS EMTs. The result was the Pediatric Education for Prehospital Providers (PEPP) course. The BLS course consists of a minimum of 7 hours, while the ALS course is a minimum of 13 hours. In developing course recommendations, the steering committee reviewed the most current data on efficacy, safety, and feasibility. Where scientific data were not available, the steering committee used expert opinion and clinical experience in hospitals, emergency departments (EDs), and pediatric ambulatory settings to shape the course content. The course is subject to the steering committee's ongoing review (AAP, 2005a). The first edition of the PEPP manual sold more than 100,000 copies, and the program extends into nine countries and includes more than 5,000 instructors worldwide (PEPP Program, 2006).

In the 1990s, the Maternal and Child Health Bureau (MCHB) worked with and supported NHTSA in revising the Department of Transportation's (DOT) National Standard Curricula to ensure that the needs of children would be addressed during initial EMT education and refresher courses. The curricula for first responders, EMT-Bs, EMT-Is, and EMT-Ps were all revised. Table 4-1 shows the content of the National Standard Curricula specific to pediatrics for first responders, EMT-Bs and EMT-Is. It should be noted that there are more cognitive, affective, and psychomotor objectives related to pediatrics included in other parts of the curriculum. For example, a module on assessment-based management may include instruction related to pediatrics. Still, the number of hours dedicated to pediatrics appears low.

The National Standard Curriculum for Paramedics was developed in 1998, but the hours specific to each module are not specified. Instead, the curriculum emphasizes meeting educational objectives. The curriculum

TABLE 4-1 Recommended Pediatric Education in the Current U.S. Department of Transportation National Standard Curricula

Content	Recommended Minimum Hours
First Responder (1995)	
Infants and Children	2
Practical Lab: Children and Childbirth	1
Evaluation: Children and Childbirth	1
Emergency Medical Technician-Basic (1994)	
Infants and Children	3
Practical Skills Lab: Infants and Children	3
Evaluation: Infants and Children	1
Emergency Medical Technician-Intermediate (1999)	
Neonatal Resuscitation	2
Practical Lab: Neonatal Resuscitation	2
Pediatrics	8
Practical Lab: Pediatrics	4

SOURCE: Personal communication, D. Bryson, NHTSA, 2006.

includes the following modules that address pediatric issues: pharmacology, venous access and medication administration, life span development, neonatology, pediatrics, abuse and assault, patients with special challenges, acute interventions for the chronic care patient, and assessment-based management (Personal communication, D. Bryson, January 26, 2006).

The National Standard Curricula, which many but not all states follow, are likely to be replaced in the future by the National EMS Education Standard. It will be updated on a 2- or 3-year cycle as a new national approach to EMT education is developed (NHTSA, 2006).

When the DOT National Standard Curricula were developed, there was concern that many EMS instructors did not have the knowledge or clinical experience to teach the new pediatric components of the curriculum adequately (MCHB, 1996). As a result, the EMS-C program awarded a grant to New York University to develop the Teaching Resource for Instructors in Prehospital Pediatrics (TRIPP). TRIPP, originally published in 1997, is an encyclopedic resource manual for instructors who teach the pediatric sections of the EMT-B National Standard Curriculum. In 2002, the developers of TRIPP released another version for instructors of ALS.

The National Association of Emergency Medical Technicians (NAEMT) also established its own Pediatric Prehospital Care (PPC) course in 2000 after recognizing a need by EMTs for additional training to better understand the anatomical, physiological, and communication challenges surrounding the treatment of children. The course is overseen primarily by EMTs, with strong guidance from a pediatric emergency medicine physician. Some EMS systems adopt the course as their only pediatric training program (NAEMT, 2005). However, the pediatric continuing education courses required by EMS agencies still vary considerably. Those commonly required include Pediatric Airway Management for the Prehospital Professional, Pediatric Advanced Life Support, and Advanced Pediatric Life Support. A review of the literature revealed no studies that have evaluated whether EMS training in these courses has led to changes in patient outcomes.

Perhaps the newest course for the prehospital professional is one that focuses on children with special health care needs. The EMS-C program funded the development of Special Children's Outreach and Prehospital Education (SCOPE), designed to teach EMTs how to care for children with special health care needs. This curriculum is particularly important since special needs children are frequent users of the prehospital system. The curriculum, created in 2003, provides basic information on various chronic medical conditions, as well as on the technologies and equipment that may be necessary for the survival of children with these conditions (MCHB, 2003).

Despite advances in educational opportunities and materials, pediatric issues continue to be a challenge for EMTs. According to a NREMT newsletter, in 1996, nearly one-third of individuals taking the NREMT EMT-P examination failed on their first attempt. Of those who failed, two-thirds failed the pediatric/obstetrics section; the failures related primarily to the pediatric questions within that section (Glaeser et al., 2000).

Limited studies of pediatric training for EMTs have continued to show deficiencies, though many of these studies are dated. A survey of EMS agencies in North Carolina revealed that only 11 percent of agencies provided more than 10 hours of basic training in pediatric emergency care (Zaritsky et al., 1994). A similar survey of EMS agencies in Oklahoma found that more than half did not address pediatric topics in continuing education (Graham et al., 1993). According to the 2003 EMS-C National Grantee Survey Assessment, pediatric education requirements were a condition for recertification for EMT-Bs in 24 states and for EMT-Ps in 31 states (MCHB, 2004a).

A survey of nationally registered EMTs revealed that mandatory continuing education was not required for 35 percent of EMT-Bs, 40 percent of EMT-Is, and 25 percent of EMT-Ps. In the 2 years prior to the survey, 24 percent of EMT-Bs, 20 percent of EMT-Is, and 6 percent of EMT-Ps received 0–3 hours of pediatric continuing education. Still, continuing education was the main source of pediatric knowledge and skills for 42 percent of EMT-Bs, 56 percent of EMT-Is, and 60 percent of EMT-Ps. More than three-fourths of all EMTs surveyed said they supported a state or national mandate for required continuing education in pediatrics beyond what they currently received (Glaeser et al., 2000). Of those EMTs surveyed who supported mandated pediatric continuing education, approximately half said there were no barriers to obtaining this training. However, 23 percent of EMT-Bs, 21 percent of EMT-Is, and 13 percent of EMT-Ps said that continuing education was not available. Other common barriers cited included costs of continuing education courses, which are frequently borne by the EMTs themselves rather than their EMS agency, and the distance to the courses. Only a small percentage of EMTs said their medical director was not interested in increasing pediatric continuing education or that pediatric facilities were not cooperative (Glaeser et al., 2000).

Maintenance of Pediatric Skills

Exercising skills in real life is important to reinforce training (Wood et al., 2004). One of the challenges faced by EMTs in keeping their pediatric skills sharp is that they rarely have the opportunity to practice lifesaving procedures in real situations (Gausche-Hill, 2000). Children represent only 5–10 percent of all prehospital calls (Seidel et al., 1984; Federiuk et al., 1993); of those pediatric calls, only 12 percent involve the need for pediatric ALS (PALS) (Seidel et al., 1984). Only a small percentage of EMTs identify field experience as the main source for their pediatric knowledge and skills. This is not surprising considering that fewer than 3 percent of all EMTs care for more than 15 pediatric patients during a typical month, and perhaps only 1 of these patients needs ALS care. In one survey, 87 percent of EMT-Bs, 84 percent of EMT-Is, and 60 percent of EMT-Ps said they treated fewer than 4 pediatric patients per month (Glaeser et al., 2000).

Several studies have revealed how infrequently EMTs have the opportunity to practice certain interventions in the field. In an analysis of ALS prehospital provider calls in Boston, Massachusetts, Babl and colleagues (2001) found that ALS providers delivered on average one bag mask ventilation every 1.7 years, one intubation every 3.3 years, and one intraosseous access (placement of a needle into a bone to give fluid for resuscitation) every 6.7 years (Babl et al., 2001). Similarly, Gausche (1997) concluded that it would take at least 20 years for every paramedic in 11 counties in California to perform bag-valve-mask ventilation at least once on a pediatric patient (Seidel et al., 1991).

Quality of Care

Lack of initial and continuing pediatric education, coupled with the low frequency with which EMTs encounter critical pediatric patients, results in a lower level of care than should be expected of the nation's prehospital emergency care system. Several studies have documented deficiencies in treatment for pediatric patients. In the 1980s, Seidel and colleagues (1984) found that death rates from trauma were significantly higher for children than for adults (highest for infants), and that deaths occurred more commonly in areas where there were no pediatric centers. The study findings suggest that the needs of children in the prehospital setting were not being met (Seidel et al., 1984). In a study of 100 pediatric trauma deaths, Ramenofsky and colleagues (1984) found that 53 could have survived if the EMS/trauma system had functioned properly; errors were found in nearly 80 percent of those cases (Ramenofsky et al., 1984). Several studies have shown that EMTs have greater success rates in intubating adults compared with children (Mishark et al., 1992; Boswell et al., 1995; Doran et al., 1995).

Underutilization of acquired skills can cause an EMT to feel fearful or reluctant about performing an intervention in a time of crisis (Orr et al., 2006). And in fact, children tend to be undertreated in comparison with adults (Gausche et al., 1998; Orr et al., 2006). There are several examples. A study of children in respiratory distress found that 44 percent received inappropriate interventions. Oxygen and medications were underused, while vascular access, a procedure that paramedics perform frequently, was overused (Scribano et al., 2000). Another study found that paramedics are less likely to perform basic resuscitation procedures for pediatric patients than for equally critical adults (Su et al., 1997). In one Canadian study, half of children under age 6 who required intravascular access did not receive an intravenous line (Lillis and Jaffe, 1992).

Comfort in Caring for Pediatric Patients

Studies indicate that many EMTs are less comfortable caring for pediatric patients, particularly infants, than for adult patients. An example is that paramedics reported being very comfortable terminating CPR on adults, but very uncomfortable doing so with children (Hall et al., 2004). A study that examined job satisfaction among paramedics found that pediatric calls were among the most stressful because of the low volume of pediatric cases typically encountered (Federiuk et al., 1993).

Although the majority of EMTs in the survey of Glaeser and colleagues (2000) said they were comfortable to some degree with their own and their EMS system's ability to care for a critical pediatric patient, they indicated that critical care infants were the patients of greatest concern. Indeed, 94 percent of respondents were more uncomfortable with treating infants and toddlers than any other age group (Glaeser et al., 2000). This is an important finding considering that infants tend to use prehospital and ED services at higher rates than older children. In a 1999 study of EMS transports in Kansas City, Missouri, Murdock and colleagues (1999) found that infants younger than 1 year of age had the highest transport rates (47 transports per 1,000 persons), followed by those aged 1–4 (26 per 1,000 persons),

10–14 (18 per 1,000 persons), and 5–9 (17 per 1,000 persons) (Murdock et al., 1999).

Another problem associated with the lack of practice in the field is that certain skills deteriorate rather quickly if not used. Training in pediatric resuscitation can boost knowledge and skills initially, but one study found that this knowledge and these skills decay significantly after 6 months (Su et al., 2000). Deterioration of skills is a concern even for paramedics with years of experience. Two years after taking a PALS course, a majority of experienced paramedics could not pass a test on PALS concepts (Wolfram et al., 2003).

More troubling, EMTs' confidence is not necessarily a good indication of ability. Henderson (1998) showed that 95 percent of paramedics who failed both bag-valve-mask and endotracheal intubation attempts reported a feeling of confidence in and a lack of anxiety about their ability to perform those tasks (Henderson, 1998; Orr et al., 2006). Training increases EMTs' perception of their ability, and their confidence declines slowly over time. Unfortunately, their actual skill performance declines more quickly than perceived (Gausche-Hill, 2000).

EMERGENCY DEPARTMENT CLINICIANS

A number of different types of clinicians deliver care to children in EDs. Not just physicians and nurses, but also pharmacists, nurse practitioners, physician assistants, and others play an important role in many EDs.

ED Physicians

There were approximately 32,000 physicians working in EDs in 1999, an average of nearly 8 physicians per ED (Moorhead et al., 2002). Emergency physicians evaluate the presenting problems of patients, make diagnoses, and initiate treatment. They must be prepared for a wide variety of medical emergencies and must be well versed in such diverse subjects as anesthesia, cardiology, critical care, environmental illness, neurosciences, obstetrics/gynecology, ophthalmology, pediatrics, psychiatry, neonatology, resuscitation, toxicology, trauma, and wound management. In addition, they often represent the sole source of primary care for patients whose only access to care is through EDs. ED physicians also have duties beyond their scheduled clinical time; they spend several hours per week performing unscheduled clinical duties, administrative work, teaching, and/or research (Moorhead et al., 2002). In small hospitals that lack in-house physician support at night, many emergency physicians are required to provide backup support to the hospital from the ED.

A medical specialty of emergency medicine (EM) was created to enhance the training and skills of physicians wishing to practice in the ED. EM residency training involves a minimum of 3 years of specialized training after medical school. Board certification is granted by the American Board of Emergency Medicine (ABEM) or its osteopathic equivalent, the American Osteopathic Board of Emergency Medicine (AOBEM). Largely as a result of the steady growth in EM residency training programs, the number of self-identified EM physicians in the United States has increased substantially since 1979, when EM was first recognized as a specialty. Growth in EM has been much stronger than growth in medicine overall. The number of self-identified EM physicians in the United States increased from 14,000 in 1990 to more than 25,500 in 2002, an increase of 79 percent. During the same period, the number of all physicians increased by 39 percent (AMA, 2003).

Despite the growth in EM physicians, only 38 percent of practicing ED physicians in the United States are residency trained and board certified in the specialty of EM. The majority of those ED physicians who are not residency trained or board certified in EM have completed a residency in another specialty, most often family practice or internal medicine. Only 3 percent of practicing emergency physicians are residency trained or board certified in pediatrics (Moorhead et al., 2002). Many rural hospitals hire "moonlighting" residents to provide physician coverage in their EDs. Moonlighting—traditionally the unsupervised practice of residents before the completion of their residency (Armon and Coren, 2005)—has stirred considerable controversy among medical organizations (Kaji and Stevens, 2002). In any case, moonlighting physicians are not likely to have extensive training or experience in either EM or pediatrics.

Residency-trained EM physicians and pediatricians have the option of pursuing subspecialty fellowship training and board certification in pediatric emergency medicine. Alternatively, graduating medical students can enroll in a joint EM–pediatrics residency program, an option established in 1992 by the American Board of Pediatrics (ABP) and ABEM. Pediatric emergency medicine is now a recognized subspecialty of the American Board of Medical Specialties. Creation of the pediatric emergency medicine subspeciality grew from the recognition that the pediatric population is a distinct group of patients requiring trained staff to respond to their unique needs (Tamariz et al., 2000). A subspecialist in pediatric emergency medicine is a physician who has completed training in either pediatrics or EM, and then secured additional training in pediatric emergency medicine in an accredited fellowship program (ABMS, 2002). At present, the total number of pediatric emergency medicine physicians is quite small. In fact, the number of EM physicians and pediatricians choosing to subspecialize in pediatric emergency medicine has declined significantly, from a high of 355 in 1996–1997 to a low of 121 in 2002–2003. However, the large number of physicians who received their certification in the mid-1990s reflects those individuals who did so before the grandfather provision for the subspecialty ran out. The figure since that time indicates a rather stable number of trainees in pediatric emergency medicine. Most of the slots in these fellowship programs are being awarded to graduates of pediatric residency programs. As a result, the vast majority of pediatric emergency medicine subspecialists (89 percent of the total between 1994 and 2003) hold their primary board certification in pediatrics rather than EM (see Figure 4-1) (ABMS, 2003).

The average hospital is likely to have a board-certified EM physician attending, but unlikely to have a pediatric emergency medicine physician attending. Approximately 23 percent of EDs have a pediatric emergency medicine physician attending. Children's hospitals and hospitals with large volumes of pediatric patients (more than 7,500 pediatric ED visits per year) are more likely to have a pediatric emergency medicine physician attending than the average hospital (Middleton and Burt, 2006). Among those hospitals without a pediatric emergency medicine physician attending, just over half have a board-certified pediatrician attending, and 20 percent have a written protocol for calling a pediatrician; 17 percent of EDs have no EM, pediatric emergency medicine, or pediatric attending physician.

The physicians who work in the ED have varying degrees of training in pediatrics. Those with the most formal training are those who have completed a fellowship in pediatric emergency medicine. The goal of the fellowship program in this subspecialty is to produce physicians who are clinically proficient in the practice of pediatric emergency medicine, especially in the management of the acutely ill or injured child, in the ED (ACGME, 2004). The training period for pediatric emergency medicine subspecialty residents is 2 years for EM physicians and 3 for pediatricians. The Accreditation Council for Graduate Medical Education (ACGME) specifies that the curriculum must include at least 12 months of seeing children in an ED that treats children for the full spectrum of illnesses and injuries. The training

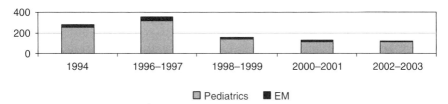

FIGURE 4-1 Number of subspecialty certificates in pediatric emergency medicine, United States, 1994–2003.
SOURCE: ABMS, 2003.

also includes 4 months in the reciprocal specialty from which the resident enters the training program. For example, pediatric graduates must spend 4 months in adult care rotations. The core content of the curriculum must include training in EMS, administration, ethics, legal issues, research, and procedures. Certification is limited according to the physician's primary board—7 years for the American Board of Pediatrics, 10 years for the American Board of Emergency Medicine (ACGME, 2004).

EM resident physicians are required to receive training in pediatric emergency care. In the early 1980s, there was considerable concern about the level and quality of pediatric emergency care training provided in these programs. Pediatric emergency care training accounted for approximately 16 percent of training time for EM residents, even though pediatric patients represented about 25 percent of all ED visits (Ludwig et al., 1982). In a survey, 42 percent of residency program directors expressed dissatisfaction with the pediatric training component of the EM residency (Ludwig et al., 1982; Christopher, 2000). Since that time, there has been increased involvement of pediatric emergency medicine physicians in EM residencies. Additionally, more EM residencies include specific training experience in pediatric emergency care, and more EM residency programs are affiliated with pediatric centers (AAP, 2000; Tamariz et al., 2000; Christopher, 2000).

Nonetheless, a more recent assessment of pediatrics in emergency medicine residency programs indicates that progress has been mixed. Pediatric training in EM residency programs continues to represent a relatively small percentage of training time. Today, approximately 13 percent of training time is spent on pediatric electives (Tamariz et al., 2000). EM residents may see children during nonpediatric rotations and certainly during their 18-plus months of supervised training on ED rotations, but the amount of pediatric contact time on these rotations is difficult to determine. At the same time, the confidence of residency directors in their pediatric curriculum has improved. The majority of directors indicated that they were either very or somewhat confident in the areas of trauma, intensive care, airway management, and urgent care. This confidence likely reflects the relatively large exposure of emergency residents to pediatric patients in EDs, pediatric EDs, pediatric intensive care units, and urgent care or fast-track clinics. In the area of neonatal resuscitation, most residency directors were somewhat confident or not very confident, suggesting that emphasis on this skill should be increased in the curriculum (Tamariz et al., 2000).

To be board certified in EM, a physician must pass an exam in that specialty. Approximately 8 percent of the EM board exam focuses on pediatric topics (ABEM, 2004). However, an individual need answer only 75 percent of the total questions correctly to pass. Therefore, an individual can answer all of the pediatric questions incorrectly and still receive a passing score on the exam.

Unfortunately, the majority of physicians practicing in the ED have not had residency training in either EM or pediatric emergency medicine (Moorhead et al., 2002). An assessment conducted in the late 1990s found that the supply of EM physicians was simply not sufficient to staff all ED physician positions, and not all EDs had access to a pediatric emergency medicine physician on staff (Holliman et al., 1997). This appears to be the case today as well (Moorhead et al., 2002). Therefore, physicians in some of the other disciplines (e.g., internal medicine, family practice) are needed to fill positions in EDs. It is difficult to determine the level of pediatric and EM training these physicians have received. Certainly those ED physicians who are pediatricians are familiar with children, but their formal training in EM may be limited. Likewise, ED physicians in such disciplines as internal medicine and family practice may have little formal training in either EM or pediatrics. Nevertheless, these ED physicians presently represent an essential component of ED staffing in many hospitals. Many may possess a high level of competency in pediatric emergency care, but it was gained through on-the-job experience rather than through formal training in a supervised setting.

As stated above, 3 percent of ED physicians are board certified in pediatrics. The committee is concerned not only about ED physicians lacking substantial training in pediatrics, but also about some pediatricians working in the ED lacking sufficient training in EM. According to the Residency Review Committee's requirements for pediatric residency programs, pediatric residents must spend a minimum of 4 months receiving training in emergency and acute illness, but only 2 of those 4 months must be in EM (National Capital Consortium Pediatrics Residency, 2004). This means that some pediatricians practicing in the ED may have spent only 5.5 percent of their 3-year residency on EM, although again, many of these physicians may possess a high level of competency in EM based on their experience in the ED. Another concern is that sick children access care through their pediatricians, who may find it difficult to detect certain emergency conditions, such as meningococcemia, among their patients. A pediatrician who received little training in EM and who spends the majority of his or her time on well-child visits may have difficulty recognizing and addressing an emergency condition.

Beyond initial specialty training, physicians have a number of opportunities to obtain training in pediatric emergency care. Different hospitals have their own requirements in terms of continuing education for ED physicians. However, the most popular pediatric continuing education courses are PALS and advanced pediatric life support (APLS). These courses are often required during initial training as well; for example, the PALS course is required in 78 percent of EM residency programs and APLS in 17 percent of programs (Tamariz et al., 2000). Additionally, professional societies help member physicians comply with continuing education requirements from state medical boards. For example, ACEP, which represents EM physicians, has a number of educational offerings designed to help members earn 150 hours of continuing education credits every 3 years. Of the 800 courses approved for credit, 23 percent are on pediatric topics, the most popular being PALS and APLS. Several other pediatric courses are offered at the ACEP annual meeting. According to a 1997 ACEP survey, however, 17 states had not offered APLS, PALS, or other similar pediatric courses in the previous 2 years (Santamaria et al., 1997). Having to travel a long distance to attend a pediatric training course naturally places an added burden on physicians who might wish to obtain the training.

Pediatric and Trauma Surgeons

The other medical specialties of particular relevance to pediatric emergency care are the surgical subspecialties of trauma surgery and pediatric surgery. In a 5-year residency training program in general surgery, surgeons receive training in a number of specialty areas, including trauma and pediatric surgery, after which they are expected to be able to manage the commonly encountered and less complex cases associated with these content areas (The American Board of Surgery, 2004). They may subsequently choose to undertake advanced training in trauma surgery or pediatric surgery (The American Board of Surgery, 2005).

Trauma surgeons perform emergent surgical procedures, usually but not exclusively involving life- or limb-threatening injuries to the neck, chest, abdomen, pelvis, and vasculature. Trauma surgeons generally complete 2 years of fellowship training in trauma surgery and surgical critical care following the completion of the 5-year surgical residency. The ACS estimates that there are about 3,000 trauma surgeons practicing in the United States today (Personal communication, C. Williams, February 17, 2006). Trauma surgeons tend to focus their practice in trauma centers.

The American Board of Surgery awards Certification in Pediatric Surgery to surgeons who complete a 2-year fellowship in pediatric surgery and pass an examination in pediatric surgery following the 5-year surgical residency (The American Board of Surgery, 2004). Pediatric surgery residents are required to meet specific curricular goals and objectives in pediatric trauma care and must help provide definitive pediatric trauma care to large numbers of pediatric trauma patients.

On-Call Specialists

Hospitals that offer specialist services, such as neurosurgery and orthopedic surgery, to inpatients must also have the same services available to patients who present at the ED (Glabman, 2005). ED physicians rely on and consult these specialists for advice or admission, as well as to arrange follow-up care after discharge, to relay information about a patient, and/or to request specific procedures or treatment for patients (Macasaet and Zun, 2005). Some of these specialist physicians have obtained advanced training in their specialty area after completing a pediatric residency (e.g., pediatric neurology or cardiology) or residency training in the specialty area followed by specialized pediatric training (e.g., pediatric surgery, orthopedics, or plastic surgery).

The salient problem with specialists is their availability. Over the past several years, many hospitals have experienced great difficulty in securing specialists for ED patients of all ages when needed. In a 2004 survey by ACEP, two-thirds of ED medical directors reported shortages of on-call specialists at their hospitals (ACEP, 2004; Vanlandingham et al., 2005). Numerous other studies and surveys have investigated the shortage of on-call specialists, finding that the problem extends across many different specialties and all regions of the country, and that it appears to be worsening (Green et al., 2005; O'Malley et al., 2005).

Part of the problem is a general shortage of pediatric subspecialists. The number and proportion of pediatric residents choosing advanced training have declined (Health Resources and Services Administration Council on Graduate Medical Education, 2002; O'Leary, 2002). This decline can be attributed at least in part to managed care's focus on primary care, which has led to reduced support for specialist fellowships and less reimbursement income for specialists (O'Leary, 2002). The American Academy of Pediatrics has called the supply of pediatric subspecialists "a pressing concern" (AAP, 2003).

In August 2001, the National Association of Children's Hospitals and Related Institutions (NACHRI) surveyed member hospitals to gauge perceptions about the supply of pediatric subspecialists, both nationally and within each hospital's own market, and to assess hospitals' physician recruitment and retention efforts. With a 34 percent response rate, the survey showed that the overall vacancy rate for pediatric subspecialists was 11.1 percent, with endocrinology, pulmonology, and neurology being the specialties with the highest vacancy rates. Respondents noted that the most difficult specialties to recruit were neurology, gastroenterology, anesthesiology, and pulmonology. The reasons given for the difficulty most frequently were an overall shortage of qualified candidates, competition from other provider organizations, and low pay relative to job demands. Reasons cited for the perceived shortage of pediatric subspecialists were residents' reduced interest in the subspecialties and reimbursement and compensation issues (O'Leary, 2002). Indeed, issues surrounding compensation are an important factor. A study by the California Medical Association showed that more than 50 percent of physicians said they had difficulty receiving reimbursement for *insured* patients at least 50 percent of the time; the problem of payment is greatly exacerbated when the patient is uninsured. To encourage subspecialists to continue taking ED call, some hospitals have begun paying for this service (Steiger, 2005).

Other forces also contribute to the shortage of on-call specialists to care for patients of all ages. Some speculate that the younger generation of specialists may be less inclined to take call than their more experienced colleagues out of a desire to improve their work–life balance (Salsberg, 2005). Hospital by-laws often require physicians to take ED call for a certain period of time, for example, 15 years, in exchange for admitting privileges. Historically, this arrangement has worked well; it allows hospitals to fill their on-call panel and gives young specialists an opportunity to build up their practices. But with the movement of specialists to large, multispecialty groups, younger physicians no longer need to rely on ED call to supply patients. Hospitals have less leverage in linking admitting privileges to ED call, and many physician groups discourage members from taking ED call (Taheri and Butz, 2004).

Still other physicians drop ED call because of liability concerns. Pediatric emergency cases are especially risky because the patient is often seriously ill or injured; medical records may be scant or nonexistent; treatment may be rendered after hours, when resources for care are less readily available; and the doctor lacks an established relationship with the child and his or her family. The rapidly rising cost of malpractice insurance is a powerful disincentive for specialists to assume liability by treating unknown emergency patients, many of whom are uninsured, may be noncompliant with discharge instructions, and may be difficult to contact regarding follow-up (Green et al., 2005). Seventy-five percent of neurosurgeons no longer operate on children because of liability concerns, sharply reducing the availability of those services for pediatric patients (Glabman, 2005).

The availability of on-call specialists is an issue discussed at length in the committee's companion report, *Hospital-Based Emergency Care: At the Breaking Point*, which offers specific recommendations for addressing the problem. One option being discussed by specialty societies is the creation of a specialty in emergency surgery or acute care surgery in which a board-certified general surgeon would receive fellowship training in elective and emergency general surgery, trauma surgery, and surgical critical care. In addition to treating what is conventionally considered "general trauma" (neck, thoracic, and abdominal injuries), the new acute care surgical specialist could also perform selected and limited neurosurgical and orthopedic procedures, with support from fellow surgical specialists (The Committee to Develop the Reorganized Specialty of Trauma Surgical Critical Care and Emergency Surgery, 2005). It is anticipated that acute care surgeons would treat both adult and pediatric patients. The proposed curriculum for the new specialty was under development at the time of this writing, but pediatric surgery is likely to be an elective option within the fellowship training.

Nurses

There are between 75,000 and 100,000 nurses working in EDs. According to the Emergency Nurses Association (ENA), emergency RNs perform the following tasks: triage, assessment, analysis, nursing diagnosis, planning, implementation of interventions and procedures, administration of medications and other therapies, monitoring of patient status, outcome identification, evaluation of responses, triage and prioritization, preparedness for emergency operations, stabilization and resuscitation, patient education, and crisis intervention for unique patient populations (e.g., sexual assault survivors) (ENA, 1999).

Nurses in EDs are predominantly female (86 percent), have a median age of 40, and are largely non-Hispanic white (88.5 percent). They generally have worked in nursing for less time than other nurses; approximately 30 percent graduated in the last 5 years, compared with 20.6 percent of other nurses. Only 11 percent graduated 26 or more years ago, compared with 22.6 percent of all nurses (DHHS, 2000). Nurses in EDs report feeling that they are under great stress significantly more often than do RNs in other settings: in one study, 37 percent of ED RNs reported feeling under great stress "almost every day," compared with 30 percent of other RNs. Surveys show that nurses in the ED tend to be more pressed for time and have heavier workloads than those working in other settings (New York State Education Department, 2003).

Training

To become a nurse, an individual typically completes one of two courses of study, an associate degree nurse (ADN) or a bachelor of science nurse (BSN). The ADN course is typically a 2-year degree program focused on the practical applications of nursing. The BSN is a 4-year program that expands into the theoretical realms of patient care. In recent years there has been a push to mandate that the BSN be a minimum requirement for being a professional nurse; this issue is still under debate. After graduation from one of these programs, nurses must take the board examination to become an RN.

Courses mandated at the basic level include hazardous materials awareness, fire and safety, CPR, and infection control. Requirements for more advanced coursework vary from hospital to hospital, although almost all require advanced cardiac life support for ED nurses working in resuscitation areas or administering intravenous (IV) sedation. Some hospitals require new ED hires to take a critical care course, depending upon their previous experience.

ED nurses wishing to obtain additional credentials in emergency nursing may become certified emergency nurses (CENs), awarded to nurses that pass the qualifying examination by the Board of Certification for Emergency Nursing. However, most nurses working in EDs are not certified as CENs. In 2004, 13,115 nurses nationwide were credentialed as CENs. There are also other advanced degree options for nurses, including masters and doctoral degree programs with various areas of specialization and practice. Many nursing management positions require advanced degrees.

Some ED nurses specialize in caring for children and may work in pediatric EDs, but there is no certification available in pediatric emergency nursing, and very little data exist regarding these nurses. State boards of nursing may require PALS or APLS for nurses providing sedation. Pediatric EDs are likely to require advanced pediatric courses for their nurses, and may even require advanced training in neonatal resuscitation. Some ED nurses may participate in a number of other pediatric continuing education courses, including the emergency nursing pediatric course. It is unclear how many nurses are required to participate in pediatric continuing education and how often.

Staffing Challenges

The nursing shortage in both hospital and nonhospital settings has been the subject of press reports and research articles for years (GAO, 2001; Gerson and Oliver, 2005). Although there have been nursing shortages in the past, many believe that the current one is different in that it is not rooted in cyclical changes (Schriver et al., 2003). Today, fewer individuals are choosing nursing as a profession than in the past, in part because of the increased professional opportunities for women and the limited number of nursing education slots resulting from a shortage of nursing faculty. The nursing shortage has led to problems for hospitals and medical centers in all units, and the problem is only expected to worsen in the future as the demand for nursing services increases with the aging of the population. The importance of an adequate-sized nursing staff cannot be overstated. A number of robust research studies have shown a direct link between nurse staffing levels and patient outcomes (Aiken et al., 2002a,b; Needleman et al., 2002).

EDs are not immune to the nursing shortage. Nationwide, it is estimated that 12 percent of nursing positions for which hospitals are actively recruiting are in EDs. This makes the ED the third most common source of nursing position openings in hospitals (following general medical/surgical and critical care units). In a survey of hospitals in New York City, 83 percent reported that they were actively recruiting for nurses in their ED (Greater New York Hospital Association, 2004). A 2005 survey of EDs by the ENA found that 26 percent of EDs had an RN vacancy rate of 10 percent or higher (ENA, 2006).

The impact of the nursing shortage on ED patient care has not been effectively evaluated; however, many speculate that the shortage has a negative impact for two reasons. First, as with other areas of the hospital, if the ED lacks appropriate nursing levels, patients will not receive the proper care or attention. For example, a triage nurse may be overwhelmed by the number of patients he or she has to evaluate and may miss an important sign of a severe illness or injury. Moreover, procedures performed on children less than 5 years of age, for example, IV starts and catheterizations, generally require more staffing to keep the child calm and manageable. Second, the nursing shortage adds to the problem of ED crowding. If nurses are not available to staff inpatient beds, admitted patients from the ED may become boarders, waiting for an available bed.

Other Medical Professionals in the ED

A number of other medical professionals may deliver care to children in the ED. Some might be surprised to hear that nearly 9 percent of ED patients are seen by an EMT (McCaig and Burt, 2005). These EMT-trained ED technicians are able to perform basic emergency care in the ED setting, allowing nurses and physicians more time to treat complex cases and perform more intensive procedures. The scope of practice for such personnel is limited, but has increased in some EDs to include intravenous infusions, splinting, and phlebotomy (Franks et al., 2004).

Approximately 7 percent of ED patients are seen by a physician assistant (PA), generally in addition to seeing a physician and/or nurse. PAs provide medical care to patients under the supervision of a physician, and their specialty is the same as that of their supervising physician. PAs must be granted clinical privileges at the hospital in which they work and can prescribe medication in most states. There are three PA educational programs in the United States offering specializations in emergency medicine, although PAs do not need to graduate from such a program to practice in EDs. In 2003, approximately 4,508 PAs (9.8 percent) worked in EDs. More than 4,600 PAs had a primary specialty in emergency medicine (10 percent). The majority of PAs working in EDs are emergency medicine specialists (93.6 percent); fewer than 1 percent are pediatric specialists (2003 Physician Assistant Census Survey, calculations by American Association of Physician Assistants staff).

Only about 2 percent of patients see a nurse practitioner (NP) during their ED visit (McCaig and Burt, 2005). NPs are master's-prepared RNs who provide significant medical care to patients. Some states require NPs to work under the supervision of a physician, while others do not. There is no national certification in emergency care for NPs, but they may obtain training in emergency care skills through university-based programs, continuing education, and work experiences (Cole et al., 1999). Advanced practice nurses (APNs) in emergency settings were most likely to report certification as a family NP (43 percent), acute care NP (13 percent), adult care NP (12 percent), critical nurse specialist (CNS) (9 percent), or pediatric NP (7 percent) (ENA, 2003).

In the 1970s, a limited number of hospitals began integrating pharmacists into their ED staff. Clinical pharmacy specialists (CPSs) who work in EDs typically have a doctor of pharmacy degree and have completed a 1-year residency. Traditionally, CPSs in EDs helped with medication billing and inventory control, but in recent years their role in the ED has expanded. With the growing number of drugs available and the increased complexity of drug selection, administration, and monitoring, some EDs use a pharmacist as part of the care team. Such use of pharmacists offers the potential to reduce the high number of medication errors that occur in that environment.

Still, the prevalence of pharmacists, particularly full-time pharmacists, in EDs remains low. A 2001 survey of directors of pharmacy in hospitals with at least one accredited pharmacy residency program was conducted to ascertain the prevalence and characteristics of pharmaceutical services in EDs nationwide. Only 3 percent of respondents reported having a dedicated pharmacist in an ED satellite pharmacy, while 14 percent reported having a dedicated pharmacist who provided services to ED patients (Thomasset and Faris, 2003). But the demand for pharmacists may grow over the next few years as a result of the Joint Commission on Accreditation of Health Care Organizations' (JCAHO) 2005 National Patient Safety Goals and Requirements, which call for complete and accurate medication reconciliation across the continuum of care (JCAHO, 2005).

Efforts to integrate clinical pharmacists into the ED care team have shown some success. For example, one study assessed the impact of having a clinical pharmacist integrated into the care team at a level I trauma center. Responsibilities of this pharmacist included clinical consultations, patient education, order screening, dispensing of drugs, medication preparation, resuscitation response, staff education, patient care, and emergency preparedness. Inclusion of the clinical pharmacist on the care team resulted in improved medical care (reduction in voluntary reporting of medical errors) and the imparting of knowledge to ED personnel. It also reduced institutional expenditures; by encouraging physicians to modify prescribing practices, the pharmacist reduced the ordering of high-cost medications, for an estimated savings of $100,000 over 1 year (Fairbanks et al., 2004).

Another study compared the effectiveness of having a pharmacist collect patients' medication histories with that of the institution's standard approach of a nurse-obtained medication history. Results showed that when the pharmacist obtained the history, more discrepancies between patients' reported home medications and initial hospital orders were identified, and a higher percentage of patients received clinical interventions. Having pharmacists take medical histories was also more time-efficient (Nester and Hale, 2002). At another hospital, ED cost savings were realized when pharmacists performed clinical interventions, such as medication selection and dosing changes. Cost savings were also realized by reducing the ED satellite inventory; pharmacists noted that duplicate medications in the same drug class were unwarranted for a single- or double-dose regimen (Levy, 1993).

Some pediatric facilities (typically children's hospitals and general hospitals with advanced pediatric capabilities) also employ suture technicians to assist with pediatric wound repair (Apolo and DiCocco, 1988). These technicians, often EMTs or nurses, receive training with general, reconstructive, and plastic surgeons on wound repair and use a variety of techniques to reduce pain and anxiety in children needing suturing. Because these technicians provide a large number of sutures (one hospital estimated that suture technicians provided 450–700 sutures per month), they are able to attain a high skill level in suturing. Additionally, the use of suture technicians helps free up the time of ED physicians so they can provide care to other patients (Akron Children's Hospital, 2005).

Skill Retention and Performance

As with EMTs, skill retention for ED providers can be a problem. Only about 10 percent of pediatric patients in the ED are classified as "emergent," meaning that care must be provided within 15 minutes (McCaig and Burt, 2005). Therefore, only a small percentage of ED visits are critical pediatric cases. As a result, deterioration of skills can be a problem. Many ED providers have infrequent contact with and rarely perform life support interventions for children. Research confirms this concern; 1 year after CPR training, for example, physician and nurse retention of CPR skills deteriorates and can even fall to pretraining levels (Gass and Curry, 1983; Mancini and Kaye, 1985).

It is difficult to say precisely how well ED providers deliver care to pediatric patients in the absence of reliable data. The limited information available on physician performance tends to focus on intubation of pediatric patients in the ED. Some findings indicate that EM and pediatric emergency medicine fellows are generally successful in performing pharmacologically assisted intubation, an airway intervention that is frequently used in the ED (Tayal et al., 1999; Sagarin et al., 2002). However, success rates for

ORDER CARD
(Customers in North America Only)

Emergency Care for Children:
Growing Pains

Use this card to order additional copies of **Emergency Care for Children**. All orders must be prepaid. Prices apply only in the United States, Canada, and Mexico and are subject to change without notice. For shipping in the U.S., please add $4.50 for shipping and handling for the first copy ordered and $0.95 for each additional copy. For Canada, please add $7.00/$0.95. For Mexico, $10.50/$2.00. If you live in CA, CT, DC, FL, MD, NY, TX, VA, WI, or Canada, add applicable sales tax or GST.

PLEASE SEND ME:

Qty.	Title	Price
	Emergency Care for Children (10171)	$43.95
	Subtotal	
	Shipping	
	Tax	
	Total	

___ I am enclosing a U.S. check or money order.

___ Please charge my VISA/MasterCard/American Express account.

Number: _____

Expiration date: _____

Signature: _____

Please print.

Name _____

Address _____

City _____ State _____ Zip Code _____ BLWC

FOUR EASY WAYS TO ORDER

- **Electronically:** Order from our secure website at: www.nap.edu
- **By phone:** Call toll-free 1-888-624-8422 or (202) 334-3313 or call your favorite bookstore.
- **By fax:** Copy the order card and fax to (202) 334-2451.
- **By mail:** Return this card with your payment to NATIONAL ACADEMIES PRESS, 500 Fifth Street NW, Lockbox 285, Washington, DC 20055.

All international customers please contact National Academies Press for export prices and ordering information.

THE NATIONAL ACADEMIES PRESS

Publisher for The National Academies

National Academy of Sciences ◆ National Academy of Engineering ◆ Institute of Medicine ◆ National Research Council

THE NATIONAL ACADEMIES
Advisers to the Nation on Science, Engineering, and Medicine

Visit our web site at

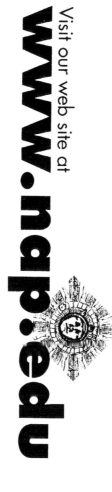

www.nap.edu

Use the form on the reverse of this card to order additional copies, or order online and receive a 10% discount.

neonatal endotracheal intubation were found to be low, despite providers' high levels of confidence in performing the procedure (Falck et al., 2003; Leone et al., 2005). Additionally, a study of pediatric patient encounters during EM residents' pediatric emergency medicine rotation found deficiencies in critical care procedures, resuscitations, child abuse evaluations, and neonatal evaluations (Chen et al., 2004). Again, though, the majority of ED physicians are not EM or pediatric emergency medicine physicians, and it is difficult to assess their performance.

As mentioned in Chapter 2, it is known that the care children receive in the ED can vary considerably. Substantial variations exist among physicians of different specialties in the management of a number of illnesses and injuries, including fever (Isaacman et al., 2001), croup (Hampers and Faries, 2002), splenic injury (Davis et al., 2005), diabetic ketoacidosis (Glaser et al., 1997), bronchiolitis (Mansbach et al., 2005), and febrile seizures (Hampers et al., 2000), as well as in sedation treatment (Babl et al., 2005). These variations may be due to differences in specialty training. In some cases, guidelines are available to help in treatment decisions, but most are not used by the physician (Isaacman et al., 2001; Han et al., 2003; Orr et al., 2006).

SUPPORTING THE WORKFORCE TO IMPROVE PEDIATRIC EMERGENCY CARE

The committee is concerned about the problem of ensuring an adequate supply of highly trained professionals for every category of emergency care provider. In its companion reports on prehospital and ED care, the committee recommends that that the federal government undertake a detailed assessment of the capacity, trends, and future needs of the emergency care workforce, including providers with pediatric expertise. In this report, however, the committee focuses on the need to support providers in their ability to deliver appropriate pediatric emergency care, for which it proposes a three-pronged approach.

Increasing Pediatric Training

There are no national standards for the core competencies of training in pediatric emergency care. Residency programs, medical schools, nursing schools, states, EMS agencies, and hospitals have varying pediatric education and training requirements and opportunities for providers. In some cases, pediatric training is intensive; as discussed above, however, pediatric training often makes up a small portion of total training time.

The committee believes all emergency care providers should possess a certain level of competency to deliver care to children. Research has shown that pediatric training works, at least initially, to improve both the competency and confidence of providers in caring for pediatric patients. Improving the confidence of providers may reduce the reluctance of some to administer treatment to children, thereby eliminating some of the disparities in care between adult and pediatric patients. But continuing education is also essential to maintain these skills and competencies. To increase the pediatric emergency care training that providers receive, the committee recommends that **every pediatric- and emergency care–related health professional credentialing and certification body define pediatric emergency care competencies and require practitioners to receive the level of initial and continuing education necessary to achieve and maintain those competencies (4.1).** The major professional organizations that create and update core content specific to the emergency medicine curriculum (ACEP, Society for Academic Emergency Medicine [SAEM], Council of Emergency Medicine Residency Directors [CORD], ABEM, Emergency Medicine Residents Association [EMRA], and Residency Review Committee for Emergency Medicine [RRC-EM]) should ensure that EM residents receive the training necessary to meet a defined pediatric competency level considering the frequency with which children seek care in EDs. Similar improvements are needed in the EM curriculum for pediatric residents. The ENA should define a pediatric competency level, review the amount of pediatric training nurses currently receive, and address any gaps. States should adopt the national standard curriculum developed by NHTSA, which includes pediatric training and pediatric continuing education components. Residency programs, medical and nursing schools, and states should ensure that individuals with pediatric expertise conduct the pediatric training. Further, states and provider organizations should ensure that all certification examinations are designed to test providers' pediatric competencies. Individuals who answer all pediatric questions incorrectly should not receive certification. All of these organizations should also explore ways to test pediatric competencies at regular intervals.

Despite the strong growth of EM residency programs, a large number of emergency physicians, particularly in rural EDs, have not undergone EM residency training. Many nurses working in EDs, particularly in rural settings, have not sought CEN certification and have not taken the emergency nursing pediatric course. To ensure that these professionals receive proper pediatric emergency medicine education, JCAHO and state licensing bodies should evaluate ED staff's pediatric training for certification; similarly, pediatricians working in the ED should be assessed on their EM training.

Provider organizations, such as hospitals and EMS agencies, must also ensure that their workforce is well prepared to handle pediatric patients. Strategies for continuing education should be developed by provider organizations and should reflect the type of setting in which providers work. For example, the continuing education needed at a dedicated pediatric ED may be very different from that needed at a general ED. Continuing education classes must be conducted regularly, as skill maintenance declines over a relatively short time period. Furthermore, courses should include a major focus on the care of infants and young children, given that they constitute the largest single group making pediatric ED visits and require care that is most different from that of adults.

Continuing education courses are critical for all emergency care providers, particularly those who rarely see children, as well as for hospitals that lack pediatric specialists. Even if critically ill pediatric patients are transported to dedicated pediatric EDs, ED staff at all hospitals need to maintain a basic level of competency to recognize and stabilize those who are critically ill or injured until transport to a higher level of care is available. High-fidelity simulation models, to the extent available, should be used for continuing education to provide as realistic an event as possible.

Developing Clinical Practice Guidelines for Pediatric Emergency Care

Treatment patterns for pediatric patients can vary widely among providers. In some cases, this variation is due to providers' lack of education. Often, however, it is the result of the absence of evidence-based clinical guidelines for pediatric patients.

Clinical practice guidelines assist providers in decision making regarding the appropriate care for specific clinical circumstances, and their use has been shown to improve the quality of care (Grimshaw and Russell, 1993). Ideally, practice guidelines are based on scientific evidence or predictability. The Institute of Medicine's (IOM) Committee on Clinical Practice recommended the implementation of evidence-based clinical practice guidelines because of their potential to improve care. However, only a limited number of nationally recognized pediatric emergency care practice guidelines exist; a 2001 review of the 1,053 practice guidelines in the national Guidelines Clearinghouse found only 15 (Moody-Williams et al., 2002).

The committee believes clinical guidelines should be science-based through use of an evidence evaluation process for several reasons. First, research indicates that clinical guidelines based on research evidence are more likely to be used than those developed in the absence of such evidence (Grol et al., 1998). Moreover, an evidence evaluation process helps ensure that clinical guidelines and standards are based on scientific evidence that is most likely to be correct. Under this process, all research studies in a particular area, for example, asthma care in the ED, are reviewed and ranked according to the validity of study findings. Studies using randomized controlled trials are ranked higher than those based on expert opinion. These rankings are then tied to grades of recommendations. For example, a systematic review documenting homogeneity of results from a large number of high-quality randomized controlled trials yields the least biased estimate of the effect of an intervention; those results are assigned a high recommendation grade and then used in the development of clinical practice guidelines and standards of care. Reviews of studies using less rigorous methods are given a lower recommendation grade and are not used to develop guidelines.

Use of a formal or systematic evidence evaluation process for emergency care research has been limited. In 1998 and again in 2005, however, the Neonatal Resuscitation Program Steering Committee of the AAP and the National Pediatric Resuscitation Subcommittee of the American Heart Association undertook a review of the scientific literature on pediatric resuscitation. They evaluated the quality of the evidence supporting practices employed at the time and changes to those practices. The first evidence evaluation process culminated in the publication of *Guidelines 2000 for Emergency Cardiovascular Care and Resuscitation: International Consensus on Science* (AAP, 2005b). The second set of guidelines was released in January 2006.

In 2001, the Health Resources and Services Administration (HRSA), NHTSA, and The Robert Wood Johnson Foundation convened a panel of experts in managed care, quality improvement, and EMS to review the literature and discuss critical issues related to practice guidelines and performance measurement in pediatric emergency care. The panel recommended the development of pediatric emergency care guidelines and suggested how the guidelines should be developed (e.g., a broad consensus process and a scientific approach), as well as what characteristics the guidelines should have (e.g., they should be flexible and not unduly complex). In 2002, the EMS-C program initiated the Clinical Practice Guidelines for Pediatric Emergency Care demonstration project, which provided funding for two projects to help develop practice guidelines. One project is investigating rehydration of children with moderate dehydration due to acute gastroenteritis; the other is evaluating the use of the National Heart, Lung and Blood Institute's pediatric asthma guideline in five adult EDs and investigating patient outcomes (MCHB, 2004b). The committee believes more such efforts are necessary. The committee therefore recommends that **the Department of Health and Human Services collaborate with professional organizations to convene a panel of individuals with multidisciplinary expertise to develop, evaluate, and update clinical practice guidelines and standards of care for pediatric emergency care (4.2).** A number of agencies within the Department of Health and Human Services (DHHS) could lead this effort, including the Food and Drug Administration (FDA), HRSA, and the Agency for Healthcare Research and Quality (AHRQ). Funding for the effort should be provided by DHHS. It will be up to the specialists from various professional organizations to evaluate the evidence in order to develop, evaluate, and update the clinical practice guidelines and standards for pediatric emergency care. The effort should be multidisciplinary and multiorganizational to promote consensus and uniformity. The more organizations are involved in the development, the more likely it will be that the guidelines will be used in practice in various disciplines.

Unless there is a commitment to funding pediatric emergency medicine research, however, there will not be an adequate evidence base from which to derive practice guidelines. The issue of research and research funding is discussed in depth in Chapter 7.

Providing Pediatric Leadership in EMS Agencies and EDs

Simply recommending more training and the development of guidelines is not enough. Someone must be responsible at the provider level for ensuring that continuing education opportunities are available and well attended. Similarly, the development of clinical guidelines is useless unless their widespread adoption by providers is ensured. To these ends, the committee believes pediatric leadership within each provider organization is needed. Therefore, the committee recommends that **emergency medical services agencies appoint a pediatric emergency coordinator and hospitals appoint two pediatric emergency coordinators—one a physician—to provide pediatric leadership for the organization (4.3).** Hospitals could choose personnel for the two coordinator positions based on available resources; often they will be filled by a physician and a nurse, but other models are possible (e.g., a physician and an EMT-P). The activities of the pediatric coordinators should be a component of medical oversight.

The pediatric coordinator position is not necessarily intended to be full-time, but instead a shared role. Still, the coordinators would have a number of responsibilities that would include ensuring adequate skill and knowledge among fellow ED or EMS providers; overseeing pediatric quality improvement initiatives; ensuring the availability of pediatric medications, equipment, and supplies; ensuring that fellow providers are following clinical practice guidelines; representing the pediatric perspective in the development of hospital or EMS protocols or procedures, for example, for family-centered care; participating in pediatric research efforts; and developing prevention programs for the hospital or EMS agency. The pediatric coordinator would monitor pediatric care issues and present concerns to the organization's leadership when a problem with pediatric care was identified. For example, if medication errors for children in the ED appeared to be rising, the pediatric coordinator should bring this to the attention of hospital administrators. Additionally, pediatric coordinators would liaison in quality improvement efforts and education with community hospitals lacking pediatric resources.

There are two reasons why it is important for hospitals to have two pediatric coordinators. First, as noted, the coordinator positions would not be full-time. However, the committee envisions the coordinator role as encompassing many responsibilities—enough that two coordinators would be necessary. Second, it is important for hospitals to have a physician serve as a pediatric coordinator rather than having the role filled by a lone nurse or EMT. While the nurse–physician relationship has generally evolved over time from an authoritarian to a collaborative one (Pavlovich-Danis et al., 2005), remnants of the old dynamic may prevent some physicians from taking suggestions for improving pediatric care amiably from nurses or EMTs and vice versa. Certainly both coordinators should collaborate on pediatric improvement initiatives within the ED.

The concept of a pediatric coordinator is not new. In fact, since 1983 all Los Angeles hospitals designated as emergency departments approved for pediatrics (EDAPs) have been required to have a pediatric liaison nurse (PdLN) on staff, similar to the pediatric coordinator proposed here. Additionally, the AAP/ACEP 2001 *Guidelines for Preparedness for the Care of Children in the Emergency Department* contain a recommendation regarding the use of a physician coordinator and a nurse coordinator for pediatric care. The guidelines stipulate that the physician coordinator may be a staff physician with other responsibilities in the ED, but should meet the criteria for credentialing as a specialist in emergency care, pediatric emergency medicine, or pediatrics and have a special interest, knowledge, and skill in emergency medical care of children. The guidelines stipulate further that the nurse coordinator should have an interest, knowledge, and skill in emergency care and resuscitation of infants and children as demonstrated by training, clinical experience, or focused continuing nursing education. The position includes such duties as coordinating pediatric quality improvement, serving as a liaison to in-hospital and out-of-hospital pediatric care committees, and facilitating nursing continuing education in pediatrics (AAP, 2001). Pediatric coordinators for EMS agencies appear to be less common, but are necessary to advocate for improved competencies and the availability of resources for pediatric patients. Preferably, prehospital pediatric coordinators would be EMT-Ps with the interest, knowledge, and skills necessary to deliver care to children. EMS pediatric coordinators would have many of the same responsibilities as physician and nurse pediatric coordinators.

One children's hospital currently employs two full-time coordinators who are responsible for both EMS and hospital-based emergency care services. The hospital-based coordinator, an EMT-P, spends the majority of his time coordinating the PALS and other education programs within the hospital. He also leads a task force that examines all resuscitation events and reviews policies and procedures for resuscitation. His duties include making sure that resuscitation equipment is available and that all crash carts are uniform across all hospital floors. The coordinator reports to the administrator of the ED, as well as to the division chief of emergency medicine. The second coordinator focuses primarily on coordinating PALS and other continuing education courses for prehospital providers (Personal communication, D. LaCovey, March 13, 2006).

Approximately 18 percent of hospitals have a pediatric physician coordinator on staff; 12 percent have a nurse coordinator (Gausche-Hill et al., 2004). In Los Angeles, however, the hospitals that are best prepared for pediatric emergencies—those designated as EDAPs—are required to have pediatric coordinator positions. But pediatric coordinators are arguably most important for smaller EDs and EMS agencies that lack strong pediatric expertise; these are the facilities most in need of immediate pediatric leadership. They may not be able to staff the pediatric coordinator position with a physician that is an EM physician or a physician with pediatric expertise; however, the position should be assigned to a physician with the interest and desire to improve pediatric emergency care within the facility.

SUMMARY OF RECOMMENDATIONS

4.1 Every pediatric- and emergency care–related health professional credentialing and certification body should define pediatric emergency care competencies and require practitioners to receive the level of initial and continuing education necessary to achieve and maintain those competencies.

4.2 The Department of Health and Human Services should collaborate with professional organizations to convene a panel of individuals with multidisciplinary expertise to develop, evaluate, and update clinical practice guidelines and standards of care for pediatric emergency care.

4.3 Emergency medical services agencies should appoint a pediatric emergency coordinator, and hospitals should appoint two pediatric emergency coordinators—one a physician—to provide pediatric leadership for the organization.

REFERENCES

AAP (American Academy of Pediatrics). 2000. Access to pediatric emergency medical care. *Pediatrics* 105(3 Pt. 1):647–649.

AAP. 2001. Care of children in the emergency department: Guidelines for preparedness. *Pediatrics* 107(4):777–781.

AAP. 2003. *Council of Medical Specialty Societies: Workforce Questions.* Washington, DC: AAP.

AAP. 2005a. *About PEPP: History of PEPP.* [Online]. Available: http://www.peppsite.com/ about_history.cfm [accessed October 31, 2005].

AAP. 2005b. *Evidence-based Guidelines Process.* [Online]. Available: http://www.aap.org/nrp/ science/science_evidenceguide.html [accessed March 9, 2005].

ABEM (American Board of Emergency Medicine). 2004. *Written Certification Examination Description and Content Specifications.* [Online]. Available: http://www.abem.org/public/ portal/alias_Rainbow/lang_en-US/tabID_3368/DesktopDefault.aspx#one [accessed August 23, 2004].

ABMS (American Board of Medical Specialties). 2002. *Which Medical Specialist Is for You?* Evanston, IL: ABMS.

ABMS. 2003. *ABMS Annual Report and Reference Handbook.* Evanston, IL: ABMS.

ACEP (American College of Emergency Physicians). 2004. *Two-Thirds of Emergency Department Directors Report On-Call Specialty Coverage Problems.* [Online]. Available: http://www.acep.org/1,34081,0.html [accessed September 28, 2004].

ACGME (Accreditation Council for Graduate Medical Education). 2004. *Program Requirements for Residency Education in Pediatric Emergency Medicine.* [Online]. Available: http://www.acgme.org/downloads/RRC_progReq/114pr698.pdf [accessed August 20, 2004].

Aiken LH, Clarke SP, Sloane DM. 2002a. Hospital staffing, organization, and quality of care: Cross-national findings. *International Journal for Quality in Health Care* 14(1):5–13.

Aiken LH, Clarke SP, Sloane DM, Sochalski J, Silber JH. 2002b. Hospital nurse staffing and patient mortality, nurse burnout, and job dissatisfaction. *Journal of the American Medical Association* 288(16):1987–1993.

Akron Children's Hospital. 2005. *Suture Program.* [Online]. Available: http://www. akronchildrens.org/cms/site/d0d9e25d302b66b8/index.html [accessed February 27, 2006].

AMA (American Medical Association). 2003. *Physician Characteristics and Distribution in the U.S.: 2004 Edition.* Chicago, IL: AMA.

The American Board of Surgery. 2004. *Booklet on Certification in Surgical Specialties: Information Regarding Requirements and Examinations 2004–2005.* Philadelphia, PA: The American Board of Surgery.

The American Board of Surgery. 2005. *Booklet of Information 2005.* Philadelphia, PA: The American Board of Surgery.

Apolo JO, DiCocco D. 1988. Suture technicians in a children's hospital emergency department. *Pediatric Emergency Care* 4(1):12–14.

Armon BD, Coren JS. 2005. Basking in the moonlight. *Unique Opportunities.* [Online]. Available: http://www.uoworks.com/articles/legal.moonlighting.html [accessed January 31, 2007].

Babl FE, Vinci RJ, Bauchner H, Mottley L. 2001. Pediatric per-hospital advanced life support care in an urban setting. *Pediatric Emergency Care* 17(1):5–9.

Babl FE, Puspitadewi A, Barnett P, Oakley E, Spicer M. 2005. Preprocedural fasting state and adverse events in children receiving nitrous oxide for procedural sedation and analgesia. *Pediatric Emergency Care* 21(11):736–743.

Boswell W, McElveen N, Sharp M, Boyd CR, Frantz EI. 1995. Analysis of prehospital pediatric and adult intubation. *Air Medical Journal* 14:125–127.

Bureau of Labor Statistics. 2002. *Occupational Outlook Handbook, 2002–2003 Edition: Emergency Medical Technicians and Paramedics.* Washington, DC: U.S. Department of Labor.

Bureau of Labor Statistics, U.S. Department of Labor. 2004. Emergency medical technicians and paramedics. In: *Occupational Outlook Handbook, 2004–2005 Edition.* Washington, DC: U.S. Department of Labor.

Chen EH, Shofer FS, Baren JM. 2004. Emergency medicine resident rotation in pediatric emergency medicine: What kind of experience are we providing? *Academic Emergency Medicine* 11(7):771–773.

Christopher N. 2000. Pediatric emergency medicine education in emergency medicine training programs. *Academic Emergency Medicine* 7(7):797–799.

Cole FL, Ramirez E, Luna-Gonzales H. 1999. *Scope of Practice for the Nurse Practitioner in the Emergency Setting.* Des Plaines, IL: ENA.

The Committee to Develop the Reorganized Specialty of Trauma Surgical Critical Care and Emergency Surgery. 2005. Acute care surgery: Trauma, critical care, and emergency surgery. *The Journal of Trauma* 58(3):614–616.

Davis DH, Localio AR, Stafford PW, Helfaer MA, Durbin DR. 2005. Trends in operative management of pediatric splenic injury in a regional trauma system. *Pediatrics* 115(1):89–94.

DHHS (U.S. Department of Health and Human Services). 2000. *National Sample Survey of Registered Nurses.* Rockville, MD: HRSA, Bureau of Health Professions, National Center for Health Workforce Analysis.

Doran JV, Tortella BJ, Drivet WJ, Lavery RF. 1995. Factors influencing successful intubation in the prehospital setting. *Prehospital Disaster Medicine* 10(4):259–264.

DOT (Department of Transportation). 1998. *EMT-Paramedic: National Standard Curriculum.* Washington, DC: DOT.

EMS Insider. 2005. *EMS Employers Struggle with Paramedic Shortages.* [Online]. Available: http://www.jems.com/insider/4_04.html [accessed April 4, 2005].

ENA (Emergency Nurses Association). 1999. *Scope of Emergency Nursing Practice.* Des Plains, IL: ENA.

ENA. 2003. *Advanced Practice in Emergency Nursing.* Des Plains, IL: ENA.

ENA. 2006. *ENA 2005 National Emergency Department Benchmark Guide.* Des Plaines, IL: ENA.

Fairbanks RJ, Hays DP, Webster DF, Spillane LL. 2004. Clinical pharmacy services in an emergency department. *American Journal of Health-System Pharmacy* 61(9):934–937.

Falck AJ, Escobedo MB, Baillargeon JG, Villard LG, Gunkel JH. 2003. Proficiency of pediatric residents in performing neonatal endotracheal intubation. *Pediatrics* 112(6):1242–1247.

Federiuk CS, O'Brien K, Jui J, Schmidt TA. 1993. Job satisfaction of paramedics: The effects of gender and type of agency of employment. *Annals of Emergency Medicine* 22(4):657–662.

Franks PE, Kocher N, Chapman S. 2004. *Emergency Medical Technicians and Paramedics in University of California.* San Francisco, CA: San Francisco Center for the Health Professions.

GAO (General Accountability Office). 2001. *Emerging Nurse Shortage.* Washington, DC: General Accountability Office.

Gass DA, Curry L. 1983. Physicians' and nurses' retention of knowledge and skill after training in cardiopulmonary resuscitation. *Canadian Medical Association Journal* 128(5):550–551.

Gausche M. 1997. Differences in the out-of-hospital care of children and adults: More questions than answers. *Annals of Emergency Medicine* 29(6):776–779.

Gausche M, Tadeo R, Zane M, Lewis R. 1998. Out-of-hospital intravenous access: Unnecessary procedures and excessive cost. *Academic Emergency Medicine* 5(9):878–882.

Gausche-Hill M. 2000. Pediatric continuing education for out-of-hospital providers: Is it time to mandate review of pediatric knowledge and skills? *Annals of Emergency Medicine* 36(1):72–74.

Gausche-Hill M, Lewis R, Schmitz C. 2004. *Survey of US Emergency Departments for Pediatric Preparedness: Implementation and Evaluation of Care of Children in the Emergency Department: Guidelines for Preparedness.* Unpublished results.

Gerson J, Oliver T. 1995. *Addressing the Nursing Shortage.* Washington, DC: Kaiser Family Foundation.

Glabman M. 2005. Specialist shortage shakes emergency rooms; more hospitals forced to pay for specialist care. *The Physician Executive* 6–11.

Glaeser P, Linzer J, Tunik M, Henderson D, Ball J. 2000. Survey of nationally registered emergency medical services providers: Pediatric education. *Annals of Emergency Medicine* 36(1):33–38.

Glaser NS, Kuppermann N, Yee CK, Schwartz DL, Styne DM. 1997. Variation in the management of pediatric diabetic ketoacidosis by specialty training. *Archives of Pediatrics & Adolescent Medicine* 151(11):1125–1132.

Graham CJ, Stuemky J, Lera TA. 1993. Emergency medical services preparedness for pediatric emergencies. *Pediatric Emergency Care* 9(6):329–331.

Greater New York Hospital Association. 2004. *Survey of Nurse Staffing in GNYHA Member Hospitals, 2003.* [Online]. Available: http://www.gnyha.org/pubinfo/2005_Nurse_Staffing_Survey.pdf [accessed May 2006].

Green L, Melnick GA, Nawathe A. 2005. *On-Call Physicians at California Emergency Departments: Problems and Potential Solutions.* Oakland, CA: California Healthcare Foundation.

Grimshaw JM, Russell IT. 1993. Effect of clinical guidelines on medical practice: A systematic review of rigorous evaluations. *Lancet* 342(8883):1317–1322.

Grol R, Dalhuijsen J, Thomas S, Veld C, Rutten G, Mokkink H. 1998. Attributes of clinical guidelines that influence use of guidelines in general practice: Observational study. *British Medical Journal* 317(7162):858–861.

Hall WL II, Myers JH, Pepe PE, Larkin GL, Sirbaugh PE, Persse DE. 2004. The perspective of paramedics about on-scene termination of resuscitation efforts for pediatric patients. *Resuscitation* 60(2):175–187.

Hampers LC, Faries SG. 2002. Practice variation in the emergency management of croup. *Pediatrics* 109(3):505–508.

Hampers LC, Trainor JL, Listernick R, Eddy JJ, Thompson DA, Sloan EP, Chrisler OP, Gatewood LM, McNulty B, Krug SE. 2000. Setting-based practice variation in the management of simple febrile seizure. *Academic Emergency Medicine* 7(1):21–27.

Han YY, Carcillo JA, Dragotta MA, Bills DM, Watson RS, Westerman ME, Orr RA. 2003. Early reversal of pediatric-neonatal septic shock by community physicians is associated with improved outcome. *Pediatrics* 112(4):793–799.

Health Resources and Services Administration Council on Graduate Medical Education. 2002. *2002 Summary Report.* Rockville, MD: Health Resources and Services Administration.

Henderson DP. 1998. Education of paramedics in pediatric airway management effects of different retaining methods on self-efficacy and skill retention. *Academic Emergency Medicine* 5(5):429.

Holliman CJ, Wuerz RC, Chapman DM, Hirshberg AJ. 1997. Workforce projections for emergency medicine: How many emergency physicians does the United States need? *Academic Emergency Medicine* 4(7):725–730.

Isaacman DJ, Kaminer K, Veligeti H, Jones M, Davis P, Mason JD. 2001. Comparative practice patterns of emergency medicine physicians and pediatric emergency medicine physicians managing fever in young children. *Pediatrics* 108(2):354–358.

JCAHO (Joint Council on Accreditation of Healthcare Organizations). 2005. *2005 Hospitals' National Patient Safety Goals.* [Online]. Available: http://www.jcaho.org/accredited+organizations/patient+safety/05+npsg/05_npsg_hap.htm [accessed August 9, 2005].

Kaji A, Stevens C. 2002. Moonlighting and the emergency medicine resident. *Annals of Emergency Medicine* 40(1):63–66.

Leone TA, Rich W, Finer NN. 2005. Neonatal intubation: Success of pediatric trainees. *The Journal of Pediatrics* 146(5):638–641.

Levy DB. 1993. Documentation of clinical and cost-saving pharmacy interventions in the emergency room. *Hospital Pharmacy* 28(7):624–627, 630–634.

Lillis KA, Jaffe DM. 1992. Prehospital intravenous access in children. *Annals of Emergency Medicine* 21(12):1430–1434.

Ludwig S, Fleisher G, Henretig F, Ruddy R. 1982. Pediatric training in emergency medicine residency programs. *Annals of Emergency Medicine* 11(4):170–173.

Macasaet A, Zun A. 2005. The on-call physician. *Emedicine.Com.* [Online.] Available: http://www.emedicine.com/emerg/topic878.htm [accessed January 31, 2007].

Mancini ME, Kaye W. 1985. The effect of time since training on house officers' retention of cardiopulmonary resuscitation skills. *American Journal of Emergency Medicine* 3(1):31–32.

Mansbach JM, Emond JA, Camargo CA Jr. 2005. Bronchiolitis in U.S. emergency departments 1992 to 2000: Epidemiology and practice variation. *Pediatric Emergency Care* 21(4):242–247.

McCaig LF, Burt CW. 2005. *National Hospital Ambulatory Medical Care Survey: 2003 Emergency Department Summary.* Hyattsville, MD: National Center for Health Statistics.

MCHB (Maternal and Child Health Bureau). 1996. *Emergency Medical Services for Children, Annual Report, FY 1996.* Rockville, MD: MCHB.

MCHB. 2003. *Emergency Medical Services for Children, Annual Report, FY 2003.* Rockville, MD: MCHB.

MCHB. 2004a. *Emergency Medical Services for Children. Five Year Plan 2001–2005: Midcourse Review.* Washington, DC: EMS-C National Resource Center.

MCHB. 2004b. *Emergency Medical Services for Children FY 2003 Highlights.* [Online]. Available: http://www.mchb.hrsa.gov/programs/emsc/highlights03.htm [accessed December 3, 2005].

Middleton KR, Burt CW. 2006. *Availability of Pediatric Services and Equipment in Emergency Departments: United States, 2002–03.* Hyattsville, MD: National Center for Health Statistics.

Mishark KJ, Vukov LF, Gudgell SF. 1992. Airway management and air medical transport. *Journal of Air Medical Transport* 11(3):7–9.

Moody-Williams JD, Krug S, O'Connor R, Shook JE, Athey JL, Holleran RS. 2002. Practice guidelines and performance measures in emergency medical services for children. *Annals of Emergency Medicine* 39(4):404–412.

Moorhead JC, Gallery ME, Hirshkorn C, Barnaby DP, Barsan WG, Conrad LC, Dalsey WC, Fried M, Herman SH, Hogan P, Mannle TE, Packard DC, Perina DG, Pollack CV Jr, Rapp MT, Rorrie CC Jr, Schafermeyer RW. 2002. A study of the workforce in emergency medicine: 1999. *Annals of Emergency Medicine* 40(1):3–15.

Murdock TC, Knapp JF, Dowd MD, and Campbell JP. 1999. Bridging the emergency medical services for children information gap. *Archives of Pediatric Adolescent Medicine* 153(3):281–285.

NAEMT (National Association of Emergency Medical Technicians). 2005. *About PPC.* [Online]. Available: http://www.naemt.org/PPC/aboutPPC/ [accessed November 4, 2005].

National Capital Consortium Pediatrics Residency. 2004. *Pediatric Program Requirements: Residency Review Committee.* [Online]. Available: http://www.nccpeds.com/Chief%20Files/RRC%20Requirements.doc [accessed January 11, 2006].

NHTSA (National Highway Traffic Safety Administration). 2006. *National Standard Curricula.* [Online]. Available: http://www.nhtsa.dot.gov/people/injury/ems/nsc.htm [accessed January 25, 2006].

NHTSA, MCHB (National Highway Traffic Safety Administration, Maternal and Child Health Bureau). 1995. *First Responder: National Standard Curriculum.* Washington, DC: DOT, DHHS.

Needleman J, Buerhaus P, Mattke S, Stewart M, Zelevinsky K. 2002. Nurse-staffing levels and the quality of care in hospitals. *New England Journal of Medicine* 346(22):1715–1722.

Nester TM, Hale LS. 2002. Effectiveness of a pharmacist-acquired medication history in promoting patient safety. *American Journal of Health-System Pharmacy* 59(22):2221.

New York State Education Department. 2003. *Registered Nurses in New York State, 2002, Survey Data.* Albany, NY: USNY State Education Department.

NREMT (National Registry of Emergency Medical Technicians). 2003. *Longitudinal Emergency Medical Technician Attributes and Demographics Survey (LEADS) Data.* [Online]. Available: http://www.nremt.org/about/lead_survey.asp [accessed February 24, 2006].

O'Leary K. 2002. The shortage of pediatric subspecialists. *Children's Hospitals Today.* Winter 2002. [Online]. Available: http://www.childrenshospitals.net/AM/Template.cfm?Section=Home&CONTENTID=10936&TEMPLATE=/CM/ContentDisplay.cfm [accessed January 31, 2007].

O'Malley AS, Gerland AM, Pham HH, Berenson RA. 2005. *Rising Pressure: Hospital Emergency Departments: Barometers of the Health Care System.* Washington, DC: The Center for Studying Health System Change.

Orr RA, Han YY, Roth K. 2006. Pediatric transport: Shifting the paradigm to improve patient outcome. In: Fuhrman B, Zimmerman J, eds. *Pediatric Critical Care* (3rd edition). Mosby, Elsevier Science Health. Pp. 141–150.

Pavlovich-Danis S, Forman H, Simek PP. 2005. The nurse-physician relationship: Can it be saved? *Nursing Spectrum* 8(5):14–15.

PEPP Program. 2006. What's new with PEPP 2? *PEPP Talk.* [Online]. Available: http://www.peppsite.com/newsletter/n_06_January_2006.htm [accessed January 31, 2007].

Ramenofsky ML, Luterman A, Quindlen E, Riddick L, Curreri PW. 1984. Maximum survival in pediatric trauma: The ideal system. *The Journal of Trauma* 24(9):818–823.

Sagarin MJ, Chiang V, Sakles JC, Barton ED, Wolfe RE, Vissers RJ, Walls RM. 2002. Rapid sequence intubation for pediatric emergency airway management. *Pediatric Emergency Care* 18(6):417–423.

Salsberg E. 2005. *Physician Workforce Issues and Trends: Implications for Surgical Specialties.* Presentation at the ACS Meeting on Workforce Issues, Chicago, IL.

Santamaria JP, Abrunzo TJ, Murray R. 1997. *Assessment of the Current Status of Continuing Education Training in Pediatric Emergency Care in Emergency Medicine.* Washington, DC: ACEP.

Schriver J, Talmadge R, Chuong R, Hedges J. 2003. Emergency nursing: Historical, current, and future roles. *Academic Emergency Medicine* 10(7):798–804.

Scribano PV, Baker MD, Holmes J, Shaw KN. 2000. Use of out-of-hospital interventions for the pediatric patient in an urban emergency medical services system. *Academic Emergency Medicine* 7(7):745–750.

Seidel JS. 1986. Emergency medical services and the pediatric patient: Are the needs being met? II. Training and equipping emergency medical services providers for pediatric emergencies. *Pediatrics* 78(5):808.

Seidel JS, Hornbein M, Yoshiyama K, Kuznets D, Finklestein JZ, St Geme JW Jr. 1984. Emergency medical services and the pediatric patient: Are the needs being met? *Pediatrics* 73(6):769–772.

Seidel JS, Henderson DP, Ward P, Wayland BW, Ness B. 1991. Pediatric prehospital care in urban and rural areas. *Pediatrics* 88(4):681.

State of California Employment Development Department Labor Market Information Division. 1995. *California Occupational Guide Number 550 (Interest Area 13).* [Online]. Available: http://www.calmis.ca.gov/file/occguide/PARAMED.HTM [accessed April 2005].

Steiger B. 2005. ACEP poll: Physician leaders distressed by specialist shortage; on call pay controversial. *The Physician Executive* 31(3):14–18.

Su E, Mann NC, McCall M, Hedges JR. 1997. Use of resuscitation skills by paramedics caring for critically injured children in Oregon. *Prehospital Emergency Care* 1(3):123–127.

Su E, Schmidt TA, Mann NC, Zechnich AD. 2000. A randomized controlled trial to assess decay in acquired knowledge among paramedics completing a pediatric resuscitation course. *Academic Emergency Medicine* 7(7):779–786.

Taheri PA, Butz DA. 2004. *Specialist On-Call Coverage of Palm Beach County Emergency Departments.* MD Content Report Commissioned by the Palm Beach County Medical Society Services, December 13, 2004.

Tamariz VP, Fuchs S, Baren JM, Pollack ES, Kim J, Seidel JS. 2000. Pediatric emergency medicine education in emergency medicine training programs. SAEM Pediatric Education Training Task Force. Society for Academic Emergency Medicine. *Academic Emergency Medicine* 7(7):774–778.

Tayal VS, Riggs RW, Marx JA, Tomaszewski CA, Schneider RE. 1999. Rapid-sequence intubation at an emergency medicine residency: Success rate and adverse events during a two-year period. *Academic Emergency Medicine* 6(1):31–37.

Thomasset KB, Faris R. 2003. Survey of pharmacy services provision in the emergency department. *American Journal of Health-System Pharmacy* 60(15):1561–1564.

Vanlandingham BD, Powe NR, Diener-West M, Marone B, Rubin H. 2005. *Patient Insurance Status and Specialist On-Call Coverage in U.S. Hospital Emergency Departments: A National Study.* Presentation at the Academy Health Conference, Boston, MA.

Wilber DQ. 2005, May 7. D.C. paramedic shortage causes concern. *The Washington Post.* P. B03.

Wolfram RW, Warren CM, Doyle CR, Kerns R, Frye S. 2003. Retention of pediatric advanced life support (PALS) course concepts. *Journal of Emergency Medicine* 25(4):475–479.

Wood D, Kalinowski EJ, Miller DR. 2004. Pediatric continuing education for EMTs: Recommendations for content, method, and frequency. The National Council of State Emergency Medical Services Training Coordinators. *Pediatric Emergency Care* 20(4):269–272.

Zaritsky A, French JP, Schafermeyer R, Morton D. 1994. A statewide evaluation of pediatric prehospital and hospital emergency services. *Archives of Pediatrics & Adolescent Medicine* 148(1):76–81.

5

Improving the Quality of Pediatric Emergency Care

Providing high-quality emergency care services to children requires an infrastructure designed to support care for pediatric patients. In Chapter 2 the committee discussed how many provider organizations, both emergency medical services (EMS) agencies and hospitals, lack recommended pediatric equipment and supplies for children. Addressing these basic deficiencies is an important first step. As technology improves and knowledge of quality in health care expands, however, expectations for provider preparedness extend well beyond simply having the right-sized equipment and appropriately labeled medications. We expect provider organizations to have safeguards in place to protect pediatric patients from the hazards of EMS and emergency department (ED) environments. We expect that advances in technology and information systems adopted by provider organizations will be appropriate for children as well as adults. And we expect care to be provided in a way that is evidence based, protocol driven, and respectful to children and their parents or guardians.

This chapter begins with an overview of the threats to patient safety in the EMS and ED environments and the implications for care, with a focus on pediatric patients. The committee believes emergency care provider organizations—both EMS agencies and hospitals—must take active steps to address these threats to reduce the burden of illness and injury to all patients, including children. To this end, the chapter presents the committee's recommendations for improving the safety of emergency care for pediatric patients. Finally, the chapter addresses the important topic of how to make emergency care for children more family-centered.

PATIENT SAFETY IN THE EMERGENCY CARE SETTING

Challenges of the Emergency Care Environment

Emergency care services are delivered in an environment where the need for haste, the distraction of frequent interruptions, and clinical uncertainty abound, thus potentially exposing patients to a number of threats to safety. Children are, of course, at particular risk under these circumstances because of their physical and developmental vulnerabilities and their inability to describe their symptoms and past medical history accurately, and because they may require care from providers who are not accustomed to treating pediatric patients (see Chapter 4).

EDs are high-risk environments for medical care for patients of all ages. The nature of their mission and the multiple challenges they confront increase the risk of medical errors and adverse events (Leape et al., 1991; IOM, 2000; Vinen, 2000; Weingart et al., 2000). In their study of admissions to hospitals in Colorado and Utah, Thomas and colleagues (2000) found the ED to be the hospital department with the highest proportion of negligent adverse events (52.6 percent). An earlier study by Trautlein and colleagues (1984) found that 15 to 20 percent of hospital malpractice claims were a result of errors in the ED, most of which involved serious injury or death (Trautlein et al., 1984).

There are several reasons why the ED is an area of high risk for errors. First, many EDs face excessive crowding, resulting in a noisy, even chaotic environment with frequent workflow interruptions. The large volume of patients results in many being evaluated, treated, and housed in the ED hallways, creating situations fraught with opportunities for error (Cosby, 2003; Selbst et al., 2004; Weiss et al., 2004). Moreover, ED patients do not arrive on a scheduled basis. Therefore, ED volumes can fluctuate a great deal, which makes it difficult to make staffing adjustments to meet sudden shifts in demand (Chamberlain et al., 2004).

Second, ED personnel often work under a great deal of stress. They are required to see a broad case mix of patients and make rapid clinical decisions with little time and often without sufficient patient information (Selbst et al., 2004). Most physicians manage one patient at a time (in the operating room, clinic, diagnostic suite, or outpatient surgical center); emergency physicians, by contrast, are often responsible for the simultaneous management of 10 to 20 patients or more with a variety of problems and different levels of acuity. This is such an intrinsic part of emergency medical practice that the oral board exam administered by the American Board of Emergency Medicine (ABEM) requires examinees to properly handle three hypothetical cases simultaneously. No other specialty incorporates multiple patient encounters in its board certification examination process.

In addition to caring for multiple patients, emergency care providers often face competing demands on their time; along with examining patients and providing treatment, they may have to handle EMS calls, help manage patient flow, listen to patients' and family members' complaints about waiting times and delays in care, track down missing laboratory or radiology results, and the like. ED physicians are frequently interrupted while working. In many cases, these interruptions result in a break in the physician's focus on his or her primary task (Chisholm et al., 2001).

In contrast to outpatient clinics and doctors' offices, EDs operate 24 hours a day. The social and circadian stresses involved in consistently staffing the ED on a round-the-clock basis make ED physicians, nurses, and support staff particularly subject to fatigue, further increasing opportunities for mental errors (Vinen, 2000; Weinger and Ancoli-Israel, 2002; Chamberlain et al., 2004; Selbst et al., 2004). A study of the effect of sleep deprivation on experienced emergency physicians revealed that physicians working night shifts demonstrated a decrease in the speed of intubation and subjective alertness as compared with their day-shift work (Smith-Coggins et al., 1997).

Patient hand-offs from one provider to another midtreatment can result in loss or distortion of important clinical information, thus providing increased opportunities for errors (Croskerry, 2000; Stiell et al., 2003; Chamberlain et al., 2004; Selbst et al., 2004). Physicians, nurses, and other clinicians working on the same shift often fail to communicate effectively, further increasing chances for errors to occur (Risser et al., 1999; Croskerry, 2000; Cosby, 2003; Selbst et al., 2004; White et al., 2004). In fact, poor communication and teamwork failures are a significant problem in the ED. White and colleagues (2004) noted that communication issues were associated with 30 percent of the ED risk management files they studied, and appeared to contribute directly to adverse medical outcomes in 20 percent of those cases. In addition, a 1999 study of the contribution of teamwork failures to clinical errors found that 8 of 12 deaths reviewed could have been prevented if appropriate teamwork action had been taken (Risser et al., 1999). The study authors noted that the most frequently cited primary contributor to clinical error in the ED (35 percent) was the failure to cross-monitor the actions of team members.

Another problem faced by clinicians in the ED is lack of access to complete and accurate medical histories for the patients they are treating (Schenkel, 2000; Cosby, 2003; Chamberlain et al., 2004; Selbst et al., 2004; White et al., 2004). In most cases, ED physicians lack access to a patient's medical record or even to records of previous visits to that or other area EDs. This problem can be compounded by poor information flow from patient to provider due to the patient's age, mental health status, use of debilitating drugs or alcohol, language, culture, or apprehension and anxiety about the need for emergency care.

Less research has been conducted on threats to patient safety in the EMS environment (O'Connor et al., 2002), although that environment is similar to the ED in many ways (Fairbanks, 2004): the fast-paced nature of the work, the stressful environment for providers, and the shift work and round-the-clock coverage that contribute to provider fatigue. EMTs also lack complete and/or accurate medical histories of patients. However, EMS personnel must also contend with a different set of challenges. They often have to provide patient care in unusual locations, such as on the side of a road or highway or close to a crash scene. EMS personnel also have fewer options for backup. Many EDs have physicians to make diagnosis and develop treatment plans, nurses to start intravenous (IV) treatment and administer medications, technicians to take patients' blood pressure and pulse, social workers to talk with families, a secretary to complete billing information, and specialists that can be called in to assist with complex interventions. EMTs and paramedics in the field, by contrast, have no backup, other than perhaps the muscle and moral support of first-responding firefighters or other rescue personnel. Sometimes EMTs perform all of these tasks alone as a first responder or in the back of an ambulance. Thus the EMS environment lacks even the meager redundancies and system protections found in the ED that occur with a team approach to patient care. Additionally, much of the equipment used by EMTs was designed for in-hospital use and has not been well adapted for the EMS environment (Fairbanks, 2004).

Additional Challenges for Pediatric Emergency Care

Most of the above challenges contribute to a potentially unsafe emergency care environment for all patients, not just children. However, other factors complicate care for children more than that for adults. First, some children are preverbal and cannot self-report their symptoms. Many have multiple caregivers, which increases the likelihood that providers will be given an incomplete or inaccurate medical and medication history. Also, children are likely to be accompanied by parents or guardians suffering from great anxiety, which requires staff to attend to them while also staying focused on the patient (Chamberlain et al., 2004). Young children, particularly those who are frightened or in pain, are unable to cooperate with the examiner or understand the process of care, and may actively resist the performance of painful or uncomfortable procedures. As a result, pediatric providers must use a variety of tactics, including use of short-acting sedatives and other hazardous drugs, to complete treatment successfully.

Timeliness represents another important challenge for pediatric patients in the emergency care setting. The emergency care system must be organized to eliminate unnecessary delays in triage and treatment. Because of their unique anatomical and physiological differences, children can get into trouble physiologically much more rapidly than adults. If children do not receive effective emergency care in a timely manner, certain illnesses and injuries can lead to serious consequences, even death, relatively quickly. For example, an infant or young child's thermoregulatory system is less capable of cooling the body; body temperature can rise 3 to 5 times faster than occurs with adults, making infants and young children more susceptible to heat stroke (Null, 2006). An infant left in an enclosed automobile in hot weather, for example, will become hyperthermic very quickly. If not quickly diagnosed, hyperthermia in infants and young children leads to problems with resuscitation (ACEP and AAP, 2006). Hypothermia also occurs very quickly in children because they have thin skin, less insulating body fat, and a high ratio of body surface area to mass.

Meningococcemia, or blood stream infection, is a potentially life-threatening illness that occurs abruptly and progresses rapidly. Cases are rare, but occur most often in children younger than age 5 (Kapes, 2005). Meningococcemia can lead to death more quickly than any other infectious disease, so early recognition is critical to providing prompt therapy and supportive care. Treatment must begin quickly because irreversible shock and death may occur within hours of the onset of symptoms of the disease (Tanzi and Silverberg, 2005). However, symptoms (fever, chills, sore throat) often resemble those of other conditions. Approximately 20 percent of children who develop meningococcemia do not survive (Children's Hospital Boston, 2005b).

Another example is shock. Pediatric practitioners treating acutely ill children, from neonates to young adults, are faced with multiple causes of shock (e.g., trauma, infection, anaphylaxis). Hypovolemic shock results from a deficiency of blood volume and is a leading cause of pediatric mortality in the United States. Whereas an adult can lose 500 cubic centimeters (cc) of blood without much effect, losing only half this amount of blood will result in death in infants. Delay in recognizing and quickly treating a state of shock can lead to widespread multiple system organ failure and death in pediatric patients (Schwarz, 2006). In a study of nearly 100 patients over a 10-year period, researchers were able to determine that when community hospitals, primary care physicians, and families recognized and treated children for shock before bringing them to the hospital, the mortality rate decreased dramatically. However, shock tends to be underrecognized and undertreated by emergency providers (Han et al., 2003).

Children are also more susceptible to smoke inhalation and carbon monoxide toxicity than adults because of their higher metabolic rates and smaller volume of distribution for the carbon monoxide they ingest (ACEP and AAP, 2006). They experience symptoms more quickly then adults, but carbon monoxide poisoning is often treated improperly in children because its symptoms are similar to those associated with the flu (without the fever) and food poisoning (Children's Hospital Boston, 2005a). A child's continued exposure to carbon monoxide can lead to neurological disorders, cardiac arrest, and death.

As another example, vomiting is rather common in children. Vomiting may be caused by gastroenteritis, which is generally less serious, or by many life-threatening conditions, such as meningitis, encephalitis, intussusception, or other conditions that can result in significant morbidity or mortality if not evaluated and managed quickly (D'Agostino, 2002; Fleisher et al., 2006).

Although these are but a few of the pediatric conditions that require prompt identification and treatment, one thing common to many of these examples is that diagnosis may be delayed if symptoms resemble those of other, more common problems. Because children can maintain normal physiology using compensatory mechanisms until they can no longer compensate, at which time they deteriorate quickly, they are particularly vulnerable if treatment is not started promptly. For example, infants and children may have normal blood pressure and be in compensated shock. Their bodies compensate by increasing the heart rate and clamping down on extremity arteries to shunt blood to central circulation. Therefore, subtle signs, such as an increase in heart rate and cool extremities, must be recognized promptly.

However, parents, guardians, and primary care physicians may not recognize the need for immediate emergency care for pediatric patients, and emergency care providers may not be able to determine the severity of illness or injury quickly. In fact, at least one study has shown that the level of agreement in triage assignment for pediatric patients in the ED is not high, and varies based on the level of pediatric training (Maldonado and Avner, 2004).

Another pediatric concern related to timeliness has to do with the often long wait times associated with ED visits. As discussed in Chapter 2, ED crowding has become a daily occurrence in many hospitals. National Hospital Ambulatory Medical Care Survey (NHAMCS) data indicate that in 2003, the average waiting time for all patients (children and adults) to see a physician in the ED was 46 minutes (McCaig and Burt, 2005). Data for 2000 demonstrate the differences in wait time according to patient acuity. On average, patients waited 24 minutes for a visit classified as "emergent," 38 minutes for an "urgent" visit, 56 minutes for a "semiurgent" visit, and 67 minutes for a "nonurgent" visit (McCaig and Ly, 2002). Prolonged wait times may result in protracted pain for all patients (Derlet and Richards, 2000; Derlet et al., 2001), but for pediatric patients there is another concern. In busy EDs that serve both adults and children, children may be exposed to inappropriate and frightening scenes, such as violence, severe injury, and threatening language. Adult EDs are generally not well suited to providing a comforting or reassuring environment for children.

Evidence of Compromised Safety for Pediatric Patients

Given this potentially perilous emergency care environment, how often do medical errors occur among pediatric patients? Surprisingly, the answer to that question is unknown. In fact, there is little high-quality data on the epidemiology of medical errors in children, particularly within the emergency care system. Instead, there are a few, typically small studies demonstrating that care is compromised during several different stages of an ED visit. For example, providers often triage patients inaccurately (Selbst et al., 2004). Errors in specimen collection methods (Walsh-Kelly et al., 1997) and interpretation of radiographs are also a concern (Walsh-Kelly et al., 1995). As might be expected, children with special medical needs or those who are dependent on technology are significantly more likely to experience a medical error than other children (Slonim et al., 2003).

One of the most telling studies on the quality of pediatric care comes from a recent drill conducted in 35 EDs (including 5 trauma centers) in North Carolina. Using life-size child manakins, researchers staged "mock codes" and presented each team with a vignette describing patients' symptoms. Nearly all of the EDs failed to stabilize seriously injured children properly during trauma simulations. Thirty-four hospitals failed to administer dextrose properly to a child in hypoglycemic shock (a life-threatening drop in blood sugar); 34 failed to warm a hypothermic child correctly; 31 failed to order proper administration of IV fluids; 24 failed to attempt or succeed at accessing a child's bloodstream through a bone (a critical alternative for delivering fluids and medicines rapidly to sick children); and 23 failed to provide appropriate medications, monitoring equipment, and personnel needed to transport a child safely within the hospital. On the other hand, many hospitals were successful at calling appropriate individuals for assistance, performing initial airway assessment and initial bag-mask ventilation, ordering appropriate imaging tests, and conducting initial assessment of vital signs (Hunt et al., 2006).

There have been few published studies describing the nature or extent of medical errors in the EMS environment. In one research effort, however, 15 paramedics were interviewed about adverse events and near misses; all had multiple events to report. In sum, 61 events were described, 23 percent of which involved a child. The major types of errors were mistakes in clinical judgment (54 percent), errors in skill performance (21 percent), and medication errors (15 percent). Only one-third of the errors had been reported to anyone (Fairbanks and Crittenden, 2006). In another small study, which tested the ability of 14 paramedics to use a manual defibrillator, several paramedics defibrillated when they intended to cardiovert. This is a potentially fatal error, and in some cases, participants were not aware they had made the mistake. The researchers attributed the error to the defibrillators' poor interface design (Fairbanks, 2004; Fairbanks et al., 2004).

However, the best evidence of medical errors and compromised safety concerns medication errors and adverse drug events in children. Prescribing errors occur more frequently in the ED than in any other part of the hospital and more frequently in the care of children than in that of adults. Medication errors were the most commonly reported type of error at one pediatric ED (Selbst et al., 1999). In a retrospective study of more than 1,500 charts of children treated in a pediatric ED, prescribing errors were identified in 10 percent of the charts (Kozer et al., 2002). These errors occurred more frequently during overnight hours (8:00 PM to 4:00 AM) and on weekends and were made most often by trainees. Another study evaluated medication errors with respect to antipyretics and found that 22 percent of acetaminophen doses ordered were outside the recommended 10–15 mg/kg/dose (Losek, 2004). Another study of medication errors among acutely ill and injured children presenting to rural EDs revealed errors in 48 percent of patient charts (Marcin et al., 2005). More seriously ill children are more likely to experience a prescribing error than those with less serious illnesses or injuries (Kozer et al., 2002).

Not surprisingly, the limited evidence available also indicates that medication errors occur frequently in the EMS environment. In a study that assessed the medication calculation skills of 109 paramedics, overall performance was found to be poor. On average, the paramedics answered 51 percent of the test questions correctly. Medication infusions were calculated incorrectly in one-third of cases (Hubble and Paschal, 2000; Fairbanks, 2004).

Challenges Associated with Prescribing and Administering Medications to Children in an Emergency Setting

Perhaps the foremost problem associated with providing medications to children is that many medications are frequently prescribed for children "off label," meaning they have not been approved for pediatric use by the Food and Drug Administration (FDA). Once a drug has been approved for use by the FDA, further studies to determine its safety and efficacy in infants and children are rarely conducted for the majority of drugs (Rapkin, 1999). The result is that emergency providers must prescribe medications to children without a full understanding of the risks, benefits, or implications.

One example is the use of medications to treat depression in children. Data indicate that psychiatric emergencies are on the rise for children and adolescents, yet there is only one medication, fluoxetine, approved for pediatric use. Still, others are frequently prescribed. The dosages, efficacy, and safety of these medications have not been well established for pediatric patients. Although there is some evidence that one of those drugs, paroxetine, may lead to an increased risk of suicide, the research is thin, and it is unclear why there is a greater risk associated with this and other drugs in comparison with fluoxetine.

Medications designed for adults may not be suitable for children because of differences in pharmacokinetics (what the body does to a drug) and pharmacodynamics (what a drug does to the body). Children's bodies absorb, distribute, metabolize, and eliminate medications differently from those of adults. But pharmacokinetics and pharmacodynamics also differ as children develop, so the needs of a premature infant, full-term infant, child, and adolescent can vary greatly. A good example is morphine. To achieve a morphine steady-state serum concentration of 10 nanograms (ng)/ml, the infusion rate in micrograms (µg)/kg/hr is 5 for neonates, 8.5 at 1 month of age, 13.5 at 3 months, 18 at 1 year, and 16 at ages 1–3 after noncardiac surgery in an intensive care unit (ICU) (Bouwmeester et al., 2004).

Currently, emergency care professionals have little by way of evidence-based guidelines and information to assist them with the prescribing of medications for infants, children, and adolescents (Mace et al., 2004). For example, there is currently no consensus on optimal guidelines for medications for pediatric sedation; in fact, sometimes these medications are given to children in combination with other drugs. Adverse drug events are common, particularly for antibiotics (e.g., ceftriaxone, clindamycin, amoxicillin), opioids (e.g., morphine, hydromorphone, acetaminophen with codeine), and anticonvulsants (e.g., phenytoin, phenobarbital, valproic acid); drugs in these classes are commonly prescribed to children in an emergency setting. Because of the startling knowledge gap and the frequent use of medications in children in the emergency setting, the committee recommends that the **Department of Health and Human Services fund studies of the efficacy, safety, and health outcomes of medications used for infants, children, and adolescents in emergency care settings in order to improve patient safety (5.1).** A number of different agencies within the Department of Health and Human Services (DHHS) could lead this effort, including the FDA, the Health Resources and Services Administration (HRSA), and the Agency for Healthcare Research and Quality (AHRQ). Congress has already taken some action in this area by passing two laws that provide incentives for or require drug manufacturers to conduct studies on the effects of drugs when used for pediatric patients—the Best Pharmaceuticals for Children Act of

2002 (BPCA) and the Pediatric Research Equity Act of 2003 (PREA), respectively. Under BCPA, the manufacturer takes the initiative in conducting pediatric studies and requests 6-month patent extensions from the FDA; however, this may not occur for drugs with limited market potential. PREA applies only to new molecular entities or new drugs, for which the FDA can require that the manufacturer conduct pediatric studies unless exceptions are granted. There is currently no regulation providing incentives for or requiring manufacturers to perform pediatric studies for the vast majority of drugs on the market in the generic forms used for pediatric patients.

Even for the small group of medications for which pediatric guidelines are available, a number of pitfalls exist at the prescribing, dispensing, administration, and monitoring stages that can result in medication errors and adverse drug events. Most adverse drug events for pediatric patients are a result of errors that occur at the prescribing stage, and they often involve incorrect dosing (IOM, 2000; Kaushal et al., 2001; Selbst et al., 2004; Chamberlain et al., 2004). Doses for pediatric patients must be calculated based on the patient's weight and therefore must be determined specifically for each patient. But the calculations needed to develop the dosing are complicated, and errors are common (Selbst et al., 2004). Patient weight can be and often is obtained or recorded incorrectly (Selbst et al., 1999). Among the most serious dosing errors are 10-fold errors that occur when a decimal point is missing or misread. There have been several examples of children receiving 10 or 100 times the intended dose of a medication and dying as a result. In one case, a baby was given 15 milligrams of morphine instead of the intended 0.15 milligrams—a 100-fold difference in dosing (Goldstein, 2001).

Other dosing errors can occur if there is confusion between milligrams (mg) and micrograms (µg) or mg and milliliters (ml). Additionally, errors are common with combinations of products, for example, Tylenol with codeine; it may be unclear whether the dosage is for the Tylenol or the codeine. Finally, dosage errors may occur when a product is prepared in two different ways and the concentrations are different. For example, Tylenol comes in a syrup and a drop, but the concentrations differ.

The process of dispensing and administering medications for children, compared with that for adults, relies much more heavily on manual compounding of liquid medications and administration to patients who are unable to perform their own medication safety checks. This may well make the dispensing and administering of medications for children more prone to error. Additionally, errors can occur during the dispensing stage if drugs that look or sound alike are confused, for example, Zantac and Zyrtec or Tobrex and Tobradex. Additionally, the packaging of two medications may look alike, contributing to errors at the dispensing stage (Levine et al., 2001;

Selbst et al., 2004). Most EDs do not have a pharmacist on staff to review orders or assist with medication use (Selbst et al., 2004). At the administration phase, a drug may be delivered twice if the first dosing is not promptly recorded in the medical record.

To reduce the high frequency of medication errors that occur in pediatric emergency care, the committee recommends that **the Department of Health and Human Services and the National Highway Traffic Safety Administration fund the development of medication dosage guidelines, formulations, labeling guidelines, and administration techniques for the emergency care setting to maximize effectiveness and safety for infants, children, and adolescents. Emergency medical services agencies and hospitals should incorporate these guidelines, formulations, and techniques into practice (5.2).** Agencies could commission research studies and/or convene a panel of experts to carry out these tasks. The Office of Emergency Medical Services within the National Highway Traffic Safety Administration (NHTSA) is a natural leader for this effort; within DHHS, a number of agencies could lead the effort, including the FDA, HRSA, and AHRQ. Implementing the proposed guidelines would not only improve patient safety, but also potentially reduce providers' liability claims since medication errors have been shown to be the second most frequent and second most expensive reason for such claims (Physician Insurers Association of America, 1993).

IMPROVING SAFETY FOR PEDIATRIC PATIENTS

The task of ED and EMS providers—to care for patients of all types, often with limited patient information and in a difficult, crowded environment—is enormous, and many providers and organizations are up to that task. However, there is enough evidence to suggest the need for action to improve the safety of emergency care, including that provided to pediatric patients. The committee therefore recommends that **hospitals and emergency medical services agencies implement evidence-based approaches to reducing errors in emergency and trauma care for children (5.3).** Those organizations that give guidance to providers, such as government agencies and professional organizations, should encourage providers to implement measures designed to protect patient safety. Continued research is needed to determine the best strategies for improving patient safety in prehospital and ED care; however, these strategies should focus on the factors that contribute to the deterioration of performance, such as crowding, problems with communication and information, and lack of provider resources.

Various hospitals and EMS agencies have tried several promising strategies with some success that could be replicated in other organizations. These initiatives have the potential to help all patients, not just children. Below we classify the strategies into three groups: provider policies, provider training, and technologies. Ideally, organizations would adopt all three of these strategies. A few examples of each type are given here.

Provider Policies

One of the problems associated with reducing the incidence of medical errors is that the frequency of errors and their most important triggers are unknown. Provider initiatives aimed at raising awareness of medical errors have shown some potential, although such programs must be coupled with limits on provider liability to encourage participation. For example, one hospital created and implemented the Good Catch Reporting Program. Under this program, all staff are required to report suspected and identified medical errors and near misses without fear of reprisal. Senior hospital leadership appointed a patient safety manager who reports to the chief nurse and reviews all errors and near misses. This information is used to develop system improvements for patient safety. Within the first 3 months of the program, reporting of near misses doubled (Salisbury, 2005). This approach could also be applied to the EMS environment.

EMS and hospital administrators have a number of opportunities to examine and specifically develop policies to address areas in which they believe shortcomings in patient safety exist. One hospital created the Look Alike/Sound Alike Project, in which a second person is required to verify all medications prior to their administration to a patient. Additionally, a pharmacist separated all look alike/sound alike medications in the pharmacy and clinics. Since the project was implemented, no look alike/sound alike medication errors have been identified (Salisbury, 2005).

Provider Training

Energized by successes in the aviation industry, where teamwork training has led to reductions in errors and improved performance (Risser et al., 1999; Sprague, 1999), several organizations have promoted the concept of teamwork training for health professionals. The similarities between pilots and doctors—highly trained technically, accustomed to viewing themselves as bearers of ultimate authority and responsibility, independent yet increasingly dependent on others of varying skill levels—suggest that teamwork training may be influential in reducing errors in the medical field (Sprague, 1999). Research on the impact of teamwork training in the ED is limited but promising. MedTeams, a Department of Defense (DoD) project that introduced teamwork training to health care, developed an Emergency Team Coordination Course (ETCC), an 8-hour didactic course for physicians, nurses, technicians, and support personnel. An evaluation of the course revealed considerable success. EDs using the ETCC experienced a 67 percent increase in error-averting behavior and a 58 percent reduction in observable errors (Risser et al., 1999; Shapiro et al., 2004).

Training initiatives that use simulation exercises have been shown to improve performance (Chorpra et al., 1994; Shapiro et al., 2004). Simulation training involves giving emergency care providers practice in performing tasks in lifelike circumstances using human models or virtual reality, with feedback from skilled observers, other team members, and video cameras. Some hospitals and academic medical centers use robotic human simulators (for example, an infant patient simulator used to train providers for intubation) so providers can experience high-risk, low-frequency events. These human simulators, analogous to the flight simulators used by pilots, allow providers to manage a wide range of clinical scenarios and learn from mistakes without harming a real patient (ECRI, 2005). The modern human patient simulator is extremely realistic, with anatomically correct clinical signs and the ability to communicate (Reznek et al., 2002).

Pediatric human simulators are in use in a limited number of hospitals. For example, at the University of Michigan, simulation is used to train EMTs and pediatric residents in standardized pediatric resuscitation courses. An attending physician developed the Pediatric Mock Code Program, in which the pediatric human patient simulator is used during actual pediatric code activations. Evaluation and training are provided to pediatric residents as well as other code team members, including nurses, pharmacists, and respiratory therapists. The program evaluates resuscitation skills, team interaction, and team leadership skills using a variety of scenarios representing the critically ill or injured child in the arrest and prearrest state (University of Michigan Health System, 2005).

Evidence for the effectiveness of simulation-based training is limited and has focused primarily on adult patient settings. However, use of and testing with pediatric human patient simulators could be a promising approach to pediatric training, particularly since many providers encounter critically ill or injured patients infrequently in practice; use of a simulator could help these providers maintain pediatric skills. However, there is presently limited access to simulation training technologies in hospitals, and even more so in EMS environments. Mobile simulation apparatus will be needed to bring this training to providers in the field, particularly those in rural areas (NHTSA, 2002).

Technologies

To further promote safety, attention has recently focused on identifying medications, patients, and providers with bar codes. Using technology that reads these bar codes, a computer system can confirm that the right medication is being given to the right patient at the right time and warn the provider of any safety issues. But progress on this technology remains stalled as the pharmaceutical industry tries to find a standard method of identifying medications (Kaushal and Bates, 2002). A review of the available controlled studies shows time savings and error reduction with the use of bar codes; however, further study is needed (Oren et al., 2003). There is also hope that the increased use of electronic health records, computerized physician order entry, decision-support systems, and the like will help improve patient safety, making it easier for emergency care providers to determine correct diagnoses and provide proper treatment to their patients (Cosby, 2003). Indeed, all of these technologies have been shown to be effective in reducing errors in small evaluations involving patients of all ages (Hunt et al., 1998; Bates et al., 1999; Bizovi et al., 2002; Buller-Close et al., 2003), although results have not been universally positive (Han et al., 2005). The next section describes some of these technologies and addresses the need to design them for use with pediatric patients.

ADVANCES IN TECHNOLOGY AND INFORMATION SYSTEMS

Technology is also likely to advance the way care is delivered in the prehospital and ED settings. New technologies designed to accelerate diagnosis and workflow (advanced imaging modalities, rapid diagnostic tests, laboratory automation, EMS technologies, patient tracking tools, and new triage models) and improve treatment (ultrasonography, tympanocentesis, needleless drug administration, and innovations in procedural sedation) are likely to be adopted. As these new technologies are introduced, it will be critical to consider how they help (and whether they may bring harm to) pediatric patients. While this appears to be a rather obvious consideration, history is filled with examples of medical technologies originally developed for adults and used on children with unintended consequences. Devices are typically developed for adults because they constitute a much larger share of the market for medical services than children. For similar reasons, post-market surveillance of medical devices is focused on adults, especially older adults, rather than children. Also, regulation and patient safety efforts for medical products tend to focus more on pharmaceuticals than on medical devices (IOM, 2005).

When detrimental effects on children are discovered postmarket, adjustments are eventually made to technologies, making them safer for pediatric use. One example is the infusion pump, introduced more than 30 years ago, which delivers medications and fluids intravenously. As originally designed, the devices had a wide range of acceptable programming parameters. For example, they could be programmed to deliver a drop or two every hour or a liter or more in an hour. They were designed for maximum flexibility; they could be used on an adult ICU patient one day and on a premature infant the next. Because the technology relied on human intelligence for programming, errors naturally occurred. In a neonatal ICU, for example, an infusion rate was programmed to 304 ml/hr when the physician intended the rate to be 3.4 ml/hr. In many cases, critical errors were made because a single wrong button was pressed (Reves, 2003).

Advances in infusion technology led to the introduction of "smart pumps," which are widely used today. Smart pumps utilize software that checks programmed doses. The software contains information on drugs, their usual concentrations, dosing units, and dosing limits. When the practitioner uses the pump, he or she programs it for use in a designated area (e.g., adult ICU, neonatal ICU), and the pump is automatically configured for use on adults or children. Additional safeguards are also built into the pumps, for example, alerting the user if the dosage exceeds the hospital's established limit and not allowing the user to base the dose on the patient's weight if the drug is not dosed on that basis (Reves, 2003).

A market for pediatric technologies, equipment, and supplies must be stimulated so that products will be designed initially to meet the needs of pediatric patients, instead of being adapted from products originally designed and intended for use with adult patients. The market for pediatric-designed products has not been well developed in part because providers have not been compelled to purchase pediatric-specific products. To stimulate demand for such products, emergency providers should be made aware of the potential shortcomings of products designed for adults and adapted for children. To advance this effort, the committee recommends that **federal agencies and private industry fund research on pediatric-specific technologies and equipment for use by emergency and trauma care personnel (5.4).**

This is not the first recommendation of its kind. The 2005 Institute of Medicine (IOM) report *Safe Medical Devices for Children* emphasized the need for the FDA, the National Institutes of Health (NIH), and AHRQ to define a research agenda and priorities for evaluation of the short- and long-term safety and effectiveness of medical devices for children (IOM, 2005). The report also called for the FDA to work with industry and others to focus more attention on adverse events involving the use of medical devices for children and to update product labeling promptly to reflect safety-related findings. Emergency providers should be able to take comfort in knowing that the equipment they are using on pediatric patients is safe and effective. Development and testing of new products are needed to give providers this assurance.

Federal agencies and private industry also need to take a careful look at the technologies already in place and available for use with infants, children, and adolescents. For a number of devices and technologies being used on pediatric patients, it is unclear whether they ultimately do children more good than harm. One example is the growing use of pediatric computed tomography (CT), a tool that assists ED providers in diagnosing illness and injury in children. Annually, 2–3 million CT scans are performed on children—a seven-fold increase in the past 10 years (Doheny, 2003), much of which is due to the technology's increased availability. One problem with the use of CT is radiation exposure. Children are more sensitive to radiation than adults, and they have longer life expectancy and therefore a greater opportunity to develop cancer in their lifetime. The same radiation dose when given to a neonate is several times more likely to produce cancer over the child's lifetime than when given to a 40-year-old adult (National Cancer Institute and Society for Pediatric Radiology, 2002). Indeed, research indicates that pediatric CT scans are used too liberally in the ED, frequently to appease parents or guardians who request them (Doheny, 2003). Additionally, practitioners often fail to adjust the exposure parameters when administering a CT scan to a pediatric patient. As a result, in 2002 the National Cancer Institute and the Society for Pediatric Radiology issued a guide to physicians instructing them in how to minimize children's exposure to radiation. They recommended performing CT scans only when necessary, limiting the region of the body scanned, adjusting exposure parameters based on the child's size and weight, and minimizing the use of multiple scans (National Cancer Institute and Society for Pediatric Radiology, 2002). Children scanned at adult hospitals may receive a higher dose of radiation than those scanned at children's hospitals because at the former, the machine is kept on default settings typically intended for adult patients.

Another technology that is already in use with unclear implications for children is the automated external defibrillator (AED), often used by first responders in public settings. AEDs are programmed to deliver adult-dose shocks to individuals in ventricular fibrillation (VF) cardiac arrest. None of the AEDs introduced in office buildings, airports, and other public places were designed for use in children under age 8, and none were cleared by the FDA for use in children. Additionally, there were no data regarding the safety and efficacy of AEDs in children. However, new AEDs with pediatric cables and pads have been designed to direct some of the current away so the pediatric patient receives a lower level of energy (Brown et al., 2004). The American Heart Association (AHA) and the National Association of EMS Physicians (NAEMSP) have stated that AEDs may be used together with cardiopulmonary resuscitation (CPR) in children aged 1 to 8 in cardiac arrest (Markenson and Domeier, 2003; Samson et al., 2003), and the AHA recommends the use of the two together for treatment of cardiac arrest in children above age 8 (Atkins et al., 1998). The FDA has cleared the way for the marketing of specially modified AEDs for use on infants and children younger than age 8 (Automated Defibrillator Cleared, 2001).

Today there remains uncertainty about the appropriate use of AEDs in children, however. According to a recent advisory statement from the

International Liaison Committee on Resuscitation, newer AED models with pediatric capabilities can be used on children over age 1, but only a limited number of studies have looked at the impact of AEDs on children. Although the incidence of sudden cardiac arrest among children is rare, it is estimated that AEDs could assist approximately 15 high school students with the condition per year if placed in schools (Brown et al., 2004). In 2004, a number of organizations, including the AHA, NAEMSP, the American Academy of Pediatrics (AAP), and the American College of Emergency Physicians (ACEP), developed a joint statement that outlines recommendations for the use of AEDs in schools (Hazinski et al., 2004).

One thing common to all of the examples in this section is that the technologies were not originally designed for use in children, but were used on children in practice. In the absence of pediatric-specific technologies, providers may be compelled to use adult technologies on children thinking that the benefits outweigh the risks; certainly in many cases, use of the adult technology may be better than foregoing treatment for the pediatric patient altogether (National Cancer Institute and Society for Pediatric Radiology, 2002). However, encouraging the development and testing of pediatric-specific technologies is key to ensuring that children receive the best treatment for their conditions.

A similar issue exists with the development of information technology (IT) systems. Hospitals, EMS systems, and government entities are beginning to make substantial investments in health IT systems that may improve the quality and efficiency of emergency care delivery for all patients, but there are benefits specific to pediatric patients as well. IT systems that make immunization records of children available to emergency care providers have the potential to greatly improve the efficiency and effectiveness of care. Additionally, some children with special health care needs have sizable medical records, whose details could be made available to emergency care providers with certain IT systems.

Because of the unique nature of pediatric relative to adult emergency care, specific consideration of children's needs during the design of systems is critical to ensure that the systems will be appropriate for the pediatric patient. For example, clinical decision-support systems must incorporate the various threats to children's health and diseases common to children; systems designed for adult care currently do not do so. The lack of uniform agreement on standard pediatric doses is at least part of the reason for the usual absence of pediatric-specific dosing tables powering most commercially available computerized physician order entry tools. Without standard pediatric doses and requirements for building these dosage rules into computerized prescribing tools, children will fail to fully reap the benefits of IT in the medication delivery process. Also, electronic health records must be designed to allow providers to record measurements on a sufficiently granular scale appropriate for newborns and infants (e.g., rounding to the nearest tenth of a kilogram or recording age by month rather than year) (Shiffman et al., 2001).

While studies indicate great benefits of advances in information systems, the safety, impacts, and risks of these systems for pediatric patients have received little attention (Lehmann, 2003). Pediatric experts need to be involved in the design of these products, not only to ensure that the data collected and produced by the systems are appropriate for children, but also to ensure that the systems are designed suitably for the input of data by providers of care to pediatric patients. Pediatric performance measures should be monitored before and after the implementation of new information systems. For example, at least one study revealed an increase in pediatric mortality after the implementation of a computerized physician order entry system, which was expected to reduce errors in the care of pediatric patients (Han et al., 2005).

The committee's companion report on hospital-based emergency care addresses advances in health IT in greater depth, including the need for systems to be designed appropriately for patients of all ages.

THE IMPORTANCE OF FAMILY-CENTERED CARE

One of the six aims for quality health care identified by the IOM in its seminal report *Crossing the Quality Chasm: A New Health System for the 21st Century* (IOM, 2001) is patient-centeredness. This means that care should encompass the qualities of compassion, empathy, and responsiveness to the needs, values, and preferences of the individual patient. In the case of pediatric patients, parents or guardians are recognized as the child's primary source of strength and support and play an integral role in the child's health and well-being. The aim of patient-centered care recognizes that parents and guardians must collaborate with providers in decision making regarding their child's care (Lewandowski and Tesler, 2003). Increasing recognition of the importance of meeting the psychosocial and developmental needs of children and of fostering the role of families in promoting the health and well-being of their children has led to the concept of "family-centered care" (Eichner et al., 2003). This section describes the concept of family-centered care and its benefits. Unfortunately, few EMS agencies or EDs have written policies or guidelines for family-centered care in place, and few providers are trained in offering such care (Loyacono, 2001; MacLean et al., 2003). Because the family-centered approach to care can mutually benefit the patient, family, and provider, the committee supports its widespread adoption by the emergency care system, including EMS agencies and hospitals. The committee recommends that **emergency medical services agencies and hospitals integrate family-centered care into emergency care practice (5.5).**

Entities that offer guidance to providers, such as government agencies and professional organizations, should demonstrate leadership in this area by promoting the use of family-centered guidelines.

The concept of family-centered care evolved between 1980 and 1990 under the leadership of parent advisory groups, health professionals, the Maternal and Child Health Bureau, and the Office of the Surgeon General. The concept contrasts with the more traditional medical model of health care, which is oriented toward disease and disability, the notion that health providers know best how to treat problems, and the view that family members should comply with treatment recommendations (Baren, 2001). There are several definitions of family-centered care, but they all essentially recognize that providers should acknowledge and use the family's knowledge of their child's condition and the family's skills and presence when caring for a child (Boudreaux et al., 2002). The core principles of family-centered care include the following (ENA et al., 2000):

- Treatment of patients and families with dignity and respect
- Communication of unbiased information
- Patient and family participation in experiences that enhance control and independence and build on their strengths
- Collaboration in the delivery of care, policy and program development, and professional education

Family-centered care is supported by a growing body of research showing the need to ensure the involvement of patients and families in their own health care decisions, to better inform families of treatment options, and to improve access to information by patient and families (Eichner et al., 2003). A number of studies have found some evidence of improved health outcomes, patient and family satisfaction, and provider satisfaction with the introduction of family-centered care (Meyers et al., 1998, 2000; Boie et al., 1999; Boudreaux et al., 2002; Saunders et al., 2003; Moreland, 2005). The approach is especially important when emergency providers have a pediatric patient with special health care needs; because of their frequent interactions with medical providers and deep familiarity with their child's condition, parents of such patients may be in a better position than emergency care providers to diagnose the problem. The development and implementation of family-centered care encompass multiple components of care delivery, policies and procedures, the care environment, and personnel practices.

Collaboration with Families in the EMS and ED Environments

Often a parent or guardian is present when emergency medical technicians (EMTs) arrive on scene or a child arrives at the ED. Emergency providers encounter families at a highly stressful time. The family-centered approach to care revolves around collaborating with families, keeping them informed about the child's condition, prognosis, and treatment (National Association of Emergency Medical Technicians, 2000a). For EMTs, simply explaining the function of equipment, procedures being performed, and their effects is important so that family members can be better prepared to make decisions about care, such as termination of resuscitation. Potential benefits include decreased patient and family anxiety and combativeness, decreased liability issues if parents/guardians are involved in decision making, and easing of the consent process for organ donation if parents/guardians are aware of everything that has been done (National Association of Emergency Medical Technicians, 2000b).

The family-centered approach to emergency services also includes giving families the option of being present during invasive procedures as long as the safety of the patient and medical providers is not compromised. Family members have traditionally been excluded at such times because of concerns that they could lose emotional control and interrupt care, a lack of staff to meet family needs, insufficient room at the bedside, increased risk of litigation, family-imposed limitations on the training of medical residents, and the potential that providers' skills could be affected by discomfort with the family's presence. But heightened awareness and new research have revealed that these concerns are overstated and that there are multiple benefits to the presence of family members: their presence removes doubt about what is happening to the child and reinforces that everything possible has been done, it reduces anxiety and fear (Wolfram and Turner, 1996; Wolfram et al., 1997), it engenders feelings of supporting and helping the patient, it sustains patient–family connectedness, it engenders feelings of being helpful to the health care staff, and it facilitates the grieving process (Doyle et al., 1987; MacLean et al., 2003). In addition, the existing literature indicates that family presence does not negatively impact the ability of providers to perform invasive procedures or exacerbate clinician anxiety (Bauchner and Vinci, 1996; Wolfram and Turner, 1996; Sacchetti et al., 2005), although at least one study showed that family members' presence during resuscitation was occasionally stressful and anxiety provoking for providers (Hanson and Strawser, 1992).

Research on this issue suggests that families want to be given the option to be present during invasive procedures and resuscitations, and when given the option often take it (Bauchner et al., 1991; Haimi-Cohen et al., 1996; Sacchetti et al., 1996; Boie et al., 1999; Boudreaux et al., 2002). Family members who were present for a procedure report favorable experiences and believe their presence benefited the patient and their own emotional response to the incident (Boudreaux et al., 2002).

While families overwhelmingly support family-centered policies, providers have mixed opinions about family presence. Often inclusion of parents or guardians goes against the culture of emergency care providers. An example is Children's Hospital of Philadelphia's pediatric/neonatal ground transport team, which historically had a policy of excluding parents from the transport of a child in a ground ambulance. The transport team cited a number of reasons for the policy: difficulty caring for the patient if the parent needed attention, potential trouble in dealing with a belligerent or hysterical parent, difficulty controlling the child if a parent was present, and the transport team's anxiety about performing medical interventions while being watched by a parent. In 1995, the transport team explored the idea of allowing parents to ride in ground ambulances and surveyed parents who were and were not allowed to do so. Overwhelmingly, results showed that parents preferred to accompany their child during transport. The research team also surveyed pediatric transport team managers from a number of different children's hospitals. They found diverse opinions and practices regarding parental accompaniment during transport (Woodward and Fleegler, 2000, 2001).

Provider opinions regarding family presence vary with the invasiveness of the procedure and the provider's experience. A recent survey of ED faculty, nurses, and pediatric residents at an urban children's hospital found that ED staff generally supported the presence of family members during minor procedures, but expressed concern regarding the effects on the family and the success of the procedure. Most attending physicians and nurses supported the family's presence during highly invasive procedures, but most residents did not (Fein et al., 2004). This study and others have shown that more experienced practitioners tend to be more comfortable than those with less experience with regard to allowing families to be present during procedures (Mitchell and Lynch, 1997; Meyers et al., 2000; O'Brien et al., 2002; Fein et al., 2004).

Studies also indicate that nurses are more likely than physicians to support family presence policies (Chalk, 1995; Helmer et al., 2000; Fein et al., 2004). In 1994, the Emergency Nurses Association (ENA) passed a resolution supporting the presence of family members at the bedside during invasive procedures and/or resuscitations. Other organizations that explicitly support family-centered care, including the Emergency Medical Services for Children (EMS-C) program, ACEP, and the American Association for the Surgery of Trauma (AAST), have not developed official resolutions on parental presence during invasive procedures (Boudreaux et al., 2002). A 2002 survey of critical care and emergency care nurses revealed that, despite the frequency of requests from family members to be present during invasive procedures, nearly all EDs lack written policies or guidelines for family presence (MacLean et al., 2003).

A few studies of family-centered care have found evidence of improvements in staff satisfaction, but most have focused on primary care delivery or inpatient care (Eichner et al., 2003). The exception is a 2001 study that found that when family-centered care was the cornerstone of culture in a pediatric ED, staff members had more positive feelings about their work than staff members in an ED where emotional support for families was not emphasized (Hemmelgarn et al., 2001).

The family-centered approach requires a shift in thinking for emergency providers typically trained to rapidly assess, treat, and/or transport patients (National Association of Emergency Medical Technicians, 2000b). A lack of training in why and how to communicate with families can be a barrier to the adoption of family-centered care. The committee recognizes the value of family-centered pediatric emergency care and encourages provider organizations to take steps to educate practitioners in and develop protocols for adopting this approach. Family members' presence during invasive procedures and resuscitations remains controversial (Sacchetti et al., 2005), but institutions should consider such policies. Family presence for more minor procedures, such as wound repair, is overwhelmingly supported by both patients and providers and should be reflected in providers' treatment protocols.

Resources exist to help guide EMS agencies and hospitals in the implementation of family-centered practices. For example, On the Same Team is a training tool for EMTs designed to assist them in becoming more proficient in engaging family members in the care of their loved ones. In 1997, the EMS-C National Resource Center, in collaboration with the Institute for Family-Centered Care (IFCC), developed an assessment tool for evaluating family-centered practices. There are separate tools for prehospital emergency care and care in the ED. More recently, the IFCC partnered with the AHA to produce a resource for practitioners wishing to advance the practice of family-centered care (AHA, 2005). The provision of family-centered care is also advanced in the Pediatric Advanced Life Support (PALS) manual, *Advanced Pediatric Life Support (APLS): Pediatric Emergency Medicine Resource*, and the AHA's guidelines for CPR (Knapp and Mulligan-Smith, 2005). Guidelines for implementing family-centered care were also provided in a report of the National Consensus Conference on Family Presence during Pediatric Cardiopulmonary Resuscitation and Procedures (Henderson and Knapp, 2005).

A Family-Centered ED Environment

Another important component of family-centered care is creating an environment in the ED that is both family- and child-friendly. However, a minority of hospitals have separate pediatric EDs (Gausche-Hill et al., 2004). The majority of hospitals treat both children and adults in the same area, creating an uncomfortable environment for parents or guardians and a frightening one for children if they are in the waiting room with bleeding or intoxicated adults.

Attention to creating a family-centered environment has grown in recent years. The 2001 *EMS-C Program Guide for Improving Family-Centered Care* contains a framework for improving the environment and design of EDs for children and their families. The guide encourages EDs to reflect on whether their environment is family-centered by answering a number of questions, such as the following: Is the waiting area large enough, with enough comfortable seating available, for all children and adults who may be waiting, even if several adults and children accompany one child? Are examination, treatment, and procedure rooms designed to accommodate parents or guardians who wish to remain with their child? Can families easily find their way from the ED to other areas of the hospital, including radiology, laboratories, pharmacy, admitting office, patient care units, and cafeteria?

Because of the emotional impact an ED visit can have on a patient and parent/guardian, the exterior and interior of the ED should be inviting and make the patient and family feel comfortable. Working with hospital staff, patients, and parents, designers of pediatric EDs have formulated advice for designing the interior of a pediatric ED. First, the normal environment for children does not include bright primary colors; it is often better to create a calming environment than a stimulating one. Second, lighting that is appropriate for an exam is not helpful to parents' or guardians' frayed nerves. Distractions such as a television or radio are welcome to families that are waiting. Third, children should feel that they can master an environment and not be overwhelmed or intimidated by it. One means to this end is to design the room to the scale of a child. Examples include wall sconces 24 inches above the floor and a rail system detailed to accommodate the sight-line of a 4-year old. Lower ceilings may also be appropriate (Pence, 2000; Hanson, 2001).

Many hospital inpatient units, particularly in pediatric centers, use child life programs and specialists to address the psychosocial aspects of hospitalization for the pediatric patient and parents or caregivers (AAP, 2000). These programs and services help reduce emotional disturbances in children and help them anticipate and make it through difficult procedures. Evidence has shown that these programs can reduce stress and aid recovery (Wolfer et al., 1998). It is unclear how prevalent these programs are in EDs, although a mid-1990s survey of large children's hospitals found that 6 of 44 EDs had at least one full-time child life specialist on staff (Krebel et al., 1996). Evidence is limited as to the impact of having child life services available in the ED setting, though the practice appears to have potential.

Cultural Competency

Another component of family-centered care is cultural competency. According to the EMS-C program, "cultural competence includes possessing the appropriate knowledge, skills, and capacity to provide emergency services to children in a manner that demonstrates respect, sensitivity, and understanding of the unique cultural differences within, among, and between groups" (EMS-C National Resource Center, 1999).

Only a few studies have been able to draw a direct link between cultural competence and health care improvement, although expert opinion strongly suggests a connection among cultural competence, quality of care, and reduced racial and ethnic disparities (Betancourt et al., 2002). These studies are not specific to pediatric patients, but cultural competency is an important issue for the emergency care system in general, not just services for children, particularly because the racial/ethnic distribution of emergency care providers is not well matched to the racial/ethnic distribution of the population, and is even less well matched to the population that uses emergency services most frequently. This disparity can only be expected to increase as the U.S. population continues to diversify at a much faster rate than most health professions and occupations (Heron and Haley, 2001; Cone et al., 2003).

One of the biggest challenges for emergency care providers is language barriers. Professional interpreters are often not available in the field or at an ED. Indeed, interpreters are frequently not used in the ED, even when thought necessary by a patient or provider (Baker et al., 1996). When providers cannot obtain adequate information from a patient interview, they tend to use more resources, such as laboratory and radiographic investigations. One study of language barriers in a pediatric ED revealed that a physician–family language barrier was associated with a higher rate of resource utilization for diagnostic studies and increased ED visit times (Hampers et al., 1999).

One special concern is the use of children as interpreters for their own care or the care of their parents/guardians when they speak English but their parents/guardians do not. Use of children as medical interpreters is common practice in many areas with large immigrant populations (Burke, 2005), often, however, the information that needs to be interpreted is beyond children's comprehension and may be inappropriate for them (Yee, 2005). Children assuming this role take on a heavy emotional responsibility. Additionally, use of an untrained interpreter can lead to medical errors. In one study, the error rate was highest for the youngest interpreter, an 11-year-old (Flores et al., 2003). Some states have regulations that prevent children from serving as medical interpreters for their parents/guardians, but these rules may not apply in emergency situations. The traditional subordinate role of children can be reversed when they are used as interpreters, and in some cultures, their assumption of this role can be seen as a threat to parental authority and therefore serve as a barrier to care (National Association of Emergency Medical Technicians, 2000b).

The challenge goes beyond language barriers, however. Providers need to be aware of the various cultures residing in their catchment area so as to be prepared to serve them. Also, understanding different family structures can help avoid hostile reactions resulting from inadvertent disrespect toward families (National Association of Emergency Medical Technicians, 2000b). Providers' actions can affect patient perceptions of care. A survey of adult patients presenting to an ED with one of six chief complaints found that non–English speakers were less satisfied with their care in the ED, were less willing to return to the same ED if they had a problem they felt required emergency care, and reported more problems with emergency care (Carrasquillo et al., 1999).

Failure to appreciate the importance of culture and language during pediatric emergencies can result in multiple adverse consequences, including difficulties with informed consent; miscommunication; inadequate understanding of diagnosis and treatment by families; dissatisfaction with care; preventable morbidity and mortality; unnecessary child abuse evaluations; lower-quality care; clinician bias; and ethnic disparities in prescriptions, analgesia, test ordering, and diagnostic evaluation (Flores et al., 2002). The National Association of Emergency Medical Technicians emphasizes the use of communication strategies to combat some of the cultural barriers to care that may arise. Examples of these strategies include identifying providers to the patient and family members, identifying a team member to interact with the family members on each call, asking how the patient and family would like to be addressed, using courtesy titles, and watching for verbal and nonverbal cues from families about the amount of information they want and whether they understand what is being explained to them (National Association of Emergency Medical Technicians, 2000b).

Care of Adolescents

Less research on patient- and family-centered care has been conducted for adolescents than for younger children. In fact, relatively little is known about adolescents' health care preferences or expectations (Britto et al., 2004). Results of a study of adolescents with chronic illness suggest that aspects of interpersonal care are most important to their judgment of quality. Physicians' honesty and attention to pain are deemed of critical importance. Adolescents also want to participate in their own care and have their views taken seriously by providers (Britto et al., 2004).

Adolescents tend to find the ED a fast-paced, confusing, and frightening place according to results from a focus group of teens in four cities.

Respondents reacted negatively to the idea of emergency care personnel approaching them at the hospital and engaging them in discussions of violence or personal safety (Dowd et al., 2000). This finding presents a real challenge to emergency care providers since teens often present with conditions resulting from violence or alcohol or drug use. Most EDs do not provide preventive screenings or counseling for adolescents (Wilson and Klein, 2000). Physicians tend to find adolescent patients "frustrating," and according to one study, adolescents receive less-than-optimal care in the emergency room (March and Jay, 1993). Yet brief interventional counseling for adolescents may be of value. A prevention effort at one ED targeting injured adolescents resulted in greater use of seat belts and bicycle helmets (Johnston et al., 2002).

Certainly more research is necessary to provide adolescents with emergency services in a way that is both patient-centered and effective. Clearly, however, an understanding of the psychosocial and developmental issues that characterize adolescence may help staff respond more effectively to adolescent patients (March and Jay, 1993).

SUMMARY OF RECOMMENDATIONS

5.1 The Department of Health and Human Services should fund studies of the efficacy, safety, and health outcomes of medications used for infants, children, and adolescents in emergency care settings in order to improve patient safety.

5.2 The Department of Health and Human Services and the National Highway Traffic Safety Administration should fund the development of medication dosage guidelines, formulations, labeling guidelines, and administration techniques for the emergency care setting to maximize effectiveness and safety for infants, children, and adolescents. Emergency medical services agencies and hospitals should incorporate these guidelines, formulations, and techniques into practice.

5.3 Hospitals and emergency medical services agencies should implement evidence-based approaches to reducing errors in emergency and trauma care for children.

5.4 Federal agencies and private industry should fund research on pediatric-specific technologies and equipment for use by emergency and trauma care personnel.

5.5 Emergency medical services agencies and hospitals should integrate family-centered care into emergency care practice.

REFERENCES

AAP (American Academy of Pediatrics). 2000. Access to pediatric emergency medical care. *Pediatrics* 105(3 Pt. 1):647–649.

ACEP, AAP (American College of Emergency Physicians, American Academy of Pediatrics). 2006. *APLS: The Pediatric Emergency Medicine Resource* (4th edition). Elk Grove Village, IL/Dallas, TX: ACEP and AAP.

AHA (American Hospital Association). 2005. *Strategies for Leadership: Patient-and Family-Centered Care*. [Online]. Available: http://www.aha.org/aha/key_issues/patient_safety/resources/patientcenteredcare.html [accessed January 25, 2006].

Atkins DL, Hartley LL, York DK. 1998. Accurate recognition and effective treatment of ventricular fibrillation by automated external defibrillators in adolescents. *Pediatrics* 101(3 Pt. 1):393–397.

Automated defibrillator cleared for use in infants and children. 2001. *FDA Consumer* 35(4):4.

Baker DW, Parker RM, Williams MV, Coates WC, Pitkin K. 1996. Use and effectiveness of interpreters in an emergency department. *Journal of the American Medical Association* 275(10):783–788.

Baren JM. 2001. Rising to the challenge of family-centered care in emergency medicine. *Academic Emergency Medicine* 8(12):1182–1185.

Bates DW, Teich JM, Lee J, Seger D, Kuperman GJ, Ma'Luf N, Boyle D, Leape L. 1999. The impact of computerized physician order entry on medication error prevention. *Journal of the American Medical Informatics Association* 6(4):313–321.

Bauchner H, Vinci R. 1996. Parents and procedures: A randomized controlled trial. *Pediatrics* 861.

Bauchner H, Waring C, Vinci R. 1991. Parental presence during procedures in an emergency room: Results from 50 observations. *Pediatrics* 87(4):544–548.

Betancourt JR, Green AR, Emilio Carillo J. 2002. *Cultural Competence in Health Care: Emerging Frameworks and Practical Approaches. Field Report*. New York: The Commonwealth Foundation.

Bizovi KE, Beckley BE, McDade MC, Adams AL, Lowe RA, Zechnich AD, Hedges JR. 2002. The effect of computer-assisted prescription writing on emergency department prescription errors. *Academic Emergency Medicine* 9(11):1168-1175.

Boie ET, Moore GP, Brummett C, Nelson DR. 1999. Do parents want to be present during invasive procedures performed on their children in the emergency department? A survey of 400 parents. *Annals of Emergency Medicine* 34(1):70–74.

Boudreaux E, Francis J, Loyacono T. 2002. Family presence during invasive procedures and resuscitations in the emergency department: A critical review and suggestions for future research. *Annals of Emergency Medicine* 40(2):193–205.

Bouwmeester NJ, Anderson BJ, Tibboel D, Holford NHG. 2004. Developmental pharmacokinetics of morphine and its metabolites in neonates, infants and young children. *British Journal of Anaesthesia* 92(2):208–217.

Britto MT, DeVellis RF, Hornung RW, DeFriese GH, Atherton HD, Slap GB. 2004. Health care preferences and priorities of adolescents with chronic illnesses. *Pediatrics* 114(5):1272–1280.

Brown L, Dietrich AM, Hostetler MA, Goldman RD, Barata IA, Higginbotham E, Finkler JH. 2004. *Automated External Defibrillators (AEDs) and Pediatric Patients*. Dallas, TX: ACEP.

Buller-Close K, Schriger DL, Baraff LJ. 2003. Heterogeneous effect of an emergency department expert charting system. *Annals of Emergency Medicine* 41(5):644–652.

Burke G. 2005, October 21. Children speaking for their parents? *Sacramento Union.* [Online]. Available: http://www.sacunion.com/pages/california/articles/6612/ [accessed January 31, 2007].

Carrasquillo O, Orav EJ, Brennan TA, Burstin HR. 1999. Impact of language barriers on patient satisfaction in an emergency department. *Journal of General Internal Medicine* 14(2):82–87.

Chalk A. 1995. Should relatives be present in the resuscitation room? *Accident and Emergency Nursing* 3(2):58–61.

Chamberlain J, Slonim A, Joseph J. 2004. Reducing errors and promoting safety in pediatric emergency care. *Ambulatory Pediatrics* 4(1):55–63.

Children's Hospital Boston. 2005a. *Carbon Monoxide Poisoning.* [Online]. Available: http://www.childrenshospital.org/az/Site649/mainpageS649P0.html [accessed April 4, 2006].

Children's Hospital Boston. 2005b. *Meningococcal Infections.* [Online]. Available: http://www.childrenshospital.org/az/Site1291/printerfriendlypageS1291PO.html [accessed April 4, 2006].

Chisholm CD, Dornfeld AM, Nelson DR, Cordell WH. 2001. Work interrupted: A comparison of workplace interruptions in emergency departments and primary care offices. *Annals of Emergency Medicine* 38(2):146–151.

Chorpra V, Gesnik BJ, de Jong J, Boville JG. 1994. Does training on an anesthesia simulator lead to improvement in performance? *British Journal of Anaesthesia* 73:293–297.

Cone DC, Richardson LD, Knox HT, Betancourt JR, Lowe RA. 2003. Health care disparities in emergency medicine. *Academic Emergency Medicine* 10(11):1176–1183.

Cosby KS. 2003. A framework for classifying factors that contribute to error in the emergency department. *Annals of Emergency Medicine* 42(6):815–823.

Croskerry P. 2000. The feedback sanction. *Academic Emergency Medicine* 7(11):1232–1238.

D'Agostino J. 2002. Common abdominal emergencies in children. *Emergency Medical Clinics of North America* 20(1):139–153.

Derlet RW, Richards JR. 2000. Overcrowding in the nation's emergency departments: Complex causes and disturbing effects. *Annals of Emergency Medicine* 35(1): 63–68.

Derlet RW, Richards JR, Kravitz R. 2001. Frequent overcrowding in U.S. emergency departments. *Academic Emergency Medicine* 8(2):151–155.

Doheny K. 2003, April 5. CT scans for kids: Not every bump warrants an X-ray. *HON News.* [Online]. Available: http://www.hon.ch/News/HSN/512003.html [accessed October, 2005].

Dowd MD, Seidel JS, Sheehan K, Barlow B, Bradbard SL. 2000. Teenagers' perceptions of personal safety and the role of the emergency health care provider. *Annals of Emergency Medicine* 36(4):346–350.

Doyle CJ, Post H, Burney RE, Maino J, Keefe M, Rhee KJ. 1987. Family participation during resuscitation: An option. *Annals of Emergency Medicine* 16(6):673–675.

ECRI (Emergency Care Research Institute). 2005, February. Teamwork takes hold to improve patient safety. *The Risk Management Reporter* 24(1):1–7.

Eichner JM, Neff JM, Hardy DR, Klein M, Percelay JM, Sigrest T, Stucky ER, Dull S, Perkins MT, Wilson JM, Corden TE, Ostric EJ, Mucha S, Johnson BH, Ahmann E, Crocker E, DiVenere N, MacKean G, Schwab WE. 2003. Family-centered care and the pediatrician's role. *Pediatrics* 691–696.

EMS-C National Resource Center (Emergency Medical Services for Children National Resource Center). 1999. *EMSC and Cultural Competence.* Washington, DC: EMS-C National Resource Center.

ENA, HRSA, EMSC (Emergency Nurses Association, Health Resources and Services Administration, Emergency Medical Services Cooperation). 2000. *Assessment of Family-Centered Care in the Emergency Department.* Des Plaines, IL: ENA.

Fairbanks RG, Crittenden CN. 2006. *The Nature of Adult and Pediatric Adverse Events.* Unpublished report. [Online]. Available: http://www.thefederationonline.org/PowerPoint/ TerryFairbanks.pdf [accessed February 2006].

Fairbanks RJ, Caplan S, Shah MN, Marks A, Bishop P. 2004. Defibrillator usability study among paramedics. *Human Factors and Ergonomics Society Meeting.* [Online.] Available: http://www.thefederationonline.org/PowerPoint/TerryFairbanks.pdf [accessed September 2005].

Fairbanks T. 2004. *Human Factors and Patient Safety in Emergency Medical Services. Science Forum on Patient Safety and Human Factors Research.* Rochester, NY: University of Rochester.

Fein JA, Ganesh J, Alpern ER. 2004. Medical staff attitudes toward family presence during pediatric procedures. *Pediatric Emergency Care* 20(4):224–227.

Fleisher GR, Ludwig S, Henretig FM, Ruddy RM, Silverman BK. 2006. *Textbook of Pediatric Emergency Medicine.* Philadelphia, PA: Lippincott Williams and Wilkins.

Flores G, Rabke-Verani J, Pine W, Sabharwal A. 2002. The importance of cultural and linguistic issues in the emergency care of children. *Pediatric Emergency Care* 18(4):271–284.

Flores G, Laws MB, Mayo SJ, Zuckerman B, Abreu M, Medina L, Hardt EJ. 2003. Errors in medical interpretation and their potential clinical consequences in pediatric encounters. *Pediatrics* 111(1):6–14.

Gausche-Hill M, Lewis R, Schmitz C. 2004. *Survey of US Emergency Departments for Pediatric Preparedness—Implementation and Evaluation of Care of Children in the Emergency Department: Guidelines for Preparedness. Emergency Medical Services for Children Partnership for Information and Communication Grant #IU93 MC 00184.* Unpublished results.

Goldstein A. 2001, April 20. Overdose kills girl at Children's Hospital. *The Washington Post.* p. B1.

Haimi-Cohen Y, Amir J, Harel L, Straussberg R, Varsano Y. 1996. Parental presence during lumbar puncture: Anxiety and attitude toward the procedure. *Clinical Pediatrics* 35(1):2–4.

Hampers LC, Cha S, Gutglass DJ, Binns HJ, Krug SE. 1999. Language barriers and resource utilization in a pediatric emergency department. *Pediatrics* 103(6):1253–1256.

Han YY, Carcillo JA, Dragotta MA, Bills DM, Watson RS, Westerman ME, Orr RA. 2003. Early reversal of pediatric neonatal septic shock by community physicians is associated with improved outcome. *Pediatrics* 112(4):793–799.

Han YY, Carcillo JA, Venkataraman ST, Clark RS, Watson RS, Nguyen TC, Bayir H, Orr RA. 2005. Unexpected increased mortality after implementation of a commercially sold computerized physician order entry system. *Pediatrics* 116(6):1506–1512.

Hanson C, Strawser D. 1992. Family presence during cardiopulmonary resuscitation: Foote Hospital emergency department's nine-year perspective. *Journal of Emergency Nursing* 18(2):104–106.

Hanson T. 2001. Pediatric design—put yourself in some small shoes—design perspectives. *Healthcare Review.*

Hazinski MF, Markenson D, Neish S, Gerardi M, Hootman J, Nichol G, Taras H, Hickey R, O'Connor R, Potts J, van der Jagt E, Berger S, Schexnayder S, Garson A Jr, Doherty A, Smith S. 2004. Response to cardiac arrest and selected life-threatening medical emergencies: The medical emergency response plan for schools—a statement for healthcare providers, policymakers, school administrators, and community leaders. *Annals of Emergency Medicine* 43(1):83–99.

Helmer SD, Smith RS, Dort JM, Shapiro WM, Katan BS. 2000. Family presence during trauma resuscitation: A survey of American Association for the Surgery of Trauma and Emergency Nurses Association members. *The Journal of Trauma* 48(6):1015–1022; discussion 1023–1024.

Hemmelgarn A, Glisson C, Dukes D. 2001. Emergency room culture and the emotional support component of family-centered care. *Childrens Health Care* 30(2):93–110.

Henderson DP, Knapp JF. 2005. Report of the national consensus conference on family presence during pediatric cardiopulmonary resuscitation and procedures. *Pediatric Emergency Care* 21(11):787–791.

Heron S, Haley L Jr. 2001. Diversity in emergency medicine: A model program. *Academic Emergency Medicine* 8(2):192–195.

Hubble MW, Paschal KR. 2000. Medication calculation skills of practicing paramedics. *Prehospital Emergency Care* 4(3):253–260.

Hunt DL, Haynes RB, Hayward RS, Pim MA, Horsman J. 1998. Patient-specific evidence-based care recommendations for diabetes mellitus: Development and initial clinic experience with a computerized decision support system. *International Journal of Medical Informatics* 51(2–3):127–135.

Hunt EA, Hohenhaus SM, Luo X, Frush KS. 2006. Simulation of pediatric trauma stabilization in 35 North Carolina emergency departments: Identification of targets for performance improvement. *Pediatrics* 117(3):641–648.

IOM (Institute of Medicine). 2000. *To Err Is Human: Building a Safer Health System.* LT Kohn, JM Corrigan, MS Donaldson, eds. Washington, DC: National Academy Press.

IOM. 2001. *Crossing the Quality Chasm: A New Health System for the 21st Century.* Washington, DC: National Academy Press.

IOM. 2005. *Safe Medical Devices for Children.* Washington, DC: The National Academies Press.

Johnston BD, Rivara FP, Droesch RM, Dunn C, Copass MK. 2002. Behavior change counseling in the emergency department to reduce injury risk: A randomized, controlled trial. *Pediatrics* 110(2 Pt. 1):267–274.

Kapes B. 2005, April 1. Accurate, timely diagnosis of dermatoses in children critical. *Dermatology Times.* [Online]. Available: http://www.highbeam.com/doc/1G1-135648502.html [accessed September, 2005].

Kaushal R, Bates DW. 2002. Information technology and medication safety: What is the benefit? *Quality & Safety in Health Care* 11(3):261–265.

Kaushal R, Bates DW, Landrigan C, McKenna KJ, Clapp MD, Federico F, Goldmann DA. 2001. Medication errors and adverse drug events in pediatric inpatients. *Journal of the American Medical Association* 285(16):2114–2120.

Knapp J, Mulligan-Smith D. 2005. Death of a child in the emergency department. *Pediatrics* 115(5):1432–1437.

Kozer E, Scolnik D, Macpherson A, Keays T, Shi K, Luk T, Koren G. 2002. Variables associated with medication errors in pediatric emergency medicine. *Pediatrics* 110(4):737–742.

Krebel MS, Clayton C, Graham C. 1996. Child life programs in the pediatric emergency department. *Pediatric Emergency Care* 12(1):13–15.

Leape LL, Brennan TA, Laird N, Lawthers AG, Localio AR, Barnes BA, Hebert L, Newhouse JP, Weiler PC, Hiatt H. 1991. The nature of adverse events in hospitalized patients. Results of the Harvard Medical Practice Study II. *New England Journal of Medicine* 324(6):377–384.

Lehmann CU. 2003. Medical information systems in pediatrics. *Pediatrics* 111(3):679.

Levine SR, Cohen RM, Blanchard NR, Frederico F, Magelli M, Lomax C, Greiner G, Poole RL, Lee CKK, Lesko A. 2001. Guidelines for preventing medication errors in pediatrics. *Journal of Pediatric Pharmacological Therapy* 6:426–442.

Lewandowski LA, Tesler MD, eds. 2003. *Family Centered Care: Putting it into Action: The SPN/ANA Guide to Family-Centered Care.* Washington, DC: SPN and ANA.

Losek JD. 2004. Acetaminophen dose accuracy and pediatric emergency care. *Pediatric Emergency Care* 20(5):285–288.

Loyacono TR. 2001. Family-centered prehospital care. *Emergency Medical Services* 30(6):83.

Mace SE, Barata IA, Cravero JP, Dalsey WC, Godwin SA, Kennedy RM, Malley KC, Moss RL, Sacchetti AD, Warden CR, Wears RL. 2004. Clinical policy: Evidence-based approach to pharmacologic agents used in pediatric sedation and analgesia in the emergency department. *Journal of Pediatric Surgery* 39(10):1472–1484.

MacLean S, Guzzetta C, White C, Fontaine D, Eichhorn D, Meyers T, Desy P. 2003. Family presence during cardiopulmonary resuscitation and invasive procedures: Practices of critical care and emergency nurses. *Journal of Emergency Nursing* 29(3):208–221.

Maldonado T, Avner J. 2004. Triage of the pediatric patient in the emergency department: Are we all in agreement? *Pediatrics* 114(2):356–360.

March CA, Jay MS. 1993. Adolescents in the emergency department: An overview. *Adolescent Medicine* 4(1):1–10.

Marcin JP, Seifert S, Cho M, Cole SL, Romano PS. 2005, May 16. Medication errors among acutely ill and injured children presenting to rural emergency departments. Presentation to the *Pediatric Academic Societies Meeting*. Washington, DC.

Markenson DS, Domeier RM. 2003. The use of automated external defibrillators in children. *Prehospital Emergency Care* 7(2):258–264.

McCaig LF, Burt CW. 2005. *National Hospital Ambulatory Medical Care Survey: 2003 Emergency Department Summary*. Hyattsville, MD: National Center for Health Statistics.

McCaig LF, Ly N. 2002. *National Hospital Ambulatory Medical Care Survey: 2000 Emergency Department Summary. Advance Data from Vital and Health Statistics; No. 326*. Hyattsville, MD: National Center for Health Statistics.

Meyers TA, Eichhorn DJ, Guzzetta CE. 1998. Do families want to be present during CPR? A retrospective survey. *Journal of Emergency Nursing* 24(5):400–405.

Meyers TA, Eichhorn DJ, Guzzetta CE, Clark AP, Klein JD, Taliaferro E, Calvin A. 2000. Family presence during invasive procedures and resuscitation. *American Journal of Nursing* 100(2):32–42; quiz 43.

Mitchell MH, Lynch MB. 1997. Should relatives be allowed in the resuscitation room? *Journal of Accident & Emergency Medicine* 14(6):366–369; discussion 370.

Moreland P. 2005. Family presence during invasive procedures and resuscitation in the emergency department: A review of the literature. *Journal of Emergency Nursing* 31(1):58–72; quiz 119.

National Association of Emergency Medical Technicians. 2000a. *Family-Centered Prehospital Care: Partnering with Families to Improve Care. Fact Sheet*. Washington, DC: National Association of Emergency Medical Technicians.

National Association of Emergency Medical Technicians. 2000b. *Guidelines for Providing Family-Centered Prehospital Care*. Rockville, MD: HRSA.

National Cancer Institute and Society for Pediatric Radiology. 2002. *Radiation and Pediatric Computed Technology*. Rockville, MD: National Cancer Institute.

NHTSA (National Highway Traffic Safety Administration). 2002. *Patient Safety in Emergency Medical Services*. Washington, DC: NHTSA.

Null J. 2006. *Hyperthermia Deaths of Children in Hot Vehicles*. Unpublished report. [Online]. Available: http://funnel.sfsu.edu:16080/courses/metr100.2/null%20hyperthermia.ppt [accessed March 2006].

O'Brien MM, Creamer KM, Hill EE, Welham J. 2002. Tolerance of family presence during pediatric cardiopulmonary resuscitation: A snapshot of military and civilian pediatricians, nurses, and residents. *Pediatric Emergency Care* 18(6):409–413.

O'Connor RE, Slovis CM, Hunt RC, Pirrallo RG, Savre MR. 2002. Eliminating errors in emergency medical services: Realities and recommendations. *Prehospital Emergency Care* 6(1):107–113.

Oren E, Shaffer ER, Guglielmo BJ. 2003. Impact of emerging technologies on medication errors and adverse drug events. *American Journal of Health-System Pharmacy* 60(14):1447–1458.

Pence K. 2000. Pediatric design: Beyond big bird murals—design perspectives—design options for pediatric hospitals and clinics. *Healthcare Review.*

Physician Insurers Association of America. 1993. *Medication Error Study.* Washington, DC: Physician Insurers Association of America.

Rapkin K. 1999. Pediatric "off-label" prescribing: What every APN should know. *The Internet Journal of Advanced Nurse Practice* 3(1).

Reves JG. 2003. "Smart pump" technology reduces errors. *Anesthesia Patient Safety Foundation* 18(1).

Reznek M, Harter P, Krummel T. 2002. Virtual reality and simulation: Training the future emergency physician. *Academic Emergency Medicine* 9(1):78–87.

Risser DT, Rice MM, Salisbury ML, Simon R, Jay GD, Berns SD. 1999. The potential for improved teamwork to reduce medical errors in the emergency department. The MedTeams Research Consortium. *Annals of Emergency Medicine* 34(3):373–383.

Sacchetti A, Lichenstein R, Carraccio CA, Harris RH. 1996. Family member presence during pediatric emergency department procedures. *Pediatric Emergency Care* 12(4):268–271.

Sacchetti A, Paston C, Carraccio C. 2005. Family members do not disrupt care when present during invasive procedures. *Academic Emergency Medicine* 12(5):477–479.

Salisbury ML. 2005. *LLINK Upload: All Abstracts. Patient Safety Award Submissions, 2004.* Falls Church, VA: Department of Defense Patient Safety Program.

Samson RA, Berg RA, Bingham R. 2003. Use of automated external defibrillators for children: An update—an advisory statement from the Pediatric Advanced Life Support Task Force, International Liaison Committee on Resuscitation. *Pediatrics* 112(1 Pt. 1):163–168.

Saunders RP, Abraham MR, Crosby MJ, Thomas K, Edwards WH. 2003. Evaluation and development of potentially better practices for improving family-centered care in neonatal intensive care units. *Pediatrics* 111(4):e437–e499.

Schenkel S. 2000. Promoting patient safety and preventing medical error in emergency departments. *Academic Emergency Medicine* 7(11):1204–1222.

Schwarz A. 2006. Shock. *Emedicine.* [Online]. Available: http://www.emedicine.com/PED/topic3047.htm [accessed March 2006].

Selbst SM, Fein JA, Osterhoudt K, Ho W. 1999. Medication errors in a pediatric emergency department. *Pediatric Emergency Care* 15(1):1–4.

Selbst SM, Levine S, Mull C, Bradford K, Friedman M. 2004. Preventing medical errors in pediatric emergency medicine. *Pediatric Emergency Care* 20(10):702–709.

Shapiro MJ, Morey JC, Small SD, Langford V, Kaylor CJ, Jagminas L, Suner S, Salisbury ML, Simon R, Jay GD. 2004. Simulation based teamwork training for emergency department staff: Does it improve clinical team performance when added to an existing didactic teamwork curriculum? *Quality & Safety in Health Care* 13(6):417–421.

Shiffman RN, Spooner AS, Kwiatkowski K, Flatley Brennan P. 2001. Information technology for children's health and health care: Report on the information technology in children's health care expert meeting, September 21–22, 2000. *Journal of the American Medical Informatics Association* 8(6):546–551.

Slonim AD, LaFleur BJ, Ahmed W, Joseph JG. 2003. Hospital-reported medical errors in children. *Pediatrics* 111(3):617–621.

Smith-Coggins R, Rosekind MR, Buccino KR, Dinges DF, Moser RP. 1997. Rotating shiftwork schedules: Can we enhance physician adaptation to night shifts? *Academic Emergency Medicine* 4(10):951–961.

Sprague L. 1999. *Reducing Medical Error: Can You Be as Safe in a Hospital as You Are in a Jet?* (Issue Brief No. 740). Washington, DC: National Health Policy Forum.

Stiell A, Forster AJ, Stiell IG, van Walraven C. 2003. Prevalence of information gaps in the emergency department and the effect on patient outcomes. *Canadian Medical Association Journal* 169(10):1023–1028.

Tanzi E, Silverberg N. 2005, June 14. Meningococcemia. *Emedicine*. [Online]. Available: http://www.emedicine.com/DERM/topic261.htm [accessed January 2006].

Thomas EJ, Studdert DM, Burstin HR, Orav EJ, Zeena T, Williams EJ, Howard KM, Weiler PC, Brennan TA. 2000. Incidence and types of adverse events and negligent care in Utah and Colorado. *Medical Care* 38(3):261–271.

Trautlein JJ, Lambert RL, Miller J. 1984. Malpractice in the emergency department: Review of 200 cases. *Annals of Emergency Medicine* 13(9 Pt. 1):709–711.

University of Michigan Health System. 2005. *Pediatric Human Patient Simulator*. [Online]. Available: http://www.med.umich.edu/em/children/edu/pedshumansim.htm [accessed January 25, 2006].

Vinen J. 2000. Incident monitoring in emergency departments: An Australian model. *Academic Emergency Medicine* 7(11):1290–1297.

Walsh-Kelly CM, Melzer-Lange MD, Hennes HM, Lye P, Hegenbarth M, Sty J, Starshak R. 1995. Clinical impact of radiograph misinterpretation in a pediatric ED and the effect of physician training level. *American Journal of Emergency Medicine* 13(3):262–264.

Walsh-Kelly CM, Hennes HM, Melzer-Lange MD. 1997. False-positive preliminary radiograph interpretations in a pediatric emergency department: Clinical and economic impact. *American Journal of Emergency Medicine* 15(4):354–356.

Weingart SN, Wilson RM, Gibberd RW, Harrison B. 2000. Epidemiology of medical error. *British Medical Journal* 320(7237):774–777.

Weinger MB, Ancoli-Israel S. 2002. Sleep deprivation and clinical performance. *Journal of the American Medical Association* 287(8):955–957.

Weiss SJ, Derlet R, Arndahl J, Ernst AA, Richards J, Fernandez-Frackelton M, Schwab R, Stair TO, Vicellio P, Levy D, Brautigan M, Johnson A, Nick TG, Fernandez-Frankelton M. 2004. Estimating the degree of emergency department overcrowding in academic medical centers: Results of the national ED overcrowding study (NEDOCS). *Academic Emergency Medicine* 11(4):408.

White AA, Wright SW, Blanco R, Lemonds B, Sisco J, Bledsoe S, Irwin C, Isenhour J, Pichert JW. 2004. Cause-and-effect analysis of risk management files to assess patient care in the emergency department. *Academic Emergency Medicine* 11(10):1035–1041.

Wilson KM, Klein JD. 2000. Adolescents who use the emergency department as their usual source of care. *Archives of Pediatrics & Adolescent Medicine* 154(4):361–365.

Wolfer J, Gaynard L, Goldberger J, Laidley LN, Thompson R. 1998. An experimental evaluation of a model child life program. *Child Health Care* 16(4):244–254.

Wolfram RW, Turner ED. 1996. Effects of parental presence during children's venipuncture. *Academic Emergency Medicine* 3(1):58–64.

Wolfram RW, Turner ED, Philput C. 1997. Effects of parental presence during young children's venipuncture. *Pediatric Emergency Care* 13(5):325–328.

Woodward GA, Fleegler EW. 2000. Should parents accompany pediatric interfacility ground ambulance transports? The parent's perspective. *Pediatric Emergency Care* 16(6):383–390.

Woodward GA, Fleegler EW. 2001. Should parents accompany pediatric interfacility ground ambulance transports? Results of a national survey of pediatric transport team managers. *Pediatric Emergency Care* 17(1):22–27.

Yee LY. 2005. *AB 775 Fact Sheet*. [Online]. Available: http://www.anacalifornia.org/B%20775%20Fact%20Sheet.pdf [accessed January 2006].

6

Improving Emergency Preparedness and Response for Children Involved in Disasters

The term "disaster" denotes a low-probability but high-impact event that causes a large number of individuals to become ill or injured. The International Federation of Red Cross and Red Crescent Societies defines a disaster as an event that causes more than 10 deaths, affects more than 100 people, or leads to an appeal by those affected for assistance (Bravata et al., 2004). This report expands this definition to include any event that creates a significant, short-term spike in the demand for emergency care services that can be adequately addressed only through extraordinary measures.

During the development of this report, the most destructive natural disaster in the nation's history occurred. On August 29, 2005, Hurricane Katrina struck the Gulf Coast of Louisiana and Mississippi, leaving more than 1,300 people dead, countless injured, and more than 1 million displaced. The aftermath of the hurricane created a humanitarian crisis unparalleled in U.S. history, with federal disaster declarations covering 90,000 square miles (Associated Press 2005a,c). More than 4,500 children were reported missing to the National Center for Missing and Exploited Children after the storm; a month later, only half of those children had been located (Ong, 2005).

Hurricane Katrina is an extreme example of a disaster in terms of its scope and impact; most disaster incidents tend to be smaller in size and affect a fraction of these numbers of people. However, all disasters present special challenges for emergency providers. These types of incidents create a sharp imbalance between the supply of and demand for existing resources (Noji, 1996). The coordination of personnel, equipment, and medical capacity involved in responding to a disaster in a timely manner presents a number of difficulties. Understaffed and overcrowded emergency departments (EDs) are unlikely to be able to absorb the influx of patients from such an incident (Shute and Marcus, 2001). Emergency medical services (EMS) systems lacking sufficient resources even for day-to-day operations are overwhelmed in the event of a large-scale disaster. Deficiencies in the emergency care system for children that are evident during normal operations in the areas of pediatric equipment, medication and supplies, and pediatric training are greatly exacerbated during a disaster. The available evidence reveals that the nation's emergency care system is poorly prepared for disasters (Schur et al., 2004):

• *Surge capacity.* Surge capacity refers to a hospital's ability to manage a sudden, unexpected increase in patient volume that would otherwise severely challenge or exceed its normal capacity (Hick et al., 2004). Few American hospitals have the capacity to handle the increased volume of patients likely to result from a large-scale disaster or an epidemic, particularly if the patients are infants or small children (Kaji and Lweis, 2004; Oster and Chaffee, 2004).

• *Surveillance.* In public health parlance, surveillance refers to the ability to collect and analyze morbidity, mortality, and other relevant ED data in order to identify and control health threats. Few automatic, real-time surveillance systems are in operation across the United States that can accurately alert public health officials to an impending crisis (GAO, 2003a).

• *Coordination/communication.* In the event of a disaster or public health emergency, emergency care personnel may have to coordinate their efforts with personnel from other hospitals; EMS agencies; and public safety agencies, such as fire and police. A high level of coordination is required. However, communications systems are often not secure or reliable during such an event. Many communications systems are incompatible across regions or even across agencies within the same community (GAO, 2001).

• *Training.* The medical and nonmedical needs of victims of a disaster or public health emergency may vary from the type of care normally delivered by emergency care providers. Emergency personnel must be able to recognize and meet these needs. Overwhelmingly, research indicates that academic, on-the-job, and continuing education training in disaster response for emergency care personnel is insufficient, particularly when it comes to treating victims of chemical, biological, and nuclear events (Treat et al., 2001; GAO, 2003a; Rivera and Char, 2004).

• *Protective equipment.* Protective equipment refers to clothing and garments, respiratory equipment, and other barriers designed to shield emergency care personnel from chemical, biological, or other physical hazards. Evidence suggests that many emergency care providers are inadequately equipped for routine practice, and disasters make it difficult or impossible for providers to follow even normal safety procedures (Jackson et al., 2004).

Since September 11, 2001, much attention has been focused on disaster preparedness. While significant resources have been spent on protecting and securing the nation's infrastructure, fewer resources have been devoted to improving the readiness of the emergency care system (National Advisory Committee on Children and Terrorism, 2003; Sears, 2005). EMS systems, for example, have received only 4 to 6 percent of federal disaster preparedness funds from the Department of Homeland Security (DHS) and the Department of Health and Human Services (DHHS) (GAO, 2003b; Center for Catastrophe Preparedness and Response, 2005). Funding for hospital preparedness has been limited and slow to reach hospitals (McHugh et al., 2004). Even less has been done to safeguard the health and well-being of children (National Advisory Committee on Children and Terrorism, 2003), the most vulnerable age group in many types of disasters (National Center for Disaster Preparedness, 2003).

Though it is still too early to assemble all of the lessons learned from Hurricane Katrina, we have learned enough from this and other disasters to recognize that improved pediatric planning for disasters is necessary. In Chapter 3, the committee emphasized the importance of integrating pediatric planning for emergency care and disasters at the regional level. In this chapter, the committee focuses on concrete actions that federal agencies and regional emergency care systems should take to address pediatric needs in the event of a disaster. First, however, the chapter reviews what is known about the challenges of caring for children in a disaster and recent efforts to improve preparedness for treating these especially vulnerable disaster victims.

CARING FOR CHILDREN IN DISASTERS

Children react differently than adults to medical emergencies because of anatomical, physiological, developmental, and emotional differences. Because of these differences, children are among the most vulnerable individuals in the event of a disaster.

Children are more prone to injury in a fire or a biological or chemical attack because they take more breaths per minute, and their breathing zone is closer to the ground. They also have thinner skin, which provides less protection and allows greater absorption of toxic chemicals (AAP, 2002). They are more vulnerable to the effects of infectious agents that produce vomiting and/or diarrhea because they have less fluid reserve than adults and can become dehydrated more rapidly (Illinois EMS-C, 2005; CNN.

com, 2005). If they sustain burns, children have a greater likelihood of life-threatening fluid loss and susceptibility to secondary infections (Shannon, 2004). Additionally, if they sustain injuries that cause blood loss, children develop irreversible shock and die more quickly than adults (AAP, 2002). Finally, very young children's cognitive and motor abilities limit their ability to escape dangerous situations.

Younger patients require specialized equipment and different approaches to treatment in the event of a disaster. Children cannot be properly decontaminated in adult decontamination units (National Center for Disaster Preparedness, 2003) because they require adjustments to the water temperature and pressure (heated, high-volume, low-pressure water). Rescuers also need to have child-size clothing on-hand for use after the decontamination (NASEMSD, 2004). Children require different antibiotics and different dosages to counter many chemical and biological agents (National Center for Disaster Preparedness, 2003). Natural disasters pose similar challenges to pediatric care. Hurricane Katrina highlighted the social service needs of children during evacuation and sheltering—identification, supervision, special food (formula), clothing and sanitation (diapers), and sleeping accommodations (cribs) must be available (Foltin et al., forthcoming).

Like adults, children require mental health services after a disaster, and these services must be age appropriate. The most common indicators of distress in children are changes in their behavior—for example, a shift from being an outgoing child to being shy and withdrawn and behavior regression, in which past behaviors such as thumb sucking or baby talk reemerge. At the same time, children's reactions vary based on their age, their cognitive level, their family's proximity and reactions to the disaster, and whether their exposure to the disaster was direct. Preschool-aged children lack the skills needed to cope with stress, and the reactions of their parents strongly affect them. They worry about abandonment, whether they have lost a toy, a favorite pet, or a family member. School-aged children understand the concept of permanent change and loss and will therefore suffer from fears and anxieties. They may become preoccupied by the disaster and want to discuss its details at length, sometimes to the extent of interfering with other activities. Preadolescents want to know that their fears are appropriate and shared by others. Adolescents have childlike reactions mixed with adult responses. They may feel overwhelmed by their emotions and therefore be unable to discuss them with their family. They also may demonstrate more acting out and risk-taking behaviors than normal (NIMH, 2001).

Evidence from Previous Disasters

Only a handful of published studies address the effects of disasters on children and their specific needs during such an event (National Center for

Disaster Preparedness, 2003). Primarily, the available studies provide insight into the epidemiology of pediatric injury after a disaster. One example describes ED visits at Miami Children's Hospital in the weeks following Hurricane Andrew, which struck 30 miles south of Miami, Florida, in 1994. In the week following the hurricane, the hospital experienced a 41 percent increase in ED visits, or an average of 57 additional patients per day. The ED also saw an increase in patients over age 18 (2.4 versus 1 percent). This increase was likely due to the loss of electricity and structural damage that occurred after the storm, leaving few options for medical care beyond EDs for local residents and rescuers alike (Quinn et al., 1994).

Although Hurricane Andrew was an extraordinary event, the medical needs of children affected by hurricanes and other large-scale natural disasters are rather ordinary. In the week following the hurricane, conditions such as acute gastroenteritis, impetigo (bacterial skin infection), and open wounds were diagnosed more frequently, while genitourinary problems, nonspecific abdominal pain, and soft tissue injuries were seen less often. In the second week after the hurricane, the ED noted increases in dermatological problems, including cellulitis, and in injuries, including open wounds; a decrease was noted in respiratory problems, including upper respiratory infections. The increase in open wounds seen in the weeks following the hurricane was due largely to incidents related to the cleanup effort, and in children likely reflected their increasing curiosity about their changed environment. Open-wound management is a time-consuming task, particularly for uncooperative and frightened pediatric patients; thus although patient volume had returned to normal levels by the second week after the hurricane (Quinn et al., 1994), additional physician staffing was necessary.

Other studies of single incidents have been conducted. One such study showed that in the event of a school bus crash, head, neck, and spine injuries are common (Lapner et al., 2003). Another study, analyzing pediatric deaths and injuries after the Oklahoma City bombing in 1995, provided some information on the spectrum of pediatric injuries after a bomb blast, which in this case produced a high incidence of cranial injuries. Among the 19 children who died in the blast, the most common injuries were skull fractures, cerebral evisceration, abdominal or thoracic injuries, amputations, arm and leg fractures, and burns. All had extensive cutaneous contusions, avulsions, and lacerations. Understanding the spectrum of injuries that occur in a disaster not only helps emergency providers better anticipate what to expect from pediatric victims, but also provides insight into possible preventive measures that could mitigate the effects of such an incident. For example, changes to the design of school buses might be able to mitigate some of the injuries likely to occur in the event of a crash (Lapner et al., 2003).

Some studies also provide insight into how well the emergency care system responds to pediatric patients in a disaster. After the 1990 crash on

Long Island, New York, of a plane that carried 25 children among its 160 passengers, records were obtained on the 22 child survivors. The county had a disaster plan in place, which stated that cases involving severe burns, severe trauma, or severed limbs must be transported to hospitals capable of providing care for those injuries. The plan also called for EMS to distribute the balance of casualties with serious injuries to the closest hospitals, while individuals with minor injuries were supposed to be transported farther away. However, only 1 of the 7 critically injured children was transported to a level I pediatric center. Of the remaining 6 children, 1 was transported to a level II center and 5 to a level III center. Only two of the 5 critically injured children transported to level III facilities were subsequently transported to a high-level pediatric center. The closest level I pediatric trauma center, which was equipped with a helipad, received no patients from the crash. It is unclear why transport destinations were unrelated to the severity of injuries (van Amerongen et al., 1993).

While the majority of studies of pediatric disaster victims indicate that trauma is a major risk, the experience of Hurricane Katrina indicates that this is not always the case. Initial reports from front-line medical providers at the Astrodome in Houston, Texas, which served as a shelter for 23,000 hurricane evacuees, revealed an almost complete absence of trauma cases (Mattox, 2005). Thus disaster and mass casualty guidelines heavily based in trauma planning may not be appropriate for all disaster scenarios. In the immediate aftermath of Hurricane Katrina, emergency care providers from disaster management teams dealt with numerous cases involving exacerbation of asthma and diabetes. Reportedly, a great number of people needed prescription refills. By day 4 in the Astrodome, gastroenteritis had become a common ailment (one that is potentially more severe in infants and the elderly). Cholera was also a concern (Mattox, 2005).

Pediatric Disaster Planning and the Current State of Preparedness

The needs of children have traditionally been overlooked in disaster planning. Historically, the military was considered the only target of potential biological, chemical, and radiological attacks, so the focus for training, equipment, and facilities was on the care of healthy young adults (National Center for Disaster Preparedness, 2003). But even initial guidelines for civilian disaster preparedness were not appropriate for the care of children (National Center for Disaster Preparedness, 2003). A 1997 Federal Emergency Management Agency (FEMA) survey found that none of the states had incorporated pediatric components into their disaster plans (National Advisory Committee on Children and Terrorism, 2003; Illinois EMS-C, 2005).

Recognizing the absence of pediatric concerns in disaster planning, the first field triage model developed specifically for children was created in 1995, then revised in 2001. Triage is a primary and critical component of disaster management since resources must quickly be put to their most efficient use to do the greatest good for the greatest number of casualties. The pediatric triage model, called JumpSTART, is based on the adult triage tool START and helps prehospital providers make decisions so under- and overtriage will be minimized (Romig, 2002). JumpSTART is widely used today and allows emergency workers to triage children within 30 seconds. However, the model is the product of expert consensus; it has not been empirically validated and therefore is not evidence based (Ohio Pediatric Disaster Preparedness Committee, 2004).

Attention to the issue of pediatric disaster preparedness grew considerably after September 11, 2001. A number of initiatives to address pediatric disaster planning and preparedness began to emerge. In October 2001, the American Academy of Pediatrics (AAP) created a Task Force on Terrorism consisting of 12 pediatricians (Hicks, 2003), with the aim of ensuring that pediatricians and other providers will have the information they need as it becomes available and that children's needs will be considered in all planning efforts. In 2006, the task force published Pediatric Terrorism and Disaster Preparedness: A Resource for Pediatricians, designed to give pediatricians and other providers practical advice and information on best practices in the area of disaster preparedness.

In February 2003, a 3-day national consensus conference was held to discuss the particular vulnerabilities of children to terrorist attacks and possible responses. This represented one of the first efforts to define issues in pediatric disaster preparedness. The conference was sponsored by the Agency for Healthcare Research and Quality (AHRQ) and the Maternal and Child Health Bureau (MCHB) and was attended by nearly 70 subject matter experts, as well as representatives from government agencies and professional organizations. Conferees developed recommendations on a number of broad and specific issues and published them later that year (National Center for Disaster Preparedness, 2003). Because of a lack of evidence, however, these recommendations are largely a product of expert consensus.

At around the same time, the National Advisory Committee on Children and Terrorism (NACCT) released a report to the Secretary of Health and Human Services that contained a number of recommendations regarding areas in need of funding and program development. The NACCT was created by Congress through the Public Health Security and Bioterrorism Preparedness and Response Act of 2002. The committee's goal was to prepare a comprehensive public health strategy for ensuring the safety of children and meeting their needs in the face of the threat of terrorism. Unfortunately, the majority of the recommendations developed by the NACCT have not been implemented. In July 2005, an expert meeting on pediatric bioterrorism preparedness was convened to review the 2003 NACCT recommendations and update steps for moving forward. The meeting attendees agreed on the need to move quickly to disseminate the recommendations of the 2003 NACCT report and to elevate pediatric bioterrorism preparedness to the forefront of the national agenda.

There is some evidence of progress on pediatric disaster preparedness at the federal level. The Health Resources and Services Administration (HRSA) has set a benchmark for all states to establish a system that allows for the triage, treatment, and disposition of 500 adult and pediatric patients per 1 million population who suffer from acute illness or trauma requiring hospitalization following a biological, chemical, radiological, or explosive terrorist incident (AHRQ, 2004). Inclusion of pediatric patients in the benchmark language was a direct result of lobbying by the pediatric community. Additionally, guidance for the bioterrorism grants offered by HRSA, AHRQ, and the Office of Domestic Preparedness indicates that all projects should consider the needs of children.

Disaster preparedness has also been a key area of focus for the Emergency Medical Services for Children (EMS-C) program. The program has focused in particular on the inclusion of pediatric issues in state disaster plans, since a 1997 FEMA survey indicated that no states had done so. One of the objectives in the EMS-C 5-Year Plan, 2001–2005, was to increase to 100% the number of states, Tribal Reservations, or Federal Territories that include pediatric issues in State emergency disaster plans (DHHS et al., 2000). By 2003, at least 13 states had formally assigned a pediatric representative to their state disaster preparedness committee. More detailed information on state disaster plans was available in 2004 in a report from the National Association of State EMS Directors (NASEMSD). Through a survey of all states and territories (to which 46 of 56 state EMS directors responded), the NASEMSD found that states continued to fall short of including the needs of children in their plans. For example, only 85 percent of respondents noted that according to their state plan, hospitals were required to have sufficient pediatric equipment and medications, as well as capacity for appropriate assessment, treatment, and decontamination of children exposed to radiological, chemical, or biological agents. More troubling, only 6 states said their hospitals were currently equipped with sufficient pediatric equipment and medications (NASEMSD, 2004). Many state respondents did indicate that they were in the process of improving the pediatric components of their state plan. This effort will likely be assisted by a model pediatric component for state disaster plans being developed under an EMS-C program Targeted Issues Grant at the time of this writing.

While there is clearly more work to be done at the federal and state levels with regard to pediatric disaster preparedness, progress is needed at the regional and provider levels as well. For example, a study of EMS agencies in Arkansas revealed that only one-quarter of the agencies with a written plan for responding to mass casualty events had specific provisions in that plan for the care of children (Dick et al., 2004). Regions and providers must consider a number of important issues as they develop disaster plans. For example, in developing regional disaster plans, many planning bodies have identified shelter sites for the public. However, few have taken the necessary steps to ensure that these sites have in place the resources—diapers, formula, and other pediatric supplies—that will be required if children are sheltered at these locations. Additionally, protocols are being developed to guide emergency care providers on how to conduct a mass decontamination, but these protocols infrequently account for the needs of children—for example, the strength of the water stream, the water temperature, and who (parent versus rescuer) should carry an infant or a young child through the decontamination unit. The absence of these considerations and others points to the importance of having pediatric representation on planning bodies involved in emergency care, trauma, and disaster planning.

Another consideration is the extent to which emergency care and other medical providers should educate the public regarding the care of children in disasters. Well-meaning but misinformed parents may not act in the best interest or safety of their children. For example, after postal workers in New York City were exposed to anthrax spores in 2001, some of the workers said they intended to give the antibiotics they received (Cipro in most cases) to their children "to protect them from anthrax." Not only is anthrax not contagious, but the antibiotics given to the postal workers were never intended for use in children. Additionally, some workers said they were reluctant to hug or touch their children out of fear that they might transfer the anthrax spores (Aghababian, 2002).

IMPROVING RESPONSE TO DISASTERS FOR PEDIATRIC VICTIMS

The evidence summarized above indicates that the nation's emergency care system is not well prepared for disasters involving children and that the needs of children in disasters are frequently overlooked. This is not necessarily an indication that planners fail to recognize or appreciate the needs of children, but rather a sign that planners are overwhelmed by the number of competing needs. There are so many shortcomings in disaster preparedness that children's needs often fall to the wayside. The committee believes pediatric concerns should be in the forefront of disaster planning and recommends that **federal agencies (the Department of Health and Human Services, the National Highway Traffic Safety Administration, and the Department of Homeland Security), in partnership with states and regional** planning bodies and emergency care providers, convene a panel with multidisciplinary expertise to develop strategies for addressing pediatric needs in the event of a disaster. This effort should encompass the following:

- Development of strategies to minimize parent–child separation and improved methods for reuniting separated children with their families.
- Development of strategies to improve the level of pediatric expertise on Disaster Medical Assistance Teams and other organized disaster response teams.
- Development of disaster plans that address pediatric surge capacity for both injured and noninjured children.
- Development of and improved access to specific medical and mental health therapies, as well as social services, for children in the event of a disaster.
- Development of policies to ensure that disaster drills include a pediatric mass casualty incident at least once every 2 years. (6.1)

Minimizing Separation of Families

Hurricane Katrina highlighted a critical problem associated with evacuation and sheltering in the event of a disaster—the separation of children from their parents. As caregivers and children first fled from the impending hurricane and later were moved from evacuation shelters, many children became separated in the chaos. For almost a week, for example, 16-year-old Reshad B. was separated from his grandmother, his primary caregiver. The two were separated during the chaotic evacuation of the Louisiana Superdome, which served as a shelter for 10,000 New Orleans residents. He was taken to Texas, while she was transported to Kentucky. For nearly a week, Rashad lived in a Houston shelter not knowing what had happened to his grandmother. They were reunited through the efforts of the National Center for Missing and Exploited Children (Associated Press, 2005b).

There are hundreds of stories like that of Reshad B. Even weeks after the storm, Texas Child Protective Services workers reported caring for nearly 50 unaccompanied children in shelters (Associated Press, 2005b); others were temporarily placed in foster care. While organizations such as the National Center for Missing and Exploited Children and the Red Cross, as well as state agencies, worked actively to reunite families and could report many examples of success, too many children remained separated from their family members months after the storm. One of the challenges for officials was not knowing whether the missing child or parent had survived the storm, since many of the recovered bodies were not identified for a prolonged period of time. Another challenge was reuniting young, preverbal children with their parents, since these children were too young to give rescuers and social workers their name or identify family members in photographs.

There are currently no clear guidelines to direct planning in the event of parent–child separation (Freishtat, 2002). In developing such guidance, policy makers and planners should consider a number of issues. First, in the event of a disaster, particularly one that occurs without warning, children may be away from their parents in the custody of a school, day care center, babysitter, or other nonfamily caretaker; older children may be with friends or even alone. Disaster plans should not assume that children are in the custody of their parents when a disaster strikes. Second, during evacuation and sheltering, care should be taken to minimize the separation of children from their caretakers. Emergency workers overseeing the process should, to the extent possible, see that children remain paired with a parent or caretaker at all times. If children must be separated from their parents—for example, if they must be triaged to different medical institutions—emergency workers should obtain complete identification information on the child from the parent before the separation occurs. Emergency workers should also assign an individual to the task of overseeing the child until the government or family assumes custody.

Third, the steps taken to reunite families—registering children and adults and showing pictures of missing children on television—are reactive and should be evaluated (Foltin et al., forthcoming). Steps to make the identification of children easier in the future, such as widespread use of identification bracelets, name tags, or other means, should be considered. More sophisticated technologies should also be explored; for example, electronic tracking devices that contain a child's identification information, medical conditions, and medications would be helpful to officials trying to reunite families. Even if all children are easily identified, however, there will still be a need for reactive steps to reunify families if they are separated. Ideally, the most efficient and effective strategies should be used, but those strategies must take into account the loss of electricity and communications that may occur after a disaster. The nontraditional family structures that many children have must also be considered. Simply matching a child to a parent may not be sufficient; noncustodial parents or other relatives may need assurance of a child's whereabouts after a disaster as well.

These concerns are not hypothetical. Approximately 4,000 foster children were affected by Hurricane Katrina (Freddy Mac Foundation, 2005). One official from Louisiana's Department of Social Services reported that about a fourth of foster children in the custody of the state (approximately 500 children) had not been located almost a month after the storm (Cottman,

2005). The majority of foster children remained with their foster parents, but 1,000 of those families lost their homes and were displaced to other cities around the country (Freddy Mac Foundation, 2005).

Enhancing Pediatric Disaster Expertise

One of the major challenges of disaster planning and response for children is that the number of emergency providers specifically trained and equipped to handle children is limited (see Chapter 4). Although most community hospitals have pediatricians and ED physicians on staff, these providers may not have the specialized training and resources needed to care for children in the event of a disaster. It is speculated that most children's hospitals possess these resources, but they have done little specific planning or practice in managing chemical, biological, radiological, and nuclear exposure for children (National Advisory Committee on Children and Terrorism, 2003).

Emergency providers and other first responders who have limited experience in dealing with children may have a very difficult time performing in the event of a disaster. During such an event, for example, a provider may be drawn to give attention to a deceased child because of emotions; however, the provider must leave the child to address the medical needs of survivors, whether children or adults. All emergency providers and first responders should receive pediatric disaster training. One resource available to that end is the Pediatric Disaster Life Support (PDLS) course. A product of expert consensus, PDLS is a 2-day training program developed to enable EMS and ED providers (physicians and nurses) to better care for pediatric victims of a disaster. Created through an EMS-C grant, the course focuses heavily on the impact of natural disasters on children, but a portion is devoted to school violence (e.g., the Columbine school shootings are used as a case study) and intentional disasters, including terrorism (Aghababian, 2002). This course has not been widely adopted, however. It is estimated that several hundred providers from approximately 10 states have received PDLS training. The course is currently being revised to incorporate knowledge gained from more recent disasters involving children over the past 10 years (Personal communication, R. Aghababian, February 28, 2006). Pediatric disaster education should be widely accessible and an important component of training for all emergency care providers.

While prehospital and ED personnel who staff EMS and hospitals are key health care providers in the event of a disaster, DHHS's National Disaster Medical System (NDMS) will deploy Disaster Medical Assistance Teams (DMATs) to the site of such an incident to provide additional medical support. A DMAT is a group of professional and paraprofessional medical personnel who provide medical care during a disaster or other event

(National Disaster Medical System, 2005); it typically consists of 35 physicians, nurses, emergency medical technicians (EMTs), and support personnel (Lawrence, 2002). After arriving on site, DMATs triage and stabilize the injured, assist with the transfer of patients to hospitals in other areas, and set up temporary clinics for victims.

DMATs are organized by a sponsor, usually a major medical center, health department, or disaster organization. The sponsor signs a memorandum of agreement to recruit volunteer team members, coordinate training, and dispatch the team (National Disaster Medical System, 2005). The teams are able to provide care at a disaster site for up to 72 hours without resupply (Lawrence, 2002). In 2004, there were 43 DMATs nationwide (Mace and Bern, 2004; Mace and Jones, 2004), two of which were specialized pediatric teams. There is a standardized training program for all field teams, which includes a pediatric component (National Disaster Medical System, 2005).

The limited studies that have been conducted on DMATs have yielded two important findings with regard to pediatric patients: these patients constitute a considerable proportion of those treated by the teams, and the DMATs' pediatric training and resources need improvement. An analysis of patients treated in New Mexico's DMAT field clinics during four recent natural disasters found that pediatric patients represented a third of all patients treated by the team (Nufer and Gnauck, 2004). The median age of the pediatric patients was 4. The authors concluded that, based on the experience from these four disasters (two hurricanes, an earthquake, and a flood), DMATs should be adequately prepared to treat pediatric patients, particularly the very young (Nufer and Gnauck, 2004).

However, there is reason to be concerned that DMATs are not sufficiently prepared to treat pediatric patients. In the study of New Mexico's DMAT patient encounters, researchers found that the youngest children, those aged 0 to 2 months, had been sent to the hospital more frequently than those in other age groups and that the triage category for these children was more frequently missing. The researchers posited that these findings may signal providers' lack of comfort with caring for the very young (Nufer and Gnauck, 2004), something previous studies have also suggested (Glaeser et al., 2000).

While DMAT training includes a pediatric component, DMAT leaders do not express strong confidence in the area of pediatrics. In 2003, DMAT leaders were asked to rate their teams' pediatric training and abilities. Their responses (see Table 6-1) were not as positive as one would hope. The survey found that DMATs were not fully prepared for pediatric patients. Pediatric treatment tools most frequently lacking were backboards (62 percent of teams), a Broselow tape (46 percent), pediatric medications (38 percent), and cervical collars (38 percent). Pediatric burn management, pediatric pain management, psychosocial/mental health issues, and pediatric mock code

TABLE 6-1 Pediatric Preparedness of Disaster Medical Assistance Teams (DMATs)

Question to DMAT Leaders	Average Response (Likert Scale: 1 = not at all, 6 = a great degree)
How well does the standardized DMAT curriculum meet the needs of pediatric patients?	3.33 (+/–0.25)
How well is the team prepared for pediatric patients?	3.91 (+/–0.22)
How well does the team respond to a disaster with pediatric patients?	3.94 (+/–0.31)
How well is the team equipped to respond to a disaster with pediatric patients?	3.22 (+/–0.24)
How well is pediatric equipment organized?	3.08 (+/–0.29)
Agree that the system needs more pediatric specialty teams?	3.37 (+/–0.31)
Agree that current teams need more pediatric training?	3.68 (+/–0.34)

SOURCE: Mace and Bern, 2004.

practices were absent from the curriculum for 40 percent of DMATs (Mace and Bern, 2004).

The survey also provided insight into the DMAT members and their training and experience with regard to pediatric patients. The majority of DMAT physicians (74 percent) reported that they specialize in emergency medicine. Slightly more than half (54 percent) of physicians, 40 percent of nurses, 44 percent of midlevel providers (nurse practitioners and physician assistants), and 44 percent of paramedics reported working with children on a daily basis.

Many of the problems apparent in the emergency care system for children, particularly lack of equipment and training, are also apparent on DMATs. To address these shortcomings, strategies to improve the level of pediatric expertise on DMATs and other organized disaster response teams need to be developed. This can be accomplished by improving the pediatric training required of teams, equipping them with appropriate pediatric resources, and taking active steps to recruit pediatricians and pediatric emergency medicine physicians to serve on the teams.

Improving Pediatric Surge Capacity

While children represent approximately 25 percent of the U.S. population (U.S. Census Bureau, 2004), they consume a smaller proportion of inpatient hospital services (Freishtat, 2002). Since most children are relatively healthy, the U.S. hospital system is designed for a large number of adults, not children (Holbrook, 1991; Freishtat, 2002). As a result, compared with the resources available for adults, there are fewer pediatric hospital beds, pediatric specialists, and providers with experience caring for critically ill and injured children (Freishtat, 2002). In the event of a disaster, the capacity of the health care system to care for a large number of children is likely to be inadequate.

Although much of the focus of disaster planning has been on large-scale disasters, even modest incidents have the potential to push system resources to their limits. For example, a number of victims of the Rhode Island nightclub fire in 2003 required supplemental staff and specialized resources that overwhelmed local capacity (Hick et al., 2004). A total of 273 victims sought care at local hospitals. The closest hospital to the nightclub (3 miles away), Rhode Island's second largest, is a 359-bed acute care hospital that handles 58,000 ED visits per year. It received 82 patients, 25 percent of whom were admitted, while 25 percent were transferred to other hospitals. A level I trauma center located 12 miles away from the nightclub received 68 patients, approximately 63 percent of whom were admitted (Gutman et al., 2003). A number of other Rhode Island hospitals, as well as Mass General, University of Massachusetts Medical Center, and Shriners Hospital for Children, also received patients. It was only the second time Shriners had opened its doors to adult patients (Ginaitt, 2005).

What would have happened had the fire occurred in a venue filled with children? The hospitals most proximate to a disaster may not normally care for children but must still be ready to receive some pediatric victims. Children's hospitals, those with pediatric EDs, and others designated as having pediatric capabilities will be looked upon to provide the majority of care to children in critical condition, but their resources and capacities may be stretched to the limit. Other hospitals must be prepared to handle pediatric patients with more minor conditions and stabilize those in critical condition until they can be transported to a pediatric center. Pediatric centers should have predetermined means of communicating with one another so they can share patients in the event those in critical condition need to be evacuated. DMATs may be able to offer local emergency care providers some relief, but given that there are only two pediatric specialty DMATs nationwide, their reach would be limited in the event of a large-scale event.

A review of one pediatric disaster in England provides some insight into what could happen in the absence of regional planning for such disasters. In 1993, a double-decker bus full of school children was involved in a crash. Two children were killed and 56 injured. The local hospital received notification of the crash just as the first victims began to arrive. At that hospital, 42 injured children were taken to the ED. Most injuries were minor in nature, although 15 children were admitted; 4 had serious head injuries, and 2 required neurosurgical intervention. Although the hospital had a disaster plan in place, the lack of advance notification, the rapid influx of patients, and the lack of providers familiar with handling pediatric trauma injuries created difficulties (Wass et al., 1994). This incident also highlights the importance of all hospitals being prepared for pediatric emergencies, particularly in areas that lack pediatric centers.

Disaster planning must also take into account children who are not hurt but need evacuation and sheltering. The importance of having pediatric resources (e.g., formula, diapers) available in shelter locations was discussed earlier. Steps to ensure that these resources are on hand must be taken before a disaster strikes. Involvement of pediatric experts in disaster planning is critical to ensure that evacuation and sheltering plans can meet the needs of children, particularly those with special needs, as the plans are operationalized. Disaster plans should include protocols for schools and day care centers and other places where children congregate. Planners need to think about where children might be at different times of day. For example, had the September 11 attacks occurred a half hour earlier, while more than 500,000 New York City school children were in transit to school, where would the bus drivers have taken these children? Would the places selected have been adequately equipped to handle the surge of children?

Promoting Specific Therapies for Children

Children affected by disasters have a number of medical, mental health, and social service needs that must be met. Under the current system, however, services appropriate for children may not be available. As discussed in Chapter 5, medications appropriate for children are not always available; the same is true for antidotes in the event of a terrorist attack. Additionally, resources and therapies developed specifically for children may not be accessible when needed.

Potassium iodide prevents thyroid cancer and is highly recommended for children in the event of exposure to radioactive material. However, potassium iodide is currently available only in tablet form and therefore cannot be readily administered to infants and very young children. The pill can be dissolved in water, but since the resulting fluid is so salty, it must be mixed with something to disguise the taste. The tablet can be crushed and mixed with raspberry syrup, low-fat chocolate milk, or other drinks, but these mixtures will keep for only 7 days and must be stored in a refrigerator. Parents would have to crush a new tablet every 7 days to have the medication on hand when needed (FDA, 2006). Even if parents went through these steps every 7 days, however, the stability of potassium iodide when mixed with other liquids is not well known.

There are also issues related to the strategic national stockpile (SNS), which would be used in the event of a disaster severe enough to deplete local resources. Within the SNS are 12-hour push packages that contain pharmaceuticals, antidotes, and medical supplies designed for use during the early hours of an event. They are positioned in strategically located, secure warehouses ready for immediate deployment in the event of a disaster (CDC, 2004). Historically, the SNS did not meet the needs of most children, but that has changed somewhat. Today, there are pediatric representatives on every SNS advisory committee, and every new item for the SNS is reviewed for pediatric implications. However, the SNS must comply with Food and Drug Administration (FDA) labeling requirements, and if a medication is not approved for pediatric patients, it cannot be included in the push packages for children. Since most antidotes for terrorism agents are designed for adult use and not approved by the FDA for pediatric patients, they are not available for use in children (Markenson, 2005). Even with pediatric representation on SNS advisory committees, pediatric concerns are not fully addressed in developing the push packs because of the absence of approved antidotes for children.

There are also controversies regarding the use of Mark 1 kits for children. Mark 1 kits contain two antidotes—atropine and pralidoxime chloride—that are effective if a person is exposed to certain types of nerve gas. The consensus in the medical community is that this treatment is appropriate for infants and children with severe, life-threatening nerve agent toxicity (National Center for Disaster Preparedness, 2004). However, there are no protocols for providers with regard to using a Mark 1 kit to treat children because it is not approved by the FDA. Pediatric dosing for atropine was approved by the FDA in June 2003, but it remains unclear how emergency providers should treat children exposed to nerve gas; some may give children only the pediatric dose of atropine, while others may give them the full dose in the Mark 1 kit. The Mark 1 kit is not a unique example—no specific pediatric dosage guidelines exist for a large number of drugs used in disaster situations.

There is also some evidence that children's mental health needs often go unmet after a disaster. Based on a survey of parents, it is estimated that approximately 18 percent of children aged 6–17 in New York City had severe or very severe post-traumatic stress reactions after September 11, 2001, but only 10 percent received counseling (Fairbrother et al., 2003). A survey of New York City public school children yielded similar findings: 8–15 percent of the students showed elevated rates of post-traumatic stress disorder, major depression, separation anxiety, panic disorder, and/or conduct disorder. Approximately two-thirds of children with probable post-traumatic stress disorder may not have received mental health services (Hoven et al., 2002). The system's capacity to identify and treat the large number of children needing such services should be expanded.

Hurricane Katrina highlighted the vast social service needs of all displaced victims, regardless of age. It would be a challenge for disaster planners to address all the social service needs associated with a disaster of that magnitude. However, the development of evacuation plans should take into account how children can attend schools in different areas, the availability of health care services for children, pediatric capacity in the SNS, ways to expedite Medicaid enrollment for pediatric disaster victims, and long-term sheltering options available for children. Although difficult for disaster planners to address, these issues must be considered.

Conducting Pediatric Disaster Drills

It is widely believed that medical professionals do not receive as much disaster preparedness training as they should (AAMC, 2003; NASEMSD, 2005). The American College of Emergency Physicians (ACEP) has reported that the lack of bioterrorism training for medical responders is so severe that patient treatment could be seriously compromised (Maniece-Harrison, 2005). It is perhaps not surprising that pediatric training is particularly lacking. Most bioterrorism training initiatives, for example, make no reference to the needs of children (Maniece-Harrison, 2005).

Disaster drills have long been central to disaster preparedness efforts for all types of emergency responders. Such drills have proven to be effective in training hospital providers to respond to mass casualty incidents (Hsu et al., 2004) and indeed are required of most hospitals. The Joint Commission on Accreditation of Healthcare Organizations' (JCAHO) 2006 accreditation standards require hospitals to conduct two disaster drills per year, 4 to 8 months apart, one of which must include an influx of volunteers or simulated patients. Hospitals must also participate in at least one communitywide drill per year to assess the communications, coordination, and effectiveness of hospital and community command structures (JCAHO, 2005).

However, the JCAHO requirements do not specifically address conducting disaster drills with children, and in fact, many disaster drills do not include pediatric patients. For example, one hospital held a disaster drill for a mock earthquake, in which a pediatric patient was simulated by a 5-gallon water bottle on which was taped a list of symptoms (Fields, 2003). Obviously, this is a poor means of simulating a pediatric patient. Some disaster drills do not consider children at all. Most (68 percent) of DMATs include pediatric patients in disaster drill scenarios (Mace and Bern, 2004), but it is significant that 32 percent do not. An assessment of EMS agencies in Arkansas found that few had participated in school disaster drills or planned for school responses (Dick et al., 2004).

The exception is, of course, children's hospitals, where all drills involve an influx of critical pediatric patients. In September 2003, for example, Children's Hospital of Atlanta held a drill during which it received 20 critically injured pediatric patients. Yet while children's hospitals are among the most prepared for treating pediatric victims of a disaster, the vast majority of such patients are seen not in children's hospitals, but in general hospitals.

With few exceptions, natural and man-made disasters affect children as well as adults, and there is no better way to expose weaknesses in current preparedness than to demonstrate how poorly children fare in disaster drills. Children are often located in large groups (schools, day care centers) (Romig, 2002), and it is unclear how the system would respond if a disaster incident occurred at one of those locations and a large number of children required care. Therefore, disaster drills should include a meaningful pediatric component.

SUMMARY OF RECOMMENDATIONS

6.1 Federal agencies (the Department of Health and Human Services, the National Highway Traffic Safety Administration, and the Department of Homeland Security), in partnership with state and regional planning bodies and emergency care providers, should convene a panel with multidisciplinary expertise to develop strategies for addressing pediatric needs in the event of a disaster. This effort should encompass the following:

- Development of strategies to minimize parent–child separation and improved methods for reuniting separated children with their families.
- Development of strategies to improve the level of pediatric expertise on Disaster Medical Assistance Teams and other organized disaster response teams.
- Development of disaster plans that address pediatric surge capacity for both injured and noninjured children.
- Development of and improved access to specific medical and mental health therapies, as well as social services, for children in the event of a disaster.
- Development of policies to ensure that disaster drills include a pediatric mass casualty incident at least once every 2 years.

REFERENCES

AAMC (American Association of Medical Colleges). 2003. *Training Future Physicians About Weapons of Mass Destruction: Report of the Expert Panel on Bioterrorism Education for Medical Students.* Washington, DC: AAMC.

AAP (American Academy of Pediatrics). 2002. *The Youngest Victims: Disaster Preparedness to Meet the Needs of Children.* Washington, DC: AAP.

Aghababian R. 2002. Preparing EMS for acts of violence/terrorism involving children. *EMSC News* 15(2):1.

AHRQ (Agency for Healthcare Research and Quality). 2004. *Optimizing Surge Capacity: Hospital Assessment and Planning* (AHRQ Pub. No. 04-P008). Rockville, MD: AHRQ.

Associated Press. 2005a, September 12. Hurricane Katrina: By the numbers. *The Sun Herald.*

Associated Press. 2005b, September 13. Volunteers try to reunite children separated from parents. *Union Tribune.* Available: http://www.signonsandiego.com/news/nation/katrina/20050913-0050-katrina-missingchildren.html [accessed February 1, 2007].

Associated Press. 2005c, December 22. Katrina is voted top story of 2005. *USA Today.* [Online]. Available: http://www.usatoday.com/news/nation/2005-12-22-top-stories_x.htm [accessed February 7, 2007].

Bravata D, McKonald K, Owens D, Wilhelm ER, Brandeau ML, Zaric, GS, Holty, JC, Sundaram V. 2004. *Regionalization of Bioterrorism Preparedness and Response.* Rockville, MD: AHRQ.

CDC (Centers for Disease Control and Prevention). 2004. *Strategic National Stockpile.* [Online]. Available: http://www.bt.cdc.gov/stockpile/ [accessed December 1, 2005].

Center for Catastrophe Preparedness and Response. 2005. *Emergency Medical Services: The Forgotten First Responder—A Report on the Critical Gaps in Organization and Deficits in Resources for America's Medical First Responders.* New York: New York University.

CNN.com. 2005. *Influenza (Flu).* [Online]. Available: http://www.cnn.com/HEALTH/library/DS/00081.html [accessed November 27, 2005].

Cottman M. 2005, September 26. More than 2,000 young Katrina survivors still separated from their parents. *Blackamericaweb.Com.* [Online]. Available: http://www.blackamericaweb.com/site.aspx/bawnews/youngsurvivors927 [accessed February 1, 2007].

DHHS, HRSA, MCHB (Department of Health and Human Services, Health Resources and Services Administration, Maternal and Child Health Bureau). 2000. *Five-year Plan: Emergency Medical Services for Children, 2001–2005.* Washington, DC: EMS-C National Resource Center.

Dick RM, Liggin R, Shirm SW, Graham J. 2004. EMS preparedness for mass casualty events involving children. *Academic Emergency Medicine* 11(5):559.

Fairbrother G, Stuber J, Galea S, Fleischman AR, Pfefferbaum B. 2003, June. Traumatic stress reaction in New York City children after the September 11th terrorist attacks and subsequent use of counseling services. Presentation to the *AcademyHealth Annual Meeting.* Nashville, TN.

FDA (Food and Drug Administration). 2006. *Home Preparation Procedure for Emergency Administration of Potassium Iodide Tablets to Infants and Small Children.* [Online]. Available: http://www.fda.gov/cder/drugprepare/kiprep.htm [accessed May 2006].

Fields H. 2003, May 7. Hospital disaster drill follows mega-quake scenario. *Stanford Report.* [Online]. Available: http://news-service.stanford.edu/news/2003/may7/disaster.html [accessed February 1, 2007].

Foltin G, Schonfeld D, Shannon M. Forthcoming. *Pediatric Terrorism and Disaster Preparedness Resource.* Washington, DC: AAP.

Freddy Mac Foundation. 2005. *Freddie Mac Foundation Announces $1 Million for Foster Children Affected by Hurricane Katrina.* [Online]. Available: http://www.freddiemacfoundation.org/news/20050922_foster.html [accessed November 29, 2005].

Freishtat R. 2002. Issues in children's hospital disaster preparedness. *Clinical Pediatric Emergency Medicine* 3(4):224–230.

GAO (General Accounting Office). 2001. *Emergency Medical Services: Reported Needs Are Wide-Ranging, with a Growing Focus on Lack of Data* (GAO-2-28). Washington, DC: GAO.

GAO. 2003a. *Infectious Diseases: Gaps Remain in Surveillance Capabilities of State and Local Agencies* (GAO-03-1176T). Washington, DC: GAO.

GAO. 2003b. *Hospital Preparedness: Most Urban Hospitals Have Emergency Plans but Lack Certain Capacities for Bioterrorism Response.* Washington, DC: GAO.

Ginaitt PT. 2005. *Statewide Emergency Preparedness in Rhode Island: Lessons Learned "The Station" Nightclub Fire.* Orlando, FL: Hospital Association of Rhode Island.

Glaeser P, Linzer J, Tunik M, Henderson D, Ball J. 2000. Survey of nationally registered emergency medical services providers: Pediatric education. *Annals of Emergency Medicine* 36(1):33–38.

Gutman D, Biffl WL, Suner S, Cioffi WG. 2003. The station nightclub fire and disaster preparedness in Rhode Island. *Medicine and Health Rhode Island* 86(11):344–346.

Hick JL, Hanfling D, Burstein JL, DeAtley C, Barbisch D, Bogdan GM, Cantrill S. 2004. Health care facility and community strategies for patient care surge capacity. *Annals of Emergency Medicine* 44(3):253–261.

Hicks M. 2003. *Comprehensive Clinical and Policy Resource Guide to Assess Children's Needs.* Rockville, MD: AHRQ.

Holbrook PR. 1991. Pediatric disaster medicine. *Critical Care Clinics* 7(2):463–470.

Hoven CW, Duarte CS, Lucas CP, Mandell DJ, Cohen M, Rosen C, Wu P, Musa GJ, Gregorian N. 2002. *Effects of the World Trade Center Attack on NYC Public School Students: Initial Report to the New York City Board of Education.* New York: Columbia University Mailman School of Public Health, New York State Psychiatric Institute and Applied Research and Consulting, LLC.

Hsu EB, Jenckes MW, Catlett CL, Robinson KA, Feuerstein CJ, Cosgrove SE, Green G, Guedelhoefer OC, Bass EB. 2004. Training to hospital staff to respond to a mass casualty incident. *Evidence Report/Technology Assessment (Summary)* 95:1–3.

Illinois EMS-C (Illinois Emergency Medical Services for Children). 2005. *Pediatric Disaster Preparedness Guidelines.* Chicago, IL: Illinois Department of Public Health, Loyola University Medical Center.

Jackson BA, Baker JC, Ridgely MS, Bartis JT, Linn HI. 2004. *Safeguarding Emergency Responders during Major Disasters and Terrorist Attacks.* Santa Monica, CA: Rand Corporation.

JCAHO (Joint Commission on Accreditation of Healthcare Organizations). 2005. *2006 Hospital Accreditation Standards for Emergency Management Planning, Emergency Management Drills, Infection Control, and Disaster Privileges* (Standard EC.2.20). Oakbrook Terrace, IL: JCAHO.

Kaji AH, Lweis RJ. 2004. Hospital disaster preparedness in Los Angeles County, California. *Annals of Emergency Medicine* 44(4).

Lapner PC, Nguyen D, Letts M. 2003. Analysis of a school bus collision: Mechanism of injury in the unrestrained child. *Canadian Journal of Surgery* 46(4):269–272.

Lawrence T. 2002. EMSC comrades help NYC victims: Reflections on the 9/11 disaster. *EMSC News* 15(2):6–7.

Mace SE, Bern AI. 2004. Needs assessment of current pediatric guidelines for use by disaster medical assistance team members in response to disaster and shelter care. *Annals of Emergency Medicine* 44(4):S35.

Mace SE, Jones G. 2004. An analysis of disaster medical assistance team deployments in the United States. *Annals of Emergency Medicine* 44(4):S35.

Maniece-Harrison B. 2005. *Training.* Unpublished document of the National Advisory Committee on Children and Terrorism. [Online]. Available: http://www.bt.cdc.gov/children/word/working/training.doc [accessed October 2005].

Markenson D. 2005. *Model Pediatric Components for State Disaster Plans and Additional Resources.* 2005 EMSC Annual Grantee Meeting. Washington, DC: MCHB.

Mattox K. 2005, October. Life in astrocity, population: 23,000. *Emergency Medicine News.* p. 13.

McHugh M, Staiti AB, Felland LE. 2004. How prepared are Americans for public health emergencies? Twelve communities weigh in. *Health Affairs (Millwood)* 23(3):201–209.

NASEMSD (National Association of State Emergency Medical Services Directors). 2004. *Pediatric Disaster and Terrorism Preparedness.* Falls Church, VA: NASEMSD.

NASEMSD. 2005. *Domestic Terrorism: Issues of Preparedness. Resource Document.* Falls Church, VA: NASEMSD.

National Advisory Committee on Children and Terrorism. 2003. *Recommendations to the Secretary.* Washington, DC: DHHS.

National Center for Disaster Preparedness. 2003. *Pediatric Preparedness for Disasters and Trauma.* New York: Columbia University Mailman School of Public Health.

National Center for Disaster Preparedness. 2004. *Atropine Use in Children after Nerve Gas Exposure* (Info. Brief 1(1)). New York: Columbia Mailman School of Public Health.

National Disaster Medical System. 2005. *What Is a Disaster Medical Assistance Team (DMAT)?* [Online]. Available: http://ndms.dhhs.gov/dmat.html [accessed November 29, 2005].

NIMH (National Institute of Mental Health). 2001. *Helping Children and Adolescents Cope with Violence and Disasters* (NIH Publication No. 01-3518). Bethesda, MD: NIMH.

Noji EK. 1996. Disaster epidemiology. *Emergency Medicine Clinics of North America* 14(2):289–300.

Nufer KE, Gnauck K. 2004. Clarifying needs of the pediatric disaster patient: A descriptive analysis of pediatric patient encounters from four disaster medical assistance team deployments. *Annals of Emergency Medicine* 44(4):S40.

Ohio Pediatric Disaster Preparedness Committee. 2004. *Pediatric Issues in Disaster Preparedness.* [Online]. Available: http://www.prepareohio.com/members/pediatric/OHPedsPrep.ppt [accessed January 2006].

Ong B. 2005. Fractured families. *Newsweek Web Exclusive.* [Online]. Available: http://www.msnbc.msn.com/id/9615369/site/newsweek/ [accessed February 1, 2007].

Oster NS, Chaffee MW. 2004. Hospital preparedness analysis using the hospital emergency analysis tool (The HEAT). *Annals of Emergency Medicine* 44(4):S61.

Quinn B, Baker R, Pratt J. 1994. Hurricane Andrew and a pediatric emergency department. *Annals of Emergency Medicine* 23(4):737–741.

Rivera AF, Char DM. 2004. Emergency department disaster preparedness: Identifying the barriers. *Annals of Emergency Medicine* 44(4).

Romig L. 2002. JumpSTART: A disaster preparedness tool for the times. *EMSC News* 15(2):3–4.

Schur CL, Berk ML, Mueller CD. 2004. *Perspectives of Rural Hospitals on Bioterrorism Preparedness Planning* (W Series, No. 4). Bethesda, MD: NORC Walsh Center for Rural Health Analysis.

Sears M. 2005, January 2. Organized effort aims to improve response when a child is hurt; club supplies bags that streamline ambulance care. *Milwaukee Journal Sentinel.* [Online]. Available: http://www.findarticles.com/p/articles/mi_qn4196/is_20050102/ai_n11008378 [accessed February 1, 2007].

Shannon M. 2004. *Addressing Pediatric and School-based Surge Capacity in a Mass Casualty Event.* Rockville, MD: AHRQ.

Shute N, Marcus MB. 2001. Crisis in the ER. Turning away patients. Long delays. A surefire recipe for disaster. *US News World Report* 131(9):54–61.

Treat K, Williams J, Furbee P, Manley W, Russell F, Stamper C. 2001. Hospital preparedness for weapons of mass destruction incidents: An initial assessment. *Annals of Emergency Medicine* 38(5):562–565.

U.S. Census Bureau. 2004. *Annual Estimates of the Resident Population by Selected Age Groups for the United States and States: July 1, 2003 and April 1, 2000. Table ST-EST2003-01res.* [Online]. Available: http://cber.utk.edu/Census/03stage.xls [accessed October 2005].

van Amerongen RH, Fine JS, Tunik MG, Young GM, Foltin GL. 1993. The Avianca plane crash: An emergency medical system's response to pediatric survivors of the disaster. *Pediatrics* 92(1):105–110.

Wass AR, Williams MJ, Gibson MF. 1994. A review of the management of a major incident involving predominantly pediatric casualties. *Injury* 25(6):371–374.

7

Building the Evidence Base
for Pediatric Emergency Care

Pediatric emergency care is a young field. Even in the late 1970s, there were no pediatric emergency medicine textbooks or journals (Ludwig, 2001). Considerable progress has been made since that time, and these advances should be applauded. However, the advancement of knowledge in pediatric emergency care must not slow. Indeed, many unanswered questions remain about the best way to organize and deliver such care.

The committee decided to devote an entire chapter to research because of its great potential to improve the quality, organization, and delivery of pediatric emergency care. The payoff from increased pediatric emergency care research, while difficult to quantify, will include lives saved, decreased morbidity, and a more efficient and effective emergency care system. The chapter begins with a review of pediatric emergency care research from the 1980s through the present day and continues with a discussion of why advancing the state of knowledge remains critical today. It then turns to some of the barriers to pediatric emergency care research that hinder progress and presents the committee's recommendations for overcoming those barriers.

EARLY DEVELOPMENT OF PEDIATRIC
EMERGENCY CARE RESEARCH

As noted in Chapter 2, attention to deficiencies in the pediatric emergency care system grew in the 1980s, and as a result, a variety of organizations began to take action. A number of studies were published that provided information on the demographic characteristics of children who were using emergency services, the kinds of illnesses and injuries with which they presented, and the readiness of providers to care for them. These studies were generally single-site research projects initiated at children's hospitals, medical schools, and/or local departments of health. For example, published research described the epidemiology of cardiac arrest and resuscitation in children in suburban King County, Washington (Eisenberg et al., 1983); pediatric emergencies in Minneapolis, Minnesota; and pediatric versus adult death rates in the field in Los Angeles County (Seidel et al., 1984).

Emerging information on pediatric injuries and illnesses and early indications of inadequacies in the capacity of the emergency care system to address pediatric needs played a large part in the U.S. government's decision to create the Emergency Medical Services for Children (EMS-C) program in 1984. EMS-C was among the first government programs to support the collection of data on pediatric emergency care. Its early activities included collecting data on pediatric emergencies to assess the need for specialized pediatric programs. Some of the major pediatric emergency care research published in the late 1980s continued to show shortcomings in the emergency care system for children (Seidel, 1986a,b; Seidel et al., 1991), including differences in deaths rates for children in rural versus urban settings (Gausche et al., 1989a,b). There were also studies that focused on ways to improve the system for children, such as creation of a specialized pediatric emergency care system in Los Angeles (Henderson, 1988); creation of a new tool, the Broselow tape, for estimating pediatric weight and drug dosages (Lubitz et al., 1988); and development of an accurate pediatric trauma score (Ramenofsky et al., 1988).

The 1993 Institute of Medicine (IOM) Report *Emergency Medical Services for Children* called attention to the need for pediatric emergency care research by highlighting knowledge gaps in the field. These gaps encompassed the most basic questions about emergency care services for children:

- What is the structure of the system?
- Who uses the system?
- For what is the system used?
- What services or procedures are provided to patients?
- When are services provided?
- What are the outcomes of using the system?
- What are the global costs of the system?
- How well does the system perform?

The report noted that "research is needed to validate the clinical merit of care that is given, to identify better kinds of care, to devise better ways to deliver that care, and to understand the costs and benefits of the [emergency care system] now in place and toward which the nation should move" (IOM, 1993, p.16). The report contained a research agenda and called for the development of a uniform dataset that would be used by states to collect, analyze, and report data to EMS; include all elements of a national uniform dataset; describe the nature of EMS provided to children; and link data generated by separate components of EMS (IOM, 1993).

After the report's release, the EMS-C program established the National EMS Data Analysis Resource Center (NEDARC) to help grantees and state EMS offices develop capabilities to collect, analyze, and utilize EMS and other data to improve the delivery of emergency and trauma care. Specifically, NEDARC staff provide research design consultation, information on data collection (e.g., which elements to collect, hardware/software issues, confidentiality issues), information on statistics, general analysis of data, and probabilistic linkage (MCHB, 2004a).

Also in the 1990s, the first infrastructure for multicenter pediatric emergency care research was established when the American Academy of Pediatrics' Section on Emergency Medicine created the Pediatric Emergency Medicine Collaborative Research Committee (PEM CRC). The infrastructure of PEM CRC is privately funded and has served as the platform for many research projects, the majority of which have been clinical (PECARN, 2003; AAP, 2005). At least seven studies supported by the collaborative were published between 1994 and 2004 (AAP, 2005).

Perhaps the most significant development in pediatric emergency care research occurred when the EMS-C program created the Pediatric Emergency Care Applied Research Network (PECARN)—a collaborative research group consisting of hospital emergency departments (EDs) organized into nodes, with central coordination from a steering committee (PECARN, 2003, 2005). PECARN is focused on the conduct of multicenter, randomized trials and observational studies on a variety of pediatric emergency care issues. There are four Regional Node Centers, each of which coordinates five or six Hospital Emergency Department Affiliates. The strength of PECARN lies in the annual number of patient encounters it covers—900,000 ill and injured children (PECARN, 2006). Additionally, the research involves senior-level pediatric emergency medicine researchers and clinicians with expertise in epidemiology, statistics, and health services research. While PECARN is still young, it appears to hold significant promise for advancing research in pediatric emergency care. A research agenda specific to multi-institutional studies is being developed by the PECARN steering committee and will be available in late 2006 (Personal communication, D. Kavanaugh, May 10, 2006).

An important shortcoming of PECARN, however, is that it has conducted little research in the prehospital environment. The one exception is a current study on cervical spine injury, addressing the immobilization practices of prehospital providers. The study involves focus groups of prehospital providers to evaluate their opinions on immobilization practices and their willingness to participate in research evaluating those practices retrospectively. PECARN recently established an out-of-hospital working group to develop EMS research ideas. However, research in prehospital pediatric emergency care has lagged far behind that in ED-based pediatric emergency care, both within PECARN and in other research efforts.

Data indicate that the volume of research in pediatric emergency care has grown considerably. Spandorfer and colleagues (2003) reviewed abstracts on pediatric emergency medicine research submitted to national scientific meetings of the American Psychological Association (APA), American College of Emergency Physicians (ACEP), American Academy of Pediatrics (AAP), and Society for Academic Emergency Medicine (SAEM) and found that there had been a substantial increase in such research between 1987 and 1999. There had also been an increase in the number of population-based and multicenter clinical trials in the field. Additionally, the number of trials that were randomized and blinded had grown over time, although they still represented just 7 percent of pediatric emergency care studies published during the period. The design of studies had varied little between 1987 and 1999; there had been no increase in the proportion of studies that were prospective or used an analytic design (Spandorfer et al., 2003). However, the use of more sophisticated statistics had become more prevalent over time. Between 1993 and 2002, five journals published slightly more than half of the published articles related to pediatric emergency care: *Pediatric Emergency Care*, *Pediatrics*, *Annals of Emergency Medicine*, *Pediatric Clinics of North America*, and *Archives of Pediatrics and Adolescent Medicine* (Gough et al., 2004).

CONTINUED NEED FOR RESEARCH

Although the amount of research conducted in pediatric emergency care has increased considerably over the past 25 years, significant information gaps remains. Indeed, the gaps that exist today include many of the broad, systems-level questions identified as research priorities in the 1993 IOM report on emergency care for children. Additionally, many new, unanswered questions have emerged in the last 10 years as our understanding of the determinants of quality care delivery has improved. This section reviews progress made toward addressing the information gaps that existed in 1993 and identifies some other areas in which research could contribute to improved care. Finally, it presents the rationale for devoting resources to addressing the information gaps that persist today.

Progress Toward Closing the Information Gaps Identified in 1993

Despite the increase in research activity and funding since 1993, the questions about pediatric emergency care posed in the 1993 IOM report remain not only salient, but also largely unanswered.

What is the structure of the system? There is no central resource containing reliable information on the number and characteristics of the facilities, emergency care providers, and services available in the emergency care system. However, different organizations that represent emergency providers collect some basic information. For example, the American Hospital Association keeps a tally of the total number of EDs in the country, and the National Association of Children's Hospitals and Related Institutions keeps a list of the number of children's hospitals. Additionally, we have a general idea from surveys of the percentage of EMS agencies that are fire department–based versus stand-alone. However, this information is only the first step in understanding the structure of the emergency care system. Information on the capabilities and services available from each provider remains elusive, as does information on how the structure varies within and across states and regions.

Who uses the system?, For what is the system used?, What services or procedures are provided to patients?, and When are services provided? We are able to answer all of these questions today with regard to children's use of EDs; however, these questions remain unanswered with respect to those using the prehospital (EMS) system. One important source of information on ED utilization is the federal National Hospital Ambulatory Medical Care Survey (NHAMCS), which has collected nationally representative information on ED visits since 1992. NHAMCS allows researchers to study the use of EDs by patient characteristics including age, race, and insurance status. The data also include the reason for the visit and the triage category (for example, immediate, urgent, nonurgent); the physician's diagnosis for each patient, as well as the diagnostic, screening, surgical, counseling, educational, and therapy services provided during the visit; and when patients arrived at the ED, how long they waited, and when they left.

Another important data source is the State Emergency Department Databases (SEDD), part of the Healthcare Cost and Utilization Project (HCUP) sponsored by the Agency for Healthcare Research and Quality (AHRQ). The SEDD captures information on all ED visits that do not require admission and allows for the analysis of data at the state or, in many cases, the county level. The SEDD contains more than 100 clinical and nonclinical variables, including diagnoses, procedures, patient demographics, expected payer source, charges, hospital identifiers, and county identifiers. As of September 2005, 17 states were participating, and data from many of those states are available for the years 1999 to 2004 (AHRQ, 2005).

In contrast to these in-hospital data systems, data collection on the use of EMS has progressed slowly. At the local level, most data on EMS are collected on paper, although many systems are beginning to transition to electronic systems. Because EMS information systems are produced by a variety of vendors and each state defines its own data elements, there is little uniformity or consistency of data collection across agencies (Mears, 2005). As a result, a national database on EMS utilization does not exist, although one is in development.

The National Highway Traffic Safety Administration's (NHTSA) *Emergency Medical Services Agenda for the Future* described five goals for an EMS information system: (1) adopt uniform data elements and definitions, and incorporate them into information systems; (2) develop mechanisms for generating and transmitting data that are valid, reliable, and accurate; (3) develop information systems that are able to describe an entire EMS event; (4) develop integrated information systems with other health care providers, public safety agencies, and community resources; and (5) provide feedback to those who generate data (NHTSA, 1996). Efforts are under way to achieve each of these goals through the National EMS Information System (NEMSIS).

NEMSIS is geared toward improving data standardization and linking disparate EMS databases at the federal, state, and local levels (Mears et al., 2002). It will serve as a national EMS database that can be used to evaluate patient and EMS system outcomes, benchmark performance, facilitate research efforts, develop nationwide EMS training curricula, determine national fee schedules, and address issues related to disaster preparedness resources. NEMSIS will be able to supply information at the national level, such as the total number and types of EMS calls, average response times, and the most widely used medications and procedures. Currently, 48 states (excluding New York and Vermont) have elected to participate in the program. By the end of 2006, 6–7 states are expected to be fully operational in the program and will be submitting state-level data; by the end of 2007, an additional 17 states are expected to be doing so. Becoming fully operational means that states are collecting and submitting NEMSIS-compliant data from their individual EMS agencies.

What are the outcomes of using the system? Information on outcomes from the emergency care system is limited. Process outcomes, such as hospital admission or referral to a tertiary care facility, are important to understanding how patients move through the system. Some limited data are available on ED patients through NHAMCS, which contains information on the patients' disposition, including whether they were admitted to the hospital, the intensive care unit/critical care unit, or an observation unit. However, NHAMCS does not include data on hospital outcomes. Combining SEDD data with another data source within HCUP allows researchers to determine the percentage of patients who are admitted and the inpatient treatments received.

A great hindrance to addressing questions about outcomes is that many data systems cannot be linked. In other words, once a child's parents contact 9-1-1, a first-responding fire engine may arrive, and the child may be transported by EMS and delivered to a hospital ED, but information on the patient beyond each point in the hand-off is rarely available to those involved earlier in the chain of events. The absence of uniform incident numbers and other methods of achieving data linkage hinder researchers in gathering information on clinical outcomes, which is often of greater importance than measures of the processes of care. Clinical outcomes, based on hospital disposition, functional status at discharge, patient well-being, morbidity, and mortality are often available only when specifically studied by a supported research initiative, such as PECARN. Still, our knowledge of optimal treatment patterns for many pediatric interventions is limited, while such information for the prehospital environment is even less obtainable.

What are the global costs of the system? The global costs of the emergency care system for children are unknown. The direct and indirect economic costs of operating a pediatric emergency care system, as well as the monetary savings that could be realized over time through the successful expansion of initiatives to improve pediatric emergency care, are of key interest, but few studies have explored such questions (DHHS et al., 1997).

How well does the system perform? Information on the performance of the pediatric emergency care system is limited. Performance measurement for emergency care services has received growing attention, but as yet there are few opportunities for researchers to gather information on system performance at the local or state level, much less nationally.

The Growing Information Gap

Considerably more is known about pediatric emergency care than was the case in 1993, but the information gaps in the field have widened as more areas of importance have been identified. The quality framework developed by the IOM in *Crossing the Quality Chasm: A New Health System for the 21st Century* (IOM, 2001) is now widely used to evaluate the adequacy and safety of health care delivery. In Chapter 2, this framework was used to provide an overview of the state of pediatric emergency care under the current system. As explained in this chapter, however, the information necessary to fully evaluate the pediatric emergency care system is lacking. The information gaps of today include the following questions:

- **How safe is pediatric emergency care?** How often do medical errors occur? How often are patients harmed from the receipt of emergency care services? Which aspects of pediatric emergency care are least safe? Which aspects are most safe?

- **How effective is pediatric emergency care?** How much care being delivered is not supported by evidence? In what areas of pediatric emergency care is evidence most lacking?
- **How patient-centered is pediatric emergency care?** How often do providers consider the wishes of patients and their families in treatment decisions? What percentage of EMS agencies and hospitals have patient-centered policies? What percentage of EDs have a patient-centered environment? How often are parents/guardians satisfied with the emergency care provided to their children?
- **How timely is pediatric emergency care?** How long do pediatric patients wait for prehospital services? How quickly are they transported to EDs?
- **How efficient is pediatric emergency care?** Is pediatric emergency care cost-effective? How often is ineffective care delivered? How much waste exists in the emergency care system? What is the value of that waste?
- **How equitable is pediatric emergency care?** How do the availability and quality of care delivered vary based on patients' gender, age, race, ethnicity, income, education, geographic location, and/or disability?

Three Types of Research

Pressing gaps remain in our understanding of emergency care with respect to all three types of research: basic, translational, and health services. Because emergency medicine is defined by time and place rather than body part or disease process, research in the field is often mischaracterized as being strictly translational in nature. But emergency medicine requires both basic discoveries and translation of those discoveries to the clinical setting.

Basic research is aimed at increasing fundamental understanding of a subject. It typically involves study of anatomy, physiology, cells, molecules, and genes. Basic science investigations do not immediately provide results that are relevant for the delivery of emergency care, but they lead to a better understanding of diseases and provide knowledge that eventually helps in finding new ways to diagnose, treat, and prevent various types of illnesses or injuries. An example is recent studies demonstrating the detrimental effect of brain injury on an animal's ability to compensate for hemorrhage (Lewelt et al., 1980, 1982; Ishige et al., 1987, 1988; Yuan and Wade, 1991; Yuan et al., 1991; DeWitt et al., 1992a,b; Fulton et al., 1993). These findings have, at least in part, laid the foundation for some of the current guidelines of the Brain Trauma Foundation. Basic research projects in pediatric emergency medicine could address the pathophysiology of acute respiratory failure, ways to minimize the risk of secondary ischemic brain injury during limited resuscitation from hemorrhagic shock and traumatic brain injury, and the pathophysiology and treatment of traumatic spinal cord injury.

Translational research is the most active area of emergency care research because of the wide range of patients, diseases, and interventions seen by EMTs and physicians in emergency practice. These providers are afforded a unique window on the state of available treatment options, including their shortcomings, and therefore have both the motivation and opportunity for focused efforts to translate research into better modes of treatment. An example is recent translational work by Sanders and others that investigated alternative cardiopulmonary resuscitation (CPR) techniques to determine the optimal ratio of chest compressions to ventilations (Berg et al., 1995, 1997, 2001; Kern et al., 2002; Sanders et al., 2002). The data from these studies demonstrated improved neurological outcomes with a higher ratio of chest compressions to ventilations (100:2) as compared with standard CPR (compression:ventilation ratio of 15:2). These data, as well as other observations, led to changes in the American Heart Association's guidelines for CPR.

At the same time, it has been noted that the U.S. health care system has a poor record in incorporating demonstrated effective and safe therapies into routine clinical practice (Lenfant, 2003). With increasing recognition that simply establishing the safety and efficacy of a new therapy is insufficient to ensure its widespread use, many institutes within the National Institutes of Health (NIH), as well as AHRQ (which leads these efforts), have increasingly emphasized the importance of translating research into practice. This is an important area that deserves special emphasis within emergency care research as well.

Examples of pediatric translational research include the formulation of guidelines for the efficacy, safety, and dosage of medications for infants, children, and adolescents; the development of evidenced-based protocols for the treatment of common pediatric conditions (e.g., fever); assessment of the effectiveness of new interventions, such as ultrasonography, needleless drug administration, and innovations in procedural sedation; and evaluation of the pharmacokinetics and efficacy of promising clinical therapies for treating pediatric acute traumatic brain injury.

Emergency medicine by definition requires timely and efficient approaches to the delivery of services. The organization and mode of delivery have long been recognized as having major impacts on the quality and outcomes of care. But the organization and delivery of services is perhaps the weakest link in the emergency care evidence base. Even established doctrine, such as the value of paramedics in the field, has recently been overturned. This, then, represents a formative and essential area for health services research. Some of the key research questions in the delivery of pediatric health services include the feasibility and cost-effectiveness of implementing mental health or child abuse screening of pediatric patients in the ED; the causes and solutions for missed diagnosis in the ED; identification of which components of pediatric trauma systems impact outcomes and cost-effectiveness; and the impacts of ED crowding, boarding, and diversion on pediatric patients.

Health Promotion and Injury Prevention

Injury prevention is important for all age groups but particularly for children, whose unique needs must be taken into account (see Box 7-1) (IOM, 1985). Injury not only is the leading cause of death for children, accounting for more deaths among those aged 1–18 than all other causes combined, but also is responsible for more years of potential life lost than any other health problem (Baker et al., 1992). Injuries are the most common cause of pediatric ED visits as well (McCaig and Ly, 2002). Although emergency care providers are not commonly linked to public health prevention activities, their potential role in such efforts has been recognized (Maclean,

---

BOX 7-1
Airbags and Children

Just as new medical technologies and information systems must be designed with pediatric patients in mind, prevention efforts must consider the potential implications for children. Passenger side airbags are an example of a prevention device designed for adults that resulted in unintended harm to child passengers.

Since the early 1970s, airbags, in concert with seat belts, have saved thousands of lives (McCaffrey et al., 1999). Because of their potential to reduce the burden of injury in a crash, dual air bags were required as standard equipment in all cars and light trucks in the United States in the late 1990s. However, many children—as many as 35 percent of child passengers in the 1990s—ride unrestrained in automobiles (National Center for Statistics and Analysis and NHTSA, 2005). As the number of vehicles equipped with dual air bags increased, federal regulators noted a sharp increase in the number of fatal injuries to children resulting from airbag deployment. Many of these injuries stemmed from children being unrestrained or improperly restrained, but a small number occurred to children who were properly restrained in the front seat (CDC, 1996).

Because airbags must deploy at the moment of impact to catch an unrestrained passenger, they literally explode open, fully inflating within milliseconds. The speed of airbag deployment can exceed 140 to 200 miles per

1993). Patient encounters with EMS and ED providers offer a unique opportunity for preventive education. NHTSA's 1996 *Emergency Medical Services Agenda for the Future* emphasized the importance of engaging EMS systems in injury and illness prevention programs designed to address regional needs (NHTSA, 1996). ED providers have similarly been encouraged to play a key role in injury control and prevention (DHHS et al., 2000; Mace et al., 2001; ACEP, 2002).

While emergency providers' historical role in prevention has focused on surveillance and research, they also play a small but growing part in delivering preventive care and education. In fact, in 49 states and territories, emergency care personnel are utilized for injury prevention activities (MCHB, 2004b). The benefits of such activities (decreased health care consumption, reduced costs, lower morbidity and mortality) have been well established for certain prevention strategies; however, the extent to which prevention activities carried out by emergency care providers reduce the

hour. Children placed in the front passenger seat are at much higher risk for being harmed by airbag deployment than adults for several reasons: they are more likely to be moving around or leaning forward in their seat, even if restrained; children placed in the front seat in a forward-facing child restraint are several inches closer to the airbag than adults; children may shift closer to the airbag during precrash braking because their feet do not touch the floor, so they cannot brace themselves; a child's head and neck are more likely to be struck by the deploying airbag; and most important, infants placed in the front seat in a rear-facing child safety seat are inadvertently within striking distance of the airbag.

After reviewing the early pediatric injury and fatality data for airbags, the National Transportation Safety Board released a number of recommendations regarding the safe transport of children in automobiles with airbags. For example, infants should ride in rear-facing child safety seats in the back seat. Children under age 12 should be properly secured in the back seat as well. For older children, shoulder belts should not be worn behind the back or under the arm. Additionally, the vehicle seat should be set as far back as possible (CDC, 1996). Additionally, the National Highway Traffic Safety Administration enacted regulatory measures to address the problem, including labeling requirements for vehicles and child safety seats and specifications for airbag cutoff switches (CDC, 1995). In 2002, the American Academy of Pediatrics issued guidelines for counseling parents about the most appropriate child safety seats and positioning of child passengers (AAP, 2002).

burden of illness and injury in children and/or produce savings is currently
not well understood. Few research efforts have evaluated the effectiveness of
ED-based injury control and prevention interventions for children and their
parents (Mace et al., 2001; Johnston et al., 2002). As a result, it is difficult
to determine the extent to which emergency providers should be pressed
to undertake such activities. And because little support has been provided
for injury prevention research, it is unclear which prevention strategies are
likely to produce the greatest benefit.

Justification for Increasing Pediatric Emergency Care Research

Much is unknown about the nation's emergency care system, particularly with regard to pediatric patients. But numerous other unanswered
questions within the health care system remain unanswered. What makes
pediatric emergency care worthy of the scarce resources available for health
care research?

Rivara (1993) proposed a set of criteria for selecting research topics in
general pediatrics, but his criteria are easily applied across all health care research efforts. According to Rivara, research should focus on problems that
(1) occur frequently, (2) are severe, and (3) could potentially be alleviated
by taking action. Pediatric emergency care research meets all three of these
criteria. First, utilization data from individual EMS agencies and national
data from NHAMCS indicate heavy reliance on the emergency care system
among pediatric patients. Children visited EDs nearly 30 million times in
2003. Pediatric patients account for approximately 27 percent of all ED
visits and 5 to 10 percent of all EMS transports. The frequency with which
the emergency care system encounters pediatric patients contributes to the
need for research in this area.

Second, while the majority of calls to EMS and visits to the ED do not
involve life-threatening emergencies, the system must be well prepared for
sick and injured children. The severity of illnesses and injuries encountered
by emergency providers—some of which are life-threatening—provides
ample justification for efforts to expand research in the area.

Finally, the potential to overcome deficiencies in the emergency care
system through research is real. The EMS-C program, through its network
of grant coordinators in each state, has the infrastructure to help incorporate
changes in practice that are suggested by new research, as would the new
federal lead agency for emergency care proposed in Chapter 3. The potential
for change would be even greater in communities that adopted the regionalized system of emergency care services proposed in Chapter 3, under which
the coordination and organization of the system would be stronger.

ADDRESSING BARRIERS TO PEDIATRIC EMERGENCY CARE RESEARCH

The barriers that presently hinder emergency care research in general also apply to research in pediatric emergency care. Among the most commonly cited barriers are (1) inadequate funding (ACEP Research Committee, 2005); (2) limited availability of data, especially in the prehospital environment; and (3) a shortage of adequately trained investigators with sufficient protected time to develop a clearly defined research focus (Stern et al., 2001; Lewis, 2004). Additional barriers exist to the conduct of prehospital emergency care research. Survey data show that EMTs identify both a lack of interest and a lack of knowledge about the purpose of research as major barriers (Singh et al., 2004).

To address these barriers, the committee recommends that **the Secretary of Health and Human Services conduct a study to examine the gaps and opportunities in emergency care research, including pediatric emergency care, and recommend a strategy for the optimal organization and funding of the research effort. This study should include consideration of the training of new investigators, development of multicenter research networks, involvement of emergency care researchers in the grant review and research advisory processes, and improved research coordination through a dedicated center or institute. Congress and federal agencies involved in emergency and trauma care research (including the Department of Transportation, the Department of Health and Human Services, the Department of Homeland Security, and the Department of Defense) should implement the study's recommendations (7.1).**

Limited Funding for Pediatric Emergency Care Research

To improve the evidence base for pediatric emergency care interventions, there is a need for larger, multicenter studies that can provide greater statistical power and more complexity in terms of analytic design and questions investigated. These more sophisticated studies require significant amounts of funding support (Havel, 2004). However, funding for research in emergency medicine has traditionally been very limited and is highly competitive.

Some progress has been made by pediatric emergency medicine researchers in securing federal funding, particularly with the introduction of PECARN; nonetheless, funding continues to remain a critical barrier. Of the limited federal funds available for emergency care research, a small amount is directed toward pediatric studies. In 2004, SAEM identified a total of just 106 federal grants from various agencies covering a wide rage of emergency care topics. Of these, only 11 were focused on pediatrics and

4 on prehospital care. Of the 11 grants focused on pediatrics, only 1 was a basic science investigation (ACEP Research Committee, 2005).

A key characteristic of much emergency care research is its tendency to cut across multiple specialty domains. Emergency care research is often not based on a single disease entity, and simultaneously incorporates characteristics of both efficacy and health services research. This has made it difficult for emergency medicine researchers to obtain training grants from the siloed funding structure of NIH, the largest single source of support for biomedical research in the world (IOM, 2004). The broad nature of emergency medicine research does not fit well into the highly specific focus of individual NIH institutes. According to a 2005 ACEP report on emergency medicine research, "even institutes with a potential focus on emergency medicine, such as the National Institute of General Medical Sciences (NIGMS) [which includes a trauma research center and trauma training program], view funding emergency medicine training programs with skepticism." The ACEP Research Committee made a formal inquiry to the NIGMS program director regarding funding specifically for emergency medicine research. The program director described several barriers. For example, the NIGMS budget dedicated to training has remained constant, while trainee costs have risen. These budgetary pressures have led to a reduction in the total number of trainees the institute can support. In the absence of increased funding, it is highly unlikely that NIGMS will initiate a new category of training programs to foster the development of emergency care researchers. The program director also noted that although emergency medicine research covers medical issues that are within the missions of many individual institutes, it is doubtful that any single institute would support a generic program covering multiple research or training areas, as a training program in emergency care research would necessarily do (ACEP Research Committee, 2005). The same problems exist for pediatric emergency care research.

As recommendation 7.1 suggests, specific opportunities and funding streams for pediatric emergency care research should be identified and prioritized. This funding should target emergency medical and trauma care for both children and adults, including prehospital and ED care, disaster medicine, critical care, mental health emergencies, and prevention. Projects should encompass the full range of relevant research—basic, translational, and health services research, as well as clinical outcome studies—with an emphasis on the generation and testing of evidence-based prediction rules, health service delivery practices, behavioral/mental health studies, and education research.

One of the impediments to grant funding for emergency care research in federal agencies has been the lack of emergency care researchers involved in the development of intramural and extramural research strategies and in grant review panels. This situation is due in part to the cross-cutting nature of the discipline, as discussed above. It is also due in part to the recency of the fields of trauma and emergency medicine and the lack of a large cadre of mature investigators, as discussed in the next section. While the development of investigators is an imperative for the field, the number of mature investigators is growing, and they should have a stronger presence in grant review processes in the future. This should occur naturally as a greater effort to support emergency care research is made by NIH and other federal funders.

Enhanced cooperation is also needed among federal agencies in the development of multiagency research announcements and the coordination of funding for pediatric emergency care research projects. There is a precedent for this sort of activity. In response to the 1993 IOM report on emergency care for children, which called for an increase in funding for pediatric emergency care research, a multiagency announcement was released in 2001 that focused on improving the quality and quantity of research in this area. The announcement included AHRQ, the Health Resources and Services Administration's (HRSA) Maternal and Child Health Bureau, the Centers for Disease Control and Prevention's (CDC) National Institute for Occupational Safety and Health, and four NIH institutes—the National Institute of Child Health and Human Development, the National Institute on Drug Abuse, the National Institute on Mental Health, and the National Institute of Nursing Research. In 2002, eight funded projects cited this announcement as the point of referral for their proposals; in 2003, seven research awards were made for which the announcement was the initial contact for the investigators (data courtesy of Isabelle Melese d'Hospital, EMSC National Resource Center). The program announcement expired in January 2004, but in April 2005, an updated multiagency program announcement was released.

Collaboration should extend beyond federal agencies to include foundations and other sources of support (see Box 7-2). While the total funding available for pediatric emergency care research is limited, the dollars flow from a large number of different sources, including state block grants, private foundations, professional societies, and industry, although these funding streams are not always reliable, and they almost always tend to be fragmented. These funding organizations should coordinate resources that support pediatric emergency care research so that the dollars will be directed to the most appropriate studies, and overlap will be avoided.

Not only do nonfederal organizations represent a potential source of research support, but they may also provide essential venues for the diffusion of new pediatric research findings. For example, the annual meeting of the Pediatric Academic Societies is a venue for sharing information about interdisciplinary aspects of pediatric medicine. Similarly, the annual meetings of SAEM, the Emergency Nurses Association, and the National Association

---

BOX 7-2
Potential Sources of Support for
Pediatric Emergency Care Research

Although federal support for pediatric emergency care research is rather limited, a number of government agencies, given their mission, could be potential supporters of such research. Each of the agencies listed below should better define and expand its role in supporting pediatric emergency care research. A short description of each agency is provided. Potential foundation and industry sources are also identified.

Federal Agencies

Several government agencies are involved in clinical and health services research. Although the funding is not typically targeted specifically to pediatric emergency care research, researchers in the field may be able to tailor their research topics to match an agency's substantive area of interest, such as mental health, cardiac care, or injury. Within the federal government, the following agencies can and should play an important role in pediatric emergency care research.

National Institutes of Health (NIH). NIH is the main federal organization funding health and behavioral research. It consists of 27 separate institutes and centers that conduct and acquire the results of both basic and applied behavioral and biomedical research. NIH supports the research of nonfederal scientists in universities, medical schools, hospitals, and research institutions throughout the United States and abroad.

NIH does not have an institute or center focused specifically on emergency services. However, emergency medicine research may be appropriate for any of the individual institutes or centers, depending on the research topic. For example, the National Heart, Lung, and Blood Institute has encouraged the submission of applications for research that includes studies aimed at developing and evaluating programs in which the emergency department (ED) is used to introduce effective asthma management strategies, as well as epidemiological studies aimed at identifying risk factors for ED visits. Support for studies on pediatric emergency care could potentially be obtained from the National Institute for Child Health and Human Development (NICHD), which has encouraged applications for research examining outcomes of emergency care for acutely ill children and care of suicidal children and adolescents. As of July 2004, two-thirds of NICHD grants were for projects related to pediatric critical care and one-third for those relate to pediatric rehabilitation.

Although the NIH budget has expanded in recent years, this growth has not translated to an increase in funds for emergency medicine research. Emergency medicine has traditionally faced larger hurdles in competing for NIH funding relative to other medical fields (Marx, 2004).

Department of Health and Human Services (DHHS). A number of agencies within DHHS are potential supporters of pediatric emergency care research:

- *Agency for Healthcare Research and Quality (AHRQ).* The mission of AHRQ is to improve the quality, safety, efficiency, and effectiveness of health care. Unlike NIH, which tends to fund work that is more clinical in nature, AHRQ tends to fund health services research. In 2004, AHRQ received an allocation of $304 million to be used for funding a variety of health services and outcomes research, continued collection of key data characterizing the provision of health care in the United States, and a variety of specific activities mandated by Congress. For example, the 2005 AHRQ administration request included $84 million for patient safety research and $50 million for information technology, and may include $50 million for effectiveness evaluation of prescription drugs. Because funding for AHRQ is increasingly tied to specific activities, progressively fewer funds have been available to support investigator-initiated research and research training. Nonetheless, AHRQ remains a major source of funds for health services and outcomes research, with an intense focus on translating research into practice. The development of methods for effectively translating new research findings into clinical practice is particularly important in emergency care, and to its credit, AHRQ has funded some important studies in this area, including a pediatric airway management project (Gausche et al., 2000). A number of emergency care specialists have served on standing grant review panels and special emphasis panels for AHRQ.
- *Health Resources and Services Administration (HRSA).* HRSA's mission is to improve health care access. The agency awards grants and contracts primarily to support programs and demonstration initiatives. HRSA's Maternal and Child Health Bureau (MCHB) has a dedicated funding source for pediatric emergency services under its Emergency Medical Services for Children (EMS-C) program. The EMS-C program provides infrastructure support for the Pediatric Emergency Care Applied Research Network (PECARN), described in more detail in the text. The MCHB Research Program also funds pediatric emergency care research projects including PECARN studies. HRSA's Office of Rural Health Policy also supports research efforts through its Rural Health Research Center program. This program is dedicated entirely to producing policy-relevant research on health care in rural areas. Eight centers have cooperative agreements with HRSA to conduct this research, and each year, specific research topics for the centers are selected jointly by the research center directors and HRSA staff. Although the majority of studies are not focused on emergency

continued

care, one examined access to EMS, and others have looked at how changes in the health care system affect ED use.

- *Indian Health Service (IHS).* IHS is the federal government's primary advocate for delivery of health care services to Native Americans. IHS manages EMS-related activities through contractual arrangements with tribal groups, which direct a total of approximately 75 EMS programs involving some 600 emergency medical technicians (EMTs). The EMS-C program, MCHB, and HRSA contracted with IHS to develop a set of activities designed to obtain information on the capabilities of Native American tribes to serve children in emergency situations. IHS will conduct a national assessment of all Native American tribal EMS programs to obtain the information needed by MCHB to assess the state of readiness of tribes to serve children in emergency situations (EMS-C National Resource Center, 1999).
- *Centers for Disease Control and Prevention (CDC).* CDC is the lead federal agency for protecting the health and safety of U.S. residents. Its focus is on disease prevention and control, environmental health, and health promotion and education activities designed to improve the health of the population. CDC works with partners to detect and investigate health problems and conduct research aimed at enhancing prevention (CDC, 2004). Like NIH, CDC is organized into centers, institutes, and offices. The centers, institutes, and offices respond individually in their areas of expertise and pool their resources and expertise on cross-cutting issues and specific health threats. The National Center for Injury Prevention and Control is the lead federal agency for injury prevention. Its extramural research program funds and monitors research in all three phases of injury control: prevention, acute care, and rehabilitation. The program also funds research in the two major disciplines involved in injury control research: biomechanics and epidemiology. Research supported by the program focuses on the broad-based need to control morbidity, disability, death, and costs associated with injury. CDC's recently completed Injury Research Agenda was developed with extensive input from academic research centers, national nonprofit organizations, and other federal agencies with a stake in injury prevention. The document will guide research in seven areas of injury prevention and control. The current plan for implementation of the agenda is to seek $250 million in appropriations over 5 years to support research in six broad areas, all of which are directly relevant to emergency care research. Emergency providers are well positioned to interact with CDC on various efforts, including participating in extramural and intramural projects, serving on advisory and grant review committees, and providing input on the agency's recommendations (Carden et al., 1998).

- ***Centers for Medicare and Medicaid Services (CMS).*** CMS is responsible for administering the Medicare program and, in partnership with states, the Medicaid program and the State Children's Health Insurance Program (SCHIP). CMS supports a number of research projects in an effort to provide better services to program beneficiaries. Many of the research studies currently funded by CMS involve children enrolled in Medicaid and SCHIP, but none are specific to emergency care services.

Department of Transportation (DOT). The National Highway Traffic Safety Administration (NHTSA) within DOT has the mission of reducing deaths and disability, as well as health care costs, resulting from motor vehicle crashes, medical emergencies, or other injury incidents. NHTSA's Office of EMS works to enhance emergency medical care for those injured in motor vehicle crashes and acknowledges that to ensure optimal care for crash victims, EMS systems must be prepared to provide a comprehensive range of community health services. Therefore, the agency's EMS support is directed broadly at a range of system needs. The agency is closely aligned with MCHB in support of the EMS-C program. Together with MCHB, the Office of EMS commissioned the *National EMS Research Agenda*, which describes the history and current status of EMS research. It also describes strategies for improving the quality and quantity of EMS research, with the goal of providing a scientific foundation for current and future prehospital care.

Department of Defense (DoD). The military provides care to more than 3.5 million children. DoD and HRSA work together to explore pediatric access and quality improvement issues in emergency care in the developing managed care delivery system. Additionally, in 1990 Congress mandated that DoD conduct a special study of pediatric EMS systems within its military treatment facilities as part of a national initiative to improve the quality of children's medical services. The goals of the study continue to be relevant and include assessing EMS, evaluating the effectiveness of EMS within DoD, and identifying specific opportunities for improvement (DHHS et al., 2000).

Department of Homeland Security (DHS). The mission of DHS is to secure the homeland. Within that broad mission, the Federal Emergency Management Agency (FEMA) is the federal coordinating entity responsible for emergency preparedness, response, recovery, and mitigation. FEMA works with other federal, state, and local agencies to coordinate response and recovery operations following a major disaster. It also operates the FEMA for Kids Program, which provides resources for children and families on line. Within FEMA, the U.S. Fire Administration is involved in prevention programs, for example, a public safety campaign to reduce deaths from fire among infants and toddlers. FEMA does not appear to commission many research studies

continued

but certainly is a relevant participant in the provision of EMS for children, particularly as related to disasters.

Private Organizations

The financial support available from private organizations is typically more limited than that from federal sources; however, some private organizations have funding targeted specifically at emergency services or emergency medicine research.

The Emergency Medicine Foundation (EMF) was created in 1973 as the education and research arm of the American College of Emergency Physicians (ACEP). Organized as a not-for-profit, EMF is unique in that it awards funding for education and research solely in the area of emergency medicine. Funding for EMF grants comes from donations by individual emergency physicians, physician groups, corporations, and other foundations. ACEP underwrites all of the administrative expenses of EMF. EMF grant funding has grown considerably since the foundation's inception. During the first grant cycle in 1981–1982, EMF awarded 2 grants totaling $8,500; in 2004–2005, it awarded 18 grants totaling nearly $500,000 (Pollack and Cairns, 1999).

The Society of Academic Emergency Medicine (SAEM) operates its own Research Fund, supported by donations from members. The fund has about $2 million in reserves, and SAEM hopes to expand it to increase the number of grants awarded (SAEM, 2004). The fund supports several different types of grants designed to promote the development of research skills rather than to support any particular research project.

The National Emergency Medicine Association (NEMA) also offers grants to emergency medicine researchers. The organization is committed to trauma prevention and the delivery of quality medical services at each stage of trauma

of EMTs represent opportunities for pediatric emergency care researchers to disseminate new information to emergency care providers.

The Dearth of Well-Trained Pediatric Emergency Care Researchers

Many authors have decried the lack of a sufficient pool of well-trained laboratory and patient-oriented investigators in emergency care and have identified it as a major barrier to emergency care research. Emergency care providers who are also basic science investigators or who collaborate with such investigators may serve as an excellent bridge for translating the findings of basic investigations to the emergently ill patient and for bringing unanswered questions back to the laboratory. But medical training in pediatric emergency medicine, like that in emergency medicine generally, care, with an emphasis on first response at the time of the emergency. NEMA grants provide funding to hospitals, health clinics, trauma centers, fire departments, and physicians. Awards go to small, underfunded rural organizations as well as to well-established entities (NEMA, 2003).

For pediatric emergency medicine research, there are additional associations and foundations that may provide financial support. The American Academy of Pediatrics' (AAP) Section on Emergency Medicine offers a young investigator award of $10,000 for a research project that addresses issues pertinent to the acutely ill or injured child. It also offers several awards that recognize individuals who have made significant contributions to research in pediatric emergency medicine (AAP, 2003). The Ambulatory Pediatric Association, an organization of academic pediatric health professionals, offers a young investigator grant that provides up to $10,000 per project to new investigators for research in a number of areas, including pediatric emergency medicine (Christakis et al., 2001). Finally, researchers seeking funding for relatively small projects may be able to obtain it from their local tertiary pediatric referral center (Havel, 2004).

Industry

Industry or corporate funding constitutes a small source of support for clinical research in pediatric emergency care. The biomedical industry provides some funding for emergency medicine research, particularly evaluations of new drugs or medical devices. Emergency medicine physicians are in a good position to conduct this work since the ED is the initial site of diagnosis and treatment for many illnesses. This makes it an ideal setting for clinical trials of time-critical pharmaceutical agents, diagnostics, and medical devices (Morris and Manning, 2004).

is heavily focused on the development of clinical skills, with little time for formal training in research methodology (Biros et al., 1998). Clinical fellowships are more numerous and more likely to be funded than research fellowships. In 2003, only 12 percent of fellowships in the SAEM listing appeared to have a primary research focus, and only about 70 percent of those positions were filled. None were backed by federal funding from NIH or other agencies. In addition, only 11 percent of the advertised fellowships offered an advanced degree, such as a PhD, MS, or MPH, during the course of fellowship training, although others may offer that option (Pollack et al., 2003).

While some clinical fellowships have a research component, a research training program that does not include 2 years of dedicated research training (e.g., greater than 80 percent research time) is unlikely to result in long-term success in today's research climate (NIH, 2003). Formal fellowship training is now a well-recognized requirement for those embarking on a successful long-term research-based academic career (Stern et al., 2001).

As detailed in a report by the ACEP Research Committee, a substantial portion (27 percent) of all emergency medicine trainees intend to pursue an academic career, while paradoxically, the research and research training support devoted to emergency medicine and emergency care is very low. Of the 1,281 NIH training grants to medical school departments awarded in 2003, only 1 went to a department of emergency medicine. This lack of funding is even more striking when compared with that in other medical fields. For example, fewer than 9 percent of internal medicine trainees expressed a desire to purse an academic career, but NIH awarded 354 training grants to departments of internal medicine in 2003 (ACEP Research Committee, 2005). However, when emergency medicine trainees express a desire to pursue academics, it is likely that most envision themselves as clinical educators rather than federally funded investigators. While existing foundation support has increased the number of well-trained emergency care investigators, a significant increase in the total research training support available will be required to substantially expand the nation's emergency care research capability.

As discussed in Chapter 4, most pediatric emergency medicine physicians hold their primary board certification in pediatrics; moreover, most pediatric emergency medicine fellowships in the United States are organized under the pediatric residency review committee (RRC) governed by the rules of the American Board of Pediatrics (ABP). The ABP requires that pediatric emergency medicine fellowships include a meaningful scholarly project; however, the vast majority of pediatric emergency medicine trainees pursue clinician educator career paths that emphasize clinical service in pediatric emergency medicine and bedside teaching rather than academic research. Like pediatric emergency medicine fellowship programs organized under the emergency medicine RRC, pediatric emergency medicine fellowships under the pediatric RRC infrequently result in research-intensive academic careers. Historically, these fellowships have not provided research experiences that have led to sustained, independent research contributions following the fellowship.

While there is scarce funding for emergency and trauma care researchers, research training for EMS personnel is more limited still. Unlike the medical field, in which research fellowships exist, there is no clear path to the development of research expertise in EMS. As a result, EMS research is fostered largely by researchers trained in emergency medicine (Sayre et al., 2002).

One potential strategy for addressing this barrier is to promote and fund centers of excellence in emergency and trauma care. Such centers of excellence would provide funding that would allow experienced researchers to work with young investigators on projects, supporting mentorship. A series of 2-year "fellowship" opportunities could target promising young researchers to enable them to gain skills in research methodology. This goal could be met by establishing centers of excellence funded by NIH; expanding the availability and appropriateness of K-awards; and enhancing cooperation among federal, professional society, and foundation partners for the funding of young investigator awards.

Another strategy would be to develop training grants for emergency medicine educators, as well as to offer support for training programs to prepare midlevel providers, such as EMTs, nurse practitioners, and physician assistants, for conducting and participating in research. Presently, midlevel research development grants are restricted to primary care specialties, thereby excluding emergency physicians and other providers of emergency care. There is a pressing need for access to training grants, including K23 and K08 applications, specifically targeting emergency and trauma care researchers. T32 training grants should be offered to the relatively few academic departments or divisions of emergency medicine that have established viable lines of federally funded laboratory clinical and/or health services research. In addition, health care foundations concerned with reducing health care disparities and promoting access to care (such as The Robert Wood Johnson Foundation and The Henry J. Kaiser Family Foundation) should fund career development awards and fellowship programs for emergency care and trauma physicians.

Data Limitations

One of the challenges of conducting research on emergency care services is that no single institution is likely to have access to sample sizes large enough to answer important questions about critically ill individuals, particularly children. For example, a 10-center study of children with diabetic ketoacidosis identified only 61 cases of cerebral edema during the 15-year study period (Glaser et al., 2001). Similarly, a study intended to produce a decision rule for computed tomography (CT) scanning of the brain found that fewer than 1 percent of children with minor head injuries required a neurosurgical intervention (Atabaki et al., 1999). Decision rules based on small samples tend to suffer from unacceptably wide confidence intervals, so the validity of the findings are limited (PECARN, 2003). Discussed below are several options for overcoming these data limitations.

Research Networks

The use of research networks to overcome the challenge of data limitations has proven successful in the past. The large number of patients included in the networks allows researchers to carry out trials designed to evaluate rare conditions or complications.

There are a number of primary care research networks in existence. For example, the AAP established the Pediatric Research in Office Settings (PROS) Network in 1986. The mission of this network is to improve the health of children and enhance primary care practice by conducting national collaborative practice-based research. In 2004, the network included more than 1,900 practitioners from over 700 offices in the 50 states, Canada, and Puerto Rico. The network is currently working on a variety of projects, including studies on how practitioners diagnose child abuse in primary care settings, on a new way to help parents prevent child violence, and on how to improve practice/clinic immunization rates. The Vermont Oxford Network (VON), founded in 1988, includes more than 485 neonatal intensive care units in the United States and other countries. It maintains a database that provides unique, reliable, and confidential data to participating units for use in quality management, process improvement, internal audit, and peer review. The network disseminates the results of its research in medical journals and through a network publication. The National Cancer Institute at NIH also has a pediatric research network—the Children's Oncology Group (COG)—which was established in 2000. COG is a clinical trials cooperative group devoted exclusively to childhood and adolescent cancer research. It develops and coordinates clinical cancer trials conducted at its 238 member institutions in the United States, Canada, Europe, and Australia. COG members include more than 5,000 cancer researchers.

There are also several research networks focused on general aspects of emergency medicine. For example, Emergency ID Net is a CDC-funded, interdisciplinary, multicenter, ED-based network for research on emerging infectious diseases, established in cooperation with CDC's National Center for Infectious Diseases. The network is based at 11 university-affiliated urban hospital EDs with a combined annual patient visit census of more than 900,000 (Talan et al., 1998). The Emergency Medicine Network's Multi-Center Airway Research Collaborative (MARC) performs long-term research on airway disorders, including asthma, chronic obstructive pulmonary disease, anaphylaxis, pneumonia, and bronchiolitis. Many of the studies investigate both adults and children. The Emergency Medicine Cardiac Research and Education Group International, an industry-sponsored group centered in Cincinnati, Ohio, was established in 1989 to conduct multicenter clinical trials on serum markers for the early diagnosis of acute myocardial infarction. Since its inception, the network has grown from 18 researchers in 15 institutions to 44 researchers in 31 academic facilities worldwide. These collaboratives have a well-defined group leadership, such as a steering committee or board of directors; have produced multiple publications; and in many cases have received funding support from diverse sources, including government, private foundations, and industry. In addition, they tend to perform education and service functions along with research (Pollack et al., 2003).

PECARN is the only research network focused specifically on pediatric emergency care. It includes four regional nodes with 21 hospitals serving approximately 900,000 pediatric patients a year (PECARN, 2006). Since being established, PECARN has completed a major core data project, and several other projects have been federally funded for the evaluation of such issues as the efficacy of dexamethasone in the treatment of bronchiolitis, the factors that can contribute to a decision rule for the evaluation and treatment of minor head injuries in children, the use of lorazepam for treatment of seizures in children, and cervical spine injuries in children.

An important attribute of these research networks is that they establish an infrastructure for research in a particular area. If they receive the funding needed for sustainability, they not only generate important findings in the field, but also help train and support the development of young investigators. Recognizing the importance of research networks to the knowledge base and the research infrastructure, the committee formulated recommendation 7.1—that the Secretary of Health and Human Services conduct a study to examine research gaps and opportunities in emergency care, including pediatric emergency care, encompassing a focused look at the development of multicenter research networks. Ideally, such networks should address issues including prevention, trauma, and pediatric emergency medicine. In particular, research networks such as PECARN should expand their research into the prehospital environment.

Research networks generally should work toward expanding to more hospitals so their findings can be more representative of the care that is delivered nationally. For example, PECARN represents children's hospitals disproportionately to the volume of care these hospitals provide to pediatric emergency care patients nationally. Since children's hospitals tend to have more pediatric resources than other hospitals, certain findings from PECARN may not be reflective of the care provided at community hospitals nationally. One of the challenges to expanding PECARN beyond children's hospitals is that community hospitals often lack the infrastructure and resources to conduct clinical research. The professional reward structures in community hospitals often are not aligned with the commitment of large amounts of time and effort to research. PECARN and other research networks will have to be creative in achieving representation of the many children who receive care in community hospital EDs. As PECARN tries to expand its reach, network leaders should also consider how pediatric surgeons, health services researchers, and public health researchers might be better integrated into the network to expand the scope of research generated.

The committee's call for the development and enhancement of multicenter research networks is not new. In fact, at both the 1995 Emergency Medicine Research Directors Conference and the 1997 Future of Emergency Medicine Research Conference, participants encouraged the growth of such networks (Pollack et al., 2003).

Trauma Registries

Injury is the leading cause of death and disability in children beyond the first year of life. The optimal clinical management of pediatric injuries may differ significantly from that of similar injuries in adults. Despite the prevalence of pediatric trauma, many unanswered questions remain about optimal care for certain subsets of pediatric trauma patients. Trauma registries, used to collect, store, and retrieve data on trauma patients, could help in deriving answers to some of these questions by allowing researchers to study etiological factors, demographic characteristics, diagnoses, treatments, and clinical outcomes of pediatric patients. Registries could be used to evaluate and improve the quality of care, compare patient outcomes across providers, identify hazardous environments (e.g., dangerous intersections or devices), identify injury trends, prioritize and evaluate public health interventions, provide data for benchmarking and improvement purposes, and monitor trends in trauma systems (HRSA, 2005). Trauma registries are expensive to develop and maintain, but they are effective in decreasing morbidity and mortality (Shapiro et al., 1994).

There have been a number of different initiatives aimed at developing trauma registries. Today, 37 states maintain such a registry; these efforts have been supported by grant funding from HRSA's Trauma-EMS Systems Program, which was recently defunded (HRSA, 2005). This situation represents an improvement over that in 1992, when only 24 states operated trauma registries (Shapiro et al., 1994). State trauma registries collect pediatric-specific data; however, they have a number of shortcomings. They are not standardized nationally or even statewide in some cases. They vary in a number of ways, including patient inclusion/exclusion criteria, data definitions, and injury severity scoring (HRSA, 2005). And reporting is not mandatory in some states, so state trauma managers estimate that only 70 percent of trauma cases are reported to the registry (Guice and Cassidy, 2004).

There have been a number of efforts at the national level to develop trauma registries. In 1985, the National Pediatric Trauma Registry (NPTR) was established to study the causes, circumstances, and consequences of injuries to children. Funded by the National Institute for Disability and Rehabilitation Research, the NPTR contained data on more than 10,000 patients pooled from a number of different states. Data from the NPTR allowed researchers to investigate a number of topics, including the epidemiology of trauma deaths in rural children (Vane and Shackford, 1995), survival rates at pediatric trauma centers (Osler et al., 2001), and characteristics of bicycle-related head injuries (Li et al., 1995). However, the registry had several problems that limited the usefulness of the data and created challenges for institutions participating in the data collection process (Smith et al., 2001). For example, the registry was a voluntary system without a clear epidemiologically representative catchment area. The NPTR stopped collecting data as of February 2002 (Barnett and Saltzman, 2004).

Also in the 1980s, the American College of Surgeons (ACS) collected trauma data for its Major Trauma Outcome Study (MTOS), which was operational between 1982 and 1989. Under the MTOS, researchers from 140 hospitals used a standard collection form for data submission. During its 8-year lifetime, the MTOS collected data on 80,000 cases (Fantus and Fildes, 2003). More important, the MTOS led to the creation of the National Trauma Data Bank (NTDB). When the MTOS ended, the ACS committed to developing a national trauma registry, and the NTDB became operational in 1993 (Pollock, 1995). Today, the NTDB represents the largest aggregation of trauma registry data ever assembled, with 1.2 million records from nearly 500 trauma centers. The ACS receives support for the NTDB from HRSA, CDC, and NHTSA (ACS, 2004).

The NTDB is an impressive achievement. Numerous research efforts have been undertaken using the data bank. Additionally, the ACS releases an annual pediatric report that includes more than 235,000 pediatric records from 474 trauma centers in 43 states, territories, and the District of Columbia. The ACS also has a Pediatric Surgery Specialty Group that works with the NTDB Committee to expand the data bank for children, with the goal of receiving data on every pediatric patient treated in every trauma center in the United States (Fildes, 2005).

At the same time, the NTDB has some important drawbacks. First, it does not allow population estimates. It obtains data from approximately 61 percent of level I and 51 percent of level II trauma centers (essentially all of which submit adult and pediatric data) (Fildes, 2005), but it collects data only from those hospitals that choose to submit them (NHTSA, 2001). However, the NTDB's impressive yearly growth (500,000 new cases in 2002) offsets some of the concerns about its representativeness (NHTSA, 2001). The other problem with the NTDB is that it was not specifically designed to capture certain pediatric data elements.

The planned advances for the NTDB are promising, however. The ACS was awarded a contract from CDC's National Center for Injury Prevention and Control to develop a nationally representative sample of U.S. trauma centers that would provide data on trauma patients for the NTDB. Those data will allow researchers to compute national estimates with high confidence. An important part of this project is the inclusion of non–level I and II hospitals. The project has not yet developed a stratum for pediatric patients, but this is intended for the future. Additionally, the NTDB will implement a new set of data elements that will be more conducive to the collection of pediatric data; the original data elements were not defined to capture pediatric information. For example, the new data dictionary contains a field on safety devices so the NTDB can collect specific information on child restraints (Personal communication, M. Neal, March 1, 2006).

Recently, another initiative to create a national pediatric trauma registry began. In 2002, the EMS-C program awarded two grants aimed at designing and planning for a National Trauma Registry for Children (NTRC). The goal of the NTRC is "to develop a standardized, nation-wide model to provide accurate estimates of the scope and characteristics of pediatric trauma and to provide a national benchmark for valid comparisons" (Cassidy and Guice, 2005). The resulting data will allow clinical and epidemiological questions to be explored using a more expansive and richer source of information than could be obtained with regional and statewide systems.

Under the two grants, researchers identified existing data sources and methods of electronic transfer, defined necessary pediatric data elements and inclusion/exclusion criteria, developed secure data transfer methods, designed a nationally representative sample, and identified methods to ensure hospital participation (Cassidy and Guice, 2005). A third grant was awarded in 2005 to evaluate the quality of pediatric data from state registries that might contribute to the NTRC. However, implementation of the NTRC has not yet begun. The NTRC planning group is expected to recommend two implementation phases. The first will be a population-based injury surveillance system, which will allow researchers to draw population inferences from a statistical sample of national hospitals. The second will be a case contribution component, similar to the original NPTR (Cooper, 2005).

It is important to note the collaboration that has occurred between staff from the NTDB and the NTRC. In fact, a representative from the NTDB was on the NTRC planning committee, and a representative from the NTRC assisted NTDB planners with the development of new data elements more suitable for the collection of pediatric data (Personal communication, M. Neal, March 1, 2006).

Despite all of the efforts made to enhance the development of trauma systems with interpretive pediatric data, no single trauma registry currently provides accurate estimates of the scope and characteristics of pediatric trauma (Cassidy and Guice, 2005). However, the committee recognizes that the NTDB constitutes the largest repository of pediatric trauma data anywhere (Cooper, 2005) and is taking steps to improve its pediatric capacity. The committee supports the continued progress in this area. The committee recommends that **the administrators of state and national trauma registries** include standard pediatric-specific data elements and provide the data to the National Trauma Data Bank. Additionally, the American College of Surgeons should establish a multidisciplinary pediatric specialty committee to continuously evaluate pediatric-specific data elements for the National Trauma Data Bank and identify areas for pediatric research (7.2). The planning committee should include pediatric surgeons, pediatric emergency care researchers, and public health and health services researchers.

SUMMARY OF RECOMMENDATIONS

7.1 The Secretary of Health and Human Services should conduct a study to examine the gaps and opportunities in emergency care research, including pediatric emergency care, and recommend a strategy for the optimal organization and funding of the research effort. This study should include consideration of the training of new investigators, development of multicenter research networks, involvement of emergency and trauma care researchers in the grant review and research advisory processes, and improved research coordination through a dedicated center or institute. Congress and federal agencies involved in emergency and trauma care research (including the Department of Transportation, the Department of Health and Human Services, the Department of Homeland Security, and the Department of Defense) should implement the study's recommendations.

7.2 Administrators of state and national trauma registries should include standard pediatric-specific data elements and provide the data to the National Trauma Data Bank. Additionally, the American College of Surgeons should establish a multidisciplinary pediatric specialty committee to continuously evaluate pediatric-specific data elements for the National Trauma Data Bank and identify areas for pediatric research.

REFERENCES

AAP (American Academy of Pediatrics). 2002. Selecting and using the most appropriate car safety seats for growing children: Guidelines for counseling parents. *Pediatrics* 109(3):550–553.

AAP. 2003. *Section on Emergency Medicine, Description of Section Sponsored Awards.* [Online]. Available: http://www.aap.org/sections/PEM/awards.htm [accessed November 3, 2004].

AAP. 2005. *Section on Emergency Medicine—Collaborative Research Committee (PEM CRC).* [Online]. Available: www.aap.org/sections/PEM/pemcrc.pemcrc.htm [accessed September, 28, 2005].

ACEP (American College of Emergency Physicians). 2002. *The Role of the Emergency Physician in Injury Prevention and Control* (Policy Statement Number 400197). [Online]. Available: http://www.acep.org/webportal/PracticeResources/PolicyStatements/injprev/RoleEmergencyPhysicianInjuryPreventionControl.htm [accessed September 2005].

ACEP Research Committee (American College of Emergency Physicians Research Committee). 2005. *Report on Emergency Medicine Research*. Washington, DC: ACEP.

ACS (American College of Surgeons). 2004. *National Trauma Data Bank*. [Online]. Available: www.facs.org/trauma/ntdbwhatis.html [accessed November 15, 2005].

AHRQ (Agency for Healthcare Research and Quality). 2005. *Overview of the State Emergency Department Databases (SEDD)*. [Online]. Available: http://www.hcup-us.ahrq.gov/seddoverview.jsp [accessed September 29, 2005].

Atabaki S, Sadow KB, Berns SD, Chamberlain JM. 1999, May 3. How good are clinicians at predicting intracranial injuries? *Annual Meeting of the Ambulatory Pediatric Association*. San Francisco, CA.

Baker SP, O'Neill B, Ginsburg MJ, Guohua L. 1992. *The Injury Fact Book*. New York, NY: Oxford University Press.

Barnett SJ, Saltzman DA. 2004. Efficacy of pediatric-specific trauma centers [Abstract]. *Pediatric Critical Care Medicine* 5(1):93–94.

Berg RA, Wilcoxson D, Hilwig RW, Kern KB, Sanders AB, Otto CW, Eklund DK, Ewy GA. 1995. The need for ventilatory support during bystander CPR. *Annals of Emergency Medicine* 26(3):342–350.

Berg RA, Kern KB, Hilwig RW, Berg MD, Sanders AB, Otto CW, Ewy GA. 1997. Assisted ventilation does not improve outcome in a porcine model of single-rescuer bystander cardiopulmonary resuscitation. *Circulation* 95(6):1635–1641.

Berg RA, Sanders AB, Kern KB, Hilwig RW, Heidenreich JW, Porter ME, Ewy GA. 2001. Adverse hemodynamic effects of interrupting chest compressions for rescue breathing during cardiopulmonary resuscitation for ventricular fibrillation cardiac arrest. *Circulation* 104(20):2465–2470.

Biros MH, Barsan WG, Lewis RJ, Sanders AB. 1998. Supporting emergency medicine research: Developing the infrastructure. *Academic Emergency Medicine* 5(2):177–184.

Carden D, Dronen S, Gehrig G, Zalenski R. 1998. Funding strategies for emergency medicine research. *Annals of Emergency Medicine* 31(2):179–187.

Cassidy L, Guice KS. 2005. *National Trauma Registry for Children Planning Grants*. Washington, DC: HRSA.

CDC (Centers for Disease Control and Prevention). 1995. Air-bag-associated fatal injuries to infants and children riding in front passenger seats—United States. *Journal of the American Medical Association* 274(22):1752–1753.

CDC. 1996. Update: Fatal air bag-related injuries to children—United States, 1993–1996. *Morbidity & Mortality Weekly Report* 45(49):1073–1076.

CDC. 2004. *About CDC*. [Online]. Available: http://www.cdc.gov/aboutcdc.htm [accessed November 1, 2004].

Christakis DA, Mell L, Koepsell TD, Zimmerman FJ, Connell FA. 2001. Association of lower continuity of care with greater risk of emergency department use and hospitalization in children. *Pediatrics* 107(3):524–529.

Cooper A. 2005. *National Organization Updates*. 2005 EMSC Annual Grantee Meeting. Washington, DC: MCHB.

DeWitt DS, Prough DS, Taylor CL, Whitley JM. 1992a. Reduced cerebral blood flow, oxygen delivery, and electroencephalographic activity after traumatic brain injury and mild hemorrhage in cats. *Journal of Neurosurgery* 76(5):812–821.

DeWitt DS, Prough DS, Taylor CL, Whitley JM, Deal DD, Vines SM. 1992b. Regional cerebrovascular responses to progressive hypotension after traumatic brain injury in cats. *The American Journal of Physiology* 263(4 Pt. 2):H1276–H1284.

DHHS, HRSA, MCHB (Department of Health and Human Services, Health Resources and Services Administration, Maternal and Child Health Bureau). 1997. *5 Year Plan: Midcourse Review: Emergency Medical Services for Children, 1995–2000.* Washington, DC: EMS-C National Resource Center.

DHHS, HRSA, MCHB. 2000. *Five-year Plan: Emergency Medical Services for Children, 2001–2005.* Washington, DC: EMS-C National Resource Center.

Eisenberg M, Bergner L, Hallstrom A. 1983. Epidemiology of cardiac arrest and resuscitation in children. *Annals of Emergency Medicine* 12(11):672–674.

EMS-C National Resource Center. 1999. *EMSC and Cultural Competence* (00810). Washington, DC: EMS-C National Resource Center.

Fantus RJ, Fildes F. 2003, May. How national is the trauma data bank? *Bulletin of the American College of Surgeons.* P. 37.

Fildes JJ, ed. 2005. *National Trauma Data Bank Pediatric Report.* Chicago, IL: ACS.

Fulton RL, Flynn WJ, Mancino M, Bowles D, Cryer HM. 1993. Brain injury causes loss of cardiovascular response to hemorrhagic shock. *Journal of Investigative Surgery* 6(2):117–131.

Gausche M, Seidel JS, Henderson DP, Ness B, Ward PM, Wayland BW. 1989a. Violent death in the pediatric age group: Rural and urban differences. *Pediatric Emergency Care* 5(1):64–67.

Gausche M, Seidel JS, Henderson DP, Ness B, Ward PM, Wayland BW, Almeida B. 1989b. Pediatric deaths and emergency medical services (EMS) in urban and rural areas. *Pediatric Emergency Care* 5(3):158–612.

Gausche M, Lewis RJ, Stratton SJ, Haynes BE, Gunter CS, Goodrich SM, Poore PD, McCollough MD, Henderson DP, Pratt FD, Seidel JS. 2000. Effect of out-of-hospital pediatric endotracheal intubation on survival and neurological outcome: A controlled clinical trial. *Journal of the American Medical Association* 283(6):783–790.

Glaser N, Barnett P, McCaslin I, Nelson D, Trainor J, Louie J, Kaufman F, Quayle K, Roback M, Malley R, Kuppermann N, Pediatric Emergency Medicine Collaborative Research Committee of the American Academy of Pediatrics. 2001. Risk factors for cerebral edema in children with diabetic ketoacidosis. *New England Journal of Medicine* 344:264–269.

Gough J, Callahan J, Brown L. 2004. Where is the EMS-C literature? *Prehospital Emergency Care* 8(1):86.

Guice KS, Cassidy L. 2004. *State Trauma Registries Survey and Updated Report: December 2004 (Abstract)* (Product ID 001055). Rockville, MD: HRSA.

Havel C. 2004. *Research Funding in Pediatric Emergency Medicine.* [Online]. Available: http://www.saem.org/newsltr/2002/jan–feb/peds.pdf [accessed November 2, 2004].

Henderson DP. 1988. The Los Angeles pediatric emergency care system. *Journal of Emergency Nursing* 14(2):96–100.

HRSA (Health Resources and Services Administration). 2005. *Trauma-Emergency Medical Services Systems Trauma Registries.* [Online]. Available: http://www.hrsa.gov/trauma/registries.htm [accessed November 16, 2005].

IOM (Institute of Medicine). 1985. *Injury in America: A Continuing Health Problem.* Washington, DC: National Academy Press.

IOM. 1993. *Emergency Medical Services for Children.* Durch JS, Lohr KN, eds. Washington, DC: National Academy Press.

IOM. 2001. *Crossing the Quality Chasm: A New Health System for the 21st Century.* Washington, DC: National Academy Press.

IOM. 2004. *NIH Extramural Center Programs.* Manning, FJ, McGeary, M, Estabrook, R, eds. Washington, DC: The National Academies Press.

Ishige N, Pitts LH, Hashimoto T, Nishimura MC, Bartkowski HM. 1987. Effect of hypoxia on traumatic brain injury in rats: Part 1. Changes in neurological function, electroencephalograms, and histopathology. *Neurosurgery* 20(6):848–853.

Ishige N, Pitts LH, Berry I, Nishimura MC, James TL. 1988. The effects of hypovolemic hypotension on high-energy phosphate metabolism of traumatized brain in rats. *Journal of Neurosurgery* 68(1):129–136.

Johnston BD, Rivara FP, Droesch RM, Dunn C, Copass MK. 2002. Behavior change counseling in the emergency department to reduce injury risk: A randomized, controlled trial. *Pediatrics* 110(2 Pt. 1):267–274.

Kern KB, Hilwig RW, Berg RA, Sanders AB, Ewy GA. 2002. Importance of continuous chest compressions during cardiopulmonary resuscitation: Improved outcome during a simulated single lay-rescuer scenario. *Circulation* 105(5):645–649.

Lenfant C. 2003. Shattuck lecture—clinical research to clinical practice—lost in translation? *New England Journal of Medicine* 349(9):868–874.

Lewelt W, Jenkins LW, Miller JD. 1980. Autoregulation of cerebral blood flow after experimental fluid percussion injury of the brain. *Journal of Neurosurgery* 53(4):500–511.

Lewelt W, Jenkins LW, Miller JD. 1982. Effects of experimental fluid-percussion injury of the brain on cerebrovascular reactivity of hypoxia and to hypercapnia. *Journal of Neurosurgery* 56(3):332–338.

Lewis R J. 2004. Academic emergency medicine and the "tragedy of the commons" defined. *Academic Emergency Medicine* 11(5):423–427.

Li G, Baker SP, Fowler C, DiScala C. 1995. Factors related to the presence of head injury in bicycle-related pediatric trauma patients. *The Journal of Trauma* 38(6):871–875.

Lubitz DS, Seidel JS, Chameides L, Luten RC, Zaritsky AL, Campbell FW. 1988. A rapid method for estimating weight and resuscitation drug dosages from length in the pediatric age group. *Annals of Emergency Medicine* 17(6):576–581.

Ludwig S. 2001. Pediatric emergency medicine: What lies ahead. *Clinical Pediatric Emergency Medicine* 2:280–283.

Mace SE, Gerardi MJ, Dietrich AM, Knazik SR, Mulligan-Smith D, Sweeney RL, Warden CR. 2001. Injury prevention and control in children. *Annals of Emergency Medicine* 38(4):405–414.

Maclean CB. 1993. The future role of emergency medical services systems in prevention. *Annals of Emergency Medicine* 22(11):1743–1746.

Marx J. 2004. *Academic Emergency Medicine in the Year 2000*. [Online]. Available: http://www.saem.org/publicat/chap2.htm [accessed November 3, 2004].

McCaffrey M, German A, Lalonde F, Letts M. 1999. Air bags and children: A potentially lethal combination (Abstract). *Journal of Pediatric Orthopedics* 19(1):60–64.

McCaig LF, Ly N. 2002. *National Hospital Ambulatory Medical Care Survey: 2000 Emergency Department Summary* (Advance Data from Vital and Health Statistics; No. 326). Hyattsville, MD: National Center Health Statistics.

MCHB (Maternal and Child Health Bureau). 2004a. *Emergency Medical Services for Children: A 10-Year Retrospective Based on the Recommendations of the Committee on Pediatric Emergency Medical Services of the National Academy of Sciences Institute of Medicine*. Rockville, MD: HRSA.

MCHB. 2004b. *Emergency Medical Services for Children. Five Year Plan 2001–2005: Midcourse Review*. Washington, DC: EMS-C National Resource Center.

Mears G. 2005. *National EMS Database*. [Online]. Available: http://www.nemsis.org/PowerPoints/NEMSIS%20Overview%205–2005.ppt#362,1,National EMS Database [accessed August 2005].

Mears G, Ornato JP, Dawson DE. 2002. Emergency medical services information systems and a future EMS national database. *Prehospital Emergemcy Care* 6(1):123–130.

Morris D, Manning J. 2004. *Research in Academic Emergency Medicine*. [Online]. Available: http://www.saem.org/publicat/chap6.htm [accessed November 3, 2004].

National Center for Statistics and Analysis, NHTSA. 2005. *National Occupant Protection Use Survey: Controlled Intersection Study*. Washington, DC: NHTSA.

NEMA (National Emergency Medicine Association). 2003. *Grants Program of the National Emergency Medicine Association.* [Online]. Available: http://www.nemahealth.org/organization/grants.htm [accessed December, 2005].

NHTSA (National Highway Traffic Safety Administration). 1996. *Emergency Medical Services Agenda for the Future.* Washington, DC: NHTSA.

NHTSA. 2001. *Trauma System Agenda for the Future.* Washington, DC: NHTSA.

NIH. 2003. *Ruth L. Kirschstein National Research Service Awards for Individual Postdoctoral Fellows (F32).* [Online]. Available: http://grants1.nih.gov/grants/guide/pa-files/PA-03-067.html [accessed April 17, 2005].

Osler TM, Vane DW, Tepas JJ, Rogers FB, Shackford SR, Badger GJ. 2001. Do pediatric trauma centers have better survival rates than adult trauma centers? An examination of the National Pediatric Trauma Registry. *The Journal of Trauma* 50(1):96–101.

PECARN (Pediatric Emergency Care Applied Research Network). 2003. The Pediatric Emergency Care Applied Research Network (PECARN): Rationale, development, and first steps. *Academic Emergency Medicine* 10(6):661–668.

PECARN. 2005. *About PECARN.* [Online]. Available: http://www.pecarn.org/about_pecarn.htm [accessed April 16, 2005].

PECARN. 2006. *PECARN Brochure.* Available: http://www.pecarn.org/pdfs/PECARN%20Brochure%20Version%201-27-06%20FINAL.pdf [accessed January 2007].

Pollack C, Cairns CB. 1999. The Emergency Medicine Foundation: 25 years of advancing education and research. *Annals of Emergency Medicine* 33(4):448–450.

Pollack C, Hollander J, O'Neil B, Neumar R, Summers R, Camargo C, Younger J, Callaway C, Gallagher E, Kellermann A, Krause G, Schafermeyer R, Sloan E, Stern S. 2003. Status report: Development of emergency medicine research since the Macy report. *Annals of Emergency Medicine* 42(1):66–80.

Pollock DA. 1995. *Trauma Registries and Public Health Surveillance.* [Online]. Available: http://www.cdc.gov/nchs/data/ice/ice95v1/c11.pdf [accessed May 2006].

Ramenofsky ML, Ramenofsky MB, Jurkovich GJ, Threadgill D, Dierking BH, Powell RW. 1988. The predictive validity of the Pediatric Trauma Score. *The Journal of Trauma* 28(7):1038–1042.

Rivara FP. 1993. From the bedside to the public policy arena: The role of general pediatric research. *Pediatrics* 91(3):628–631.

SAEM (Society of Academic Emergency Medicine). 2004. *SAEM Research Fund Appeal to Members.* [Online]. Available: http://www.saem.org/newsltr/2002/nov–dec/appeal.pdf [accessed November 1, 2004].

Sanders AB, Kern KB, Berg RA, Hilwig RW, Heidenrich J, Ewy GA. 2002. Survival and neurologic outcome after cardiopulmonary resuscitation with four different chest compression-ventilation ratios. *Annals of Emergency Medicine* 40(6):553–562.

Sayre MR, White LJ, Brown LH, McHenry SD. 2002. National EMS research agenda. *Prehospital Emergency Care* 6:S1–S43.

Seidel JS. 1986a. A needs assessment of advanced life support and emergency medical services in the pediatric patient: State of the art. *Circulation* 74(6 Pt. 2):IV129–IV133.

Seidel JS. 1986b. Emergency medical services and the pediatric patient: Are the needs being met? II. Training and equipping emergency medical services providers for pediatric emergencies. *Pediatrics* 78(5):808.

Seidel JS, Hornbein M, Yoshiyama K, Kuznets D, Finklestein JZ, St Geme JW Jr. 1984. Emergency medical services and the pediatric patient: Are the needs being met? *Pediatrics* 73(6):769.

Seidel JS, Henderson DP, Lewis JB. 1991. Emergency medical services and the pediatric patient. III: Resources of ambulatory care centers. *Pediatrics* 88(2):230.

Shapiro MJ, Cole KE Jr, Keegan M, Prasad CN, Thompson RJ. 1994. National survey of state trauma registries—1992. *The Journal of Trauma* 37(5):835–840; discussion 840–842.

Singh T, Chamberlain J, Wright J. 2004. EMS provider attitudes and barriers towards pediatric research. *Prehospital Emergency Care* 8(1):86.

Smith R, Doyle C, Kavanaugh D. 2001. *Emergency Medical Services for Children: Program Highlights, Fiscal Year 2001.* Rockville, MD: EMS-C.

Spandorfer PR, Alessandrini EA, Shaw KN, Ludwig S. 2003. Pediatric emergency medicine research: A critical evaluation. *Pediatric Emergency Care* 19(5):293–301.

Stern SA, Wang X, Mertz M, Chowanski ZP, Remick DG, Kim HM, Dronen SC. 2001. Under-resuscitation of near-lethal uncontrolled hemorrhage: Effects on mortality and end-organ function at 72 hours. *Shock* 15(1):16–23.

Talan D, Moran G, Mower W, Newdow M, Ong S, Slutsker L, Jarvis W, Conn L, Pinner R. 1998. EMERGEncy ID NET: An emergency department-based emerging infections sentinel network. *Annals of Emergency Medicine* 32(6):703–711.

Vane DW, Shackford SR. 1995. Epidemiology of rural traumatic death in children: A population-based study. *The Journal of Trauma* 38(6):867–870.

Yuan XQ, Wade CE. 1991. Influences of traumatic brain injury on the outcomes of delayed and repeated hemorrhages. *Circulatory Shock* 35(4):231–236.

Yuan XQ, Wade CE, Clifford CB. 1991b. Suppression by traumatic brain injury of spontaneous hemodynamic recovery from hemorrhagic shock in rats. *Journal of Neurosurgery* 75(3):408–414.

APPENDIX
A

Committee and Subcommittee Membership

Gail Warden, MHA, *Chair*

SUBCOMMITTEES

Pediatric Emergency Care (PEDS)	Prehospital Emergency Medical Services (EMS)	Hospital-Based Emergency Care (ED)	MAIN COMMITTEE	SUBCOMMITTEE ONLY
David Sundwall, MD (Chair)	Shirley Gamble, MBA (Chair)	Benjamin Chu, MD, MPH (Chair)	Thomas Babor, PhD, MPH	
George Foltin, MD	Robert Bass, MD	Stuart Altman, PhD	Robert Gates, MPA	
Darrell Gaskin, PhD	Brent Eastman, MD	Brent Asplin, MD, MPH	William Kelley, MD	
Marianne Gausche-Hill, MD	Arthur Kellermann, MD, MPH	John Halamka, MD	Mark Smith, MD, MBA	
Richard Orr, MD	Jerry Overton, MA	Mary Jagim, RN		
	Nels Sanddal, MS, REMT-B	Peter Layde, MD, MSc		
		Eugene Litvak, PhD		
		John Prescott, MD		
		William Schwab, MD		
Rosalyn Baker	Kaye Bender, PhD, RN	Kenneth Kizer, MD		
Mary Fallat, MD	Herbert Garrison, MD	John Lumpkin, MD		
Jane Knapp, MD	Mary Beth Michos, RN	Daniel Manz, EMT		
Thomas Loyacono, EMT-P	Fred Neis, RN	Joseph Wright, MD		
Milap Nahata, PharmD	Daniel Spaite, MD			
Donna Ojanen Thomas, RN				

APPENDIX
B

Biographical Information for Main Committee and Pediatric Emergency Care Subcommittee

Gail L. Warden, M.H.A., F.A.C.H.E., *Main Committee Chair*, is president emeritus of Henry Ford Health System in Detroit, Michigan, one of the nation's leading vertically integrated health care systems. He is an elected member of the Institute of Medicine (IOM) of the National Academy of Sciences and served on its Board of Health Care Services and Committee on Quality Health Care in America, as well as serving its two terms on its Governing Council. He chairs the board of the National Quality Forum, the Healthcare Research and Development Institute, and the newly created National Center for Healthcare Leadership. Mr. Warden cochairs the National Advisory Committee on Pursuing Perfection: Raising the Bar for Health Care Performance. He is a member of The Robert Wood Johnson Foundation Board of Trustees, the Institute for Healthcare Improvement Board, and the RAND Health Board of Advisors. He is director emeritus and past chair of the Board of the National Committee on Quality Assurance. In 1997 President Clinton appointed him to the Federal Advisory Commission on Consumer Protection and Quality in the Health Care Industry. In 1995 Mr. Warden served as chair of the American Hospital Association Board of Trustees. He served as a member of the Pew Health Professions Commission and the National Commission on Civic Renewal, and is past chair of the Health Research and Education Trust Board of Directors. Mr. Warden served as president and chief executive officer of Henry Ford Health System from April 1988 until June 2003. Previously, he served as president and chief executive officer of Group Health Cooperative of Puget Sound in Seattle from 1981 to 1988. Prior to that he was executive vice president of the American Hospital Association from 1976 to 1981, and from 1965 to 1976 he served as executive vice president and chief operating officer of Rush-Presbyterian-St. Luke's Medical Center in Chicago. Mr. Warden is a graduate of Dartmouth College and holds an M.H.A. from the University of Michigan. He has an honorary doctorate in public administration from Central Michigan University and is a member of the faculty of the University of Michigan School of Public Health.

David N. Sundwall, M.D., *Pediatric Subcommittee Chair*, was nominated by Governor Jon Huntsman Jr. to serve as Executive Director of the Utah State Department of Health (UDOH) on January 3, 2005, and was confirmed for this position by the Utah Senate on January 17, 2005. In this capacity he supervises a workforce of almost 1,400 employees, and a budget of almost $1.8 billion. Previously, Sundwall served as President of the American Clinical Laboratory Association (ACLA) in September 1994, until he was appointed Senior Medical and Scientific Officer in May 2003. Prior to his position at ACLA, he was Vice President and Medical Director of American Healthcare System (AmHS), at that time the largest coalition of not-for-profit multi-hospital systems in the country.

Stuart H. Altman, Ph.D., is Sol C. Chaikin Professor of National Health Policy at the Heller Graduate School for Social Policy and Management. He served as dean of the Heller School from 1977 to a 1993. In August 2005 he again assumed the deanship of the Heller School. Dr. Altman has had extensive experience with the federal government, serving as deputy assistant secretary for planning and evaluation/health in the U.S. Department of Health, Education, and Welfare, 1971–1976; chair of the congressionally mandated Prospective Payment Assessment Commission, 1983–1996; and a member of the Bipartisan Commission on the Future of Medicare, 1999–2001. In addition, from 1973 to 1974 he served as deputy director for health of the President's Cost-of-Living Council and was responsible for developing the council's program on health care cost containment. Dr. Altman has testified before various congressional committees on the problems of rising health care costs, Medicare reform, and the need to create a national health insurance program for the United States. He chaired the IOM's Committee on the Changing Market, Managed Care, and the Future Viability of Safety Net Providers. His research activities include several studies concerning the factors responsible for the recent increases in the use of emergency departments. He holds a Ph.D. in economics from the University of California, Los Angeles, and has taught at Brown University and the University of California, Berkeley.

Brent R. Asplin, M.D., M.P.H., F.A.C.E.P., is department head of emergency medicine at Regions Hospital and HealthPartners Research Foundation in St. Paul, Minnesota, and is an associate professor and vice chair of the Department of Emergency Medicine at the University of Minnesota. After receiving his degree from Mayo Medical School, he completed the University of Pittsburgh's Affiliated Residency in Emergency Medicine. To develop his interests in research and health care policy, Dr. Asplin completed the Robert Wood Johnson Clinical Scholars Program at the University of Michigan, where he obtained an M.P.H. in health management and policy. He is currently studying methods for enhancing the reliability and efficiency of health care operations, particularly strategies for improving patient flow in hospital settings.

Thomas F. Babor, Ph.D., M.P.H., spent several years in postdoctoral research training in social psychiatry at Harvard Medical School, and subsequently served as head of social science research at McLean Hospital's Alcohol and Drug Abuse Research Center in Belmont, Massachusetts. In 1982 he moved to the University of Connecticut School of Medicine, where he has served as scientific director at the Alcohol Research Center and interim chair of the Psychiatry Department. Dr. Babor's primary interests are psychiatric epidemiology and alcohol and drug abuse. In 1998 he became chair of the Department of Community Medicine and Health Care at the University of Connecticut School of Medicine, where he directs an active research program. Dr. Babor is regional editor of the international journal *Addiction*. He previously served on two IOM committees—Prevention and Treatment of Alcohol-Related Problems: An Update on Research Opportunities, and Treatment of Alcohol Problems.

The Honorable Rosalyn H. Baker was elected to the Hawaii State Senate in 1994, where she was a member of the Senate Health Committee and served on the Joint Legislative Committee on Long Term Care Financing (1997–1998). She has chaired the Senate Committee on Health since 2002 and cochaired an Interim Legislative Working Group on Universal Healthcare (2003). Prior to serving in the State Senate, she was a member of the Hawaii State House of Representatives (1988–1993). She currently represents the 5th Senatorial District, comprising South and West Maui. The former vice chair of the Maui Service Area Board on Mental Health and Substance Abuse, Senator Baker has served the American Cancer Society both as president of the Maui, Moloka'i, Lana'i Unit (1997-2001) and as a member of the Hawaii Pacific Board of Directors (2003–2004). She is vice chair of the Hawaii Comprehensive Cancer Control Coalition. Among many awards and honors received throughout her career, she was named Legislator of the Year by the Healthcare Association of Hawaii (2004) and Hawaii Long Term Care Association (1998), as well as by the Hawaii Psychological Association for her outstanding contributions to psychology and mental health in the State of Hawaii (2003). Senator Baker has authored several laws and initiatives aimed at improving and expanding access to health care services, including emergency medical services, throughout the state of Hawaii. In the 2006 session, she authored laws establishing a statewide ban on smoking in public places and places of employment and an increase in the cigarette tax to provide dedicated funding for the Cancer Research Center of Hawaii, trauma and emergency medical services, and community health centers. Senator Baker holds a B.A. in political science and speech from Southwest Texas State University (now known as Texas State University at San Marcos) and has pursued graduate work in political studies at the University of Southwestern Louisiana (now the University of Louisiana at Lafayette).

Robert R. Bass, M.D., F.A.C.E.P., received his undergraduate and medical degrees from the University of North Carolina at Chapel Hill in 1972 and 1975, respectively. Prior to completing his undergraduate education, he was employed as a police officer in Chapel Hill, North Carolina, and served as a volunteer member of the South Orange Rescue Squad. Dr. Bass completed an internship and residency in the navy and is currently board certified in both emergency medicine and family medicine. He has served as a medical director for emergency medical services (EMS) systems in Charleston, South Carolina; Houston, Texas; Norfolk, Virginia; and Washington, D.C. Since 1994, Dr. Bass has been executive director of the Maryland Institute for EMS Systems, the state agency responsible for the oversight of Maryland's EMS and trauma system. He is clinical associate professor of surgery (emergency medicine) at the University of Maryland at Baltimore and is associate professor in the Emergency Health Services Program at the University of Maryland, Baltimore County. Dr. Bass is past president of the National Association of State EMS Officials and a founding member and the immediate past president of the National Association of EMS Physicians. Additionally, he serves on the board of directors of the American Trauma Society and the University of Maryland Medical System, and is past chair of the EMS Committee of the American College of Emergency Physicians.

Benjamin K. Chu, M.D., M.P.H., was appointed president, Kaiser Foundation Health Plan, Inc. and Kaiser Foundation Hospitals, Southern California Region, in February 2005. Before joining Kaiser Permanente, Dr. Chu was president of the New York City Health and Hospitals Corporation, with primary responsibility for management and policy implementation. Prior to that, he was senior associate dean at Columbia University College of Physicians and Surgeons. He has also served as associate dean and vice president for clinical affairs at the New York University Medical Center, managing and developing the clinical academic hospital network. Dr. Chu is a primary care internist by training, with extensive experience as a clinician, administrator, and policy advocate for the public hospital sector. He was senior vice president for medical and professional affairs at the New York City Health and Hospitals Corporation from 1990 to 1994. During that period, he also served as acting commissioner of health for the New York City Department of Health and acting executive director for Kings County Hospital Center. Dr. Chu has extensive experience in crafting public policy. He served as legislative assistant for health for Senator Bill Bradley as a 1989–1990 Robert Wood Johnson Health Policy Fellow. Earlier in his career, he served as acting director of the Kings County Hospital Adult Emergency Department. His areas of interests include health care access and insurance, graduate medical education policy, primary care, and public health issues. He has served on numerous advisory and not-for-profit boards focused on health care policy issues. Dr. Chu received a masters in public health from the Mailman School at Columbia University and his doctorate of medicine at New York University School of Medicine.

A. Brent Eastman, M.D., joined Scripps Memorial Hospital La Jolla in 1984 as director of trauma services and was appointed chief medical officer in 1998. He continues to serve in the role of director of trauma. Dr. Eastman received his medical degree from the University of California, San Francisco, where he also did his general surgical residency and served as chief surgical resident. He spent a year abroad in surgical training in England at Norfolk and Norwich Hospitals. Dr. Eastman served as chair of the Committee on Trauma for the American College of Surgeons from 1990 to 1994. This organization sets the standards for trauma care in the United States and abroad. The position led to his involvement nationally and internationally in the development of trauma systems in the United States, Canada, England, Ireland, Australia, Brazil, Argentina, Mexico, and South Africa. Dr. Eastman has authored or coauthored more than 25 publications and chapters relating principally to trauma. He has held numerous appointments and chairmanships over the last two decades, including chair, Trauma Systems Committee, for the U.S. Department of Health and Human Services; member of the board of directors, American Association for the Surgery of Trauma; and chair, Grant Review Committee, Center for Injury Prevention and Control at the U.S. Centers for Disease Control and Prevention.

Mary E. Fallat, M.D., F.A.C.S., is currently professor of surgery in the Department of Surgery, Division of Pediatric Surgery, at the University of Louisville. From 1988 to 2005, she served as trauma chief at Kosair Children's Hospital in Louisville, Kentucky, a 225-bed free-standing regional referral center and the only children's hospital in the State of Kentucky. She has been involved continuously in the Emergency Medical Services for Children

(EMS-C) program in the state of Kentucky since 1992 and is project director for the EMS-C Partnership Grant to Kentucky. In addition to her positions at the University of Louisville and Kosair Children's Hospital, Dr. Fallat completed a 6-year term as chair of the Kentucky Committee on Trauma of the American College of Surgeons and has been appointed chair of the Emergency Services-Prehospital Subcommittee of the National Committee on Trauma, for which she serves as a member of the Executive Committee. She has been a member of the governor-appointed Kentucky Board of Emergency Medical Services (KBEMS) since 2000, in addition to serving as chair of the EMS-C Subcommittee of KBEMS. On behalf of KBEMS, she has also written two successfully funded federal trauma–EMS grants for the state of Kentucky and is project director for these grants. Dr. Fallat is a member of many other organizations, including the American Academy of Pediatrics, the American Pediatric Surgical Association, the British Association of Paediatric Surgeons, and the Kentucky Pediatric Society. She has been a contributor to the Pediatric Advanced Life Support program of the American Heart Association, having served as a member of the national pediatric subcommittee for several years. Recently, she contributed as a coauthor to the Advanced Pediatric Life Support (APLS) course offered by the American College of Emergency Physicians. Dr. Fallat has written several trauma-related chapters as contributions to textbooks and has authored several trauma publications in peer-reviewed journals.

George L. Foltin, M.D., F.A.A.P., F.A.C.E.P., began his involvement with the Emergency Medical Services for Children (EMS-C) Program of the Health Resources and Services Administration in 1985. He is board certified in pediatrics, emergency medicine, and pediatric emergency medicine. Dr. Foltin served on the Medical Oversight Committee for the EMT-Basic National Standard Curriculum project and was a subject expert for the Project to Revise EMT-Intermediate and Paramedic National Standard Curriculum. He is a former board member of the National Association of EMS Physicians and served on the Committee on Pediatric Emergency Medicine of the American Academy of Pediatrics (AAP). Currently Dr. Foltin cochairs the Statewide AAP Committee on Pediatric Emergency Medicine and sits on the Regional Medical Advisory Committee of New York City. He has published extensively in the field of EMS for children, has been principal investigator for several federal grants, and serves as a consultant to the New York City and State departments of health, as well as to federal programs such as those of the Maternal and Child Health Bureau, the Agency for Healthcare Research and Quality, and the National Highway Traffic Safety Administration.

Shirley Gamble, M.B.A., served as senior advisor to The Robert Wood Johnson Foundation's Urgent Matters initiative, which is working to help hospitals eliminate emergency department crowding and help communities understand the challenges facing the health care safety net. Ms. Gamble has over 20 years of experience in the health care industry, serving as an executive with Incarnate Word Health Services, Texas Health Plans HMO, and Tampa General Hospital. As a partner in Phase 2 Consulting, a health care management and economic consulting firm, Ms. Gamble led performance improvement and strategic planning efforts for major hospital systems, managed care entities, and university faculty practice plans. She currently is chief operating officer for the United Way Capital Area in Austin, Texas. She holds an M.B.A. and B.A. from the University of Texas at Austin.

Darrell J. Gaskin, Ph.D., M.S., is associate professor of health policy and management at The Johns Hopkins Bloomberg School of Public Health and deputy director of the Morgan-Hopkins Center for Health Disparities Solutions. Dr. Gaskin's research focuses on health care disparities and access to care for vulnerable populations. Dr. Gaskin was awarded the Academy Health 2002 Article-of-the-Year Award for his *Health Services Research* article entitled "Are Urban Safety-Net Hospitals Losing Low-Risk Medicaid Maternity Patients?" Dr. Gaskin is active in professional organizations. He is a member of Academy Health, the American Economic Association, the National Economics Association (NEA), the International Health Economics Association, the American Society of Health Economists, and the American Public Health Association (APHA). He has served as a member of the board of directors of the NEA. He has been a member of the Governing Council of the APHA and is currently solicited program chair and section councilor for the APHA's Medical Care Section. He has chaired the disparities program committee for Academy Health. He is a member of the board of directors for the Maryland Citizen's Health Initiative. Dr. Gaskin earned his Ph.D. in health economics at The Johns Hopkins University, a master degree in economics from the Massachusetts Institute of Technology, and a bachelors degree in economics from Brandeis University.

Robert C. Gates, M.P.A., began his career in the County of Los Angeles Chief Administrative Office, where he was principal budget analyst for the public health, hospital, and mental health departments. He left Los Angeles to become chief operating officer for the University of California, Irvine, Medical Center in Orange County. While in Orange County, he was instrumental in creating its paramedic system. Mr. Gates then returned to Los Angeles County and spent 6 years as chief deputy director of the Department of Health Services, guiding the creation of the Los Angeles County Trauma Center system. He was then appointed director of health services for Los Angeles County and served in that capacity for over 11 years. Mr. Gates is currently serving as medical services for indigents project director for the Orange County Health Care Agency.

Marianne Gausche-Hill, M.D., F.A.C.E.P., F.A.A.P., serves as professor of clinical medicine at the David Geffen School of Medicine at the University of California, Los Angeles (UCLA). She is director of EMS and EMS fellowship and director of pediatric emergency medicine fellowship at Harbor-UCLA Medical Center. Dr. Gausche-Hill also serves as director of pediatric emergency medicine at the Little Company of Mary Hospital in Torrance, California. Board certified in both emergency medicine and pediatric emergency medicine, she earned her medical degree and completed her residency at UCLA. Dr. Gausche-Hill is the first emergency physician in the United States to have completed a pediatric emergency fellowship and passed the sub-board examination. She has done extensive research on prehospital pediatric care, authoring *Pediatric Advanced Life Support: Pearls of Wisdom* in 2001 and *Pediatric Airway Management for the Prehospital Professional* in 2004. Her research tracking the results of the use of the windpipe tube method versus the traditional bag-and-pump method as oxygen treatment for pediatric emergencies was published in the *Journal of the American Medical Association* and in *Annals of Emergency Medicine.* In May 1999, her work earned the prestigious Best Clinical Science Presentation award from the Society for Academic Emergency Medicine.

John D. Halamka, M.D., M.S., is chief information officer of the CareGroup Health System, chief information officer and associate dean for educational technology at Harvard Medical School, chair of the New England Health Electronic Data Interchange Network (NEHEN), acting chief executive officer of MA-Share, chief information officer of the Harvard Clinical Research Institute, and a practicing emergency physician. As chief information officer at CareGroup, he is responsible for all clinical, financial, administrative, and academic information technology serving 3,000 doctors, 12,000 employees, and 1 million patients. As chief information officer and associate dean for educational technology at Harvard Medical School, he oversees all educational, research, and administrative computing for 18,000 faculty and 3,000 students. As chair of NEHEN, he oversees administrative data exchange in Massachusetts. As chief executive officer of MA-Share, he oversees the clinical data exchange efforts in Massachusetts. As chair of the Healthcare Information Technology Standards Panel, he coordinates the process of harmonization of electronic standards among all stakeholders nationwide.

Mary M. Jagim, R.N., B.S.N., C.E.N., FAEN, is an experienced emergency/trauma nurse with extensive leadership background in program development and implementation, emergency department management and nursing workforce issues, emergency preparedness, government affairs, and community-based injury prevention. She is currently internal consultant for emergency preparedness and pandemic planning for MeritCare Health System in Fargo, North Dakota. Well versed in current issues affecting emergency/trauma nursing and emergency care, Ms. Jagim has served on the Emergency Nurses Association board of directors, for which she was national president in 2001. She currently serves as chair of the Emergency Nurses Association Foundation, is a member of the faculty for Key Concepts in Emergency Department Management, and is a fellow in the Academy of Emergency Nursing. She also served on the Centers for Disease Control and Prevention's (CDC) National Strategies for Advancing Child Pedestrian Safety Panel to Prevent Pedestrian Injuries and currently is cochair for Advocates for Highway and Auto Safety. Ms. Jagim received her B.S.N. from the University of North Dakota in 1984.

Arthur L. Kellermann, M.D., M.P.H., is professor and chair of the Department of Emergency Medicine at the Emory University School of Medicine and director of the Center for Injury Control at the Rollins School of Public Health at Emory University. His primary research focus is injury prevention and control. He has also conducted landmark research on prehospital cardiac care, use of diagnostic technology in emergency departments, and health care for the poor. His papers have been published in many of the nation's leading medical journals. He is a recipient of the Hal Jayne Academic Excellence Award from the Society for Academic Emergency Medicine, the Excellence in Science Award from the Injury Control and Emergency Health Services Section of the American Public Health Association, and the Scholar/Teacher Award from Emory University. A member of the IOM, Dr. Kellermann served as cochair of the IOM's Committee on the Consequences of Uninsurance from 2001 to 2004.

William N. Kelley, M.D., currently serves as professor of medicine, biochemistry, and biophysics at the University of Pennsylvania School of Medicine. Previously, he served as chief executive officer of the University of Pennsylvania Medical Center and Health System and dean of the School of Medicine from 1989 to February 2000. At the University of Pennsylvania, Dr. Kelley led the development of one of the first academic fully integrated delivery systems in the nation. He also built and implemented the largest health and disease management program in the country, with over 500 physicians and staff and 60 separate clinical sites engaged in implementing the program. Dr. Kelley holds a patent in a frequently used gene transfer technique that has allowed for numerous advances in the application of gene therapy. He received his M.D. from Emory University School of Medicine and completed his residency in internal medicine at Parkland Memorial Hospital in Dallas. After a fellowship with the National Institutes of Health and a teaching fellowship at Harvard Medical School, he began his academic career as assistant professor of medicine at Duke University School of Medicine, moving on to head Duke's Division of Rheumatic and Genetic Diseases before becoming chair of internal medicine at the University of Michigan Medical School.

Kenneth W. Kizer, M.D., M.P.H., expanded his role as chairman of the board for Medsphere Systems Corporation to become its chief executive officer in December 2005. He joined Medsphere after serving as president and chief executive officer of the National Quality Forum (NQF), a private, nonprofit, voluntary consensus standards-setting organization established in Washington, D.C., in 1999, pursuant to a presidential commission. Prior to that, he served for 5 years as under secretary for health in the U.S. Department of Veterans Affairs. In this capacity, he was the highest-ranking physician in the federal government and chief executive officer of the veterans health care system, the largest integrated health care system in the United States. Dr. Kizer also served as director of the California Department of Health Services and was California's top health official for over 6 years. Prior to that, he was chief of public health for California and director of California's Emergency Medical Services Authority. He practiced emergency medicine and toxicology in both private and academic settings for over 15 years. Dr. Kizer is an honors graduate of Stanford University and UCLA. He is board certified in six medical specialties and/or subspecialties and has authored more than 350 original articles, book chapters, and other publications in the medical literature. He is a fellow of numerous professional societies and a member of the Alpha Omega Alpha National Honor Medical Society, the Delta Omega National Honorary Public Health Society, and the IOM.

Jane F. Knapp, M.D., F.A.A.P., F.A.C.E.P., a native of Kansas City, Missouri, is professor of pediatrics at the Children's Mercy Hospital, University of Missouri-Kansas City School of Medicine. She graduated from the University of Missouri-Columbia School of Medicine in 1978 and completed a residency in pediatrics and a fellowship in pediatric emergency medicine at Children's Mercy Hospital. Dr. Knapp was one of the first two physicians to complete a 2-year fellowship in pediatric emergency medicine in the United States. Following her fellowship, she served as director of emergency services at Children's Mercy Hospital for 17 years. In 2005, she became vice chair of graduate medical education for the Department of Pediatrics at Children's Mercy Hospital. Dr. Knapp is a recognized national leader and expert in the emergency care of children. Her past national, state, and local responsibilities include serving as chair of the Section of Emergency Medicine of the American Academy of Pediatrics, chair of the Committee on Pediatric

Emergency Medicine of the American Academy of Pediatrics, member and chair of the Pediatric Emergency Medicine Subboard of the American Board of Pediatrics, chair of the Missouri Injury Control Advisory Committee, member of the Missouri Task Force on Fatal Child Abuse, and president of the Medical Staff of Children's Mercy Hospital. In 1996, she was awarded the Missouri Health Care Communicator of the Year award. Dr. Knapp was also the 2000 recipient of the Citation of Merit, the highest award given by the University of Missouri-Columbia School of Medicine Alumni Association. In January 2001, Dr. Knapp was recognized by the mayor and city council of Kansas City through a city council resolution for her devotion to the children of Kansas City. She is also the 2002 recipient of the American Academy of Pediatrics' Pediatric Emergency Medicine Distinguished Service Award. In 2005, Dr Knapp was named one of Kansas City's top doctors by *Ingram's Magazine.*

Peter M. Layde, M.D., M.Sc., is professor and interim director of the Health Policy Institute at the Medical College of Wisconsin. He has been an epidemiologist for over 25 years and an active injury control researcher for over 20 years. He has published extensively on agricultural injuries and methods for injury epidemiology, including early work on the use of case–control studies for homicide and on the epidemiological representativeness of trauma center–based studies. He has been an ad hoc reviewer for the Injury Grant Review Committee for over 10 years and served as a member of that committee from 1997 to 2000. Dr. Layde serves as codirector of the Injury Research Center at the Medical College of Wisconsin and as director of its Research Development and Support Core. He is also principal investigator for the Risk Factors for Medical Injury research project.

Eugene Litvak, Ph.D., is cofounder and director of the Program for the Management of Variability in Health Care Delivery at the Boston University Health Policy Institute. He is also a professor at the Boston University School of Management. He received his doctorate in operations research from the Moscow Institute of Physics and Technology in 1977. In 1990, he joined the faculty of the Harvard Center for Risk Analysis in the Department of Health Policy and Management at the Harvard School of Public Health, where he still teaches as adjunct professor of operations management. Prior to that time he was chief of the Operations Management Group at the Computing Center in Kiev, Ukraine. His research interests include operations management in health care delivery organizations, cost-effective medical decision making, screening for HIV and other infectious diseases, and operations research. He was leading author of cost-effective protocols for screening for HIV and is principal investigator from the United States for an international trial of these protocols, which is supported by the U.S.

Agency for International Development. Dr. Litvak was also principal investigator for the Emergency Room Diversion Study, supported by a grant from
the Massachusetts Department of Public Health. He serves as a consultant
on operations improvement to several major hospitals and is on the faculty
of the Institute for Health Care Improvement.

Thomas R. Loyacono, M.P.A., NREMT-P, is chief operations officer of the
Emergency Medical Services (EMS) Department in Baton Rouge, Louisiana.
A nationally registered Emergency Medical Technician-Paramedic with 32
years of experience in prehospital EMS, he has more than 20 years of experience as a patient care provider and has spent 15 years in EMS management.
Mr. Loyacono completed his EMS education at the University of South Alabama in 1978; he received his undergraduate degree summa cum laude from
the University of Alabama in 1992 and his master of public administration
degree from Southern University in 1998. He has had extensive training in
emergency management and has been recognized as a certified emergency
manager by the International Association of Emergency Managers. Mr.
Loyacono's professional affiliations include chairing the National Association of Emergency Medical Technicians' Pediatrics Committee and serving
as a member of the Louisiana Governor's Emergency Medical Services for
Children Advisory Council and the Board of Directors of the National Registry of Emergency Medical Technicians. Through these affiliations, he is
active on numerous local, state, and national EMS committees and panels.

John R. Lumpkin, M.D., M.P.H., is senior vice president and director,
Health Care Group at The Robert Wood Johnson Foundation. Dr. Lumpkin
joined the Illinois Department of Public Health (IDHP) in1985 as associate
director of IDPH's Office of Health Care Regulations, and later became the
first African American to hold the position of director. Dr. Lumpkin served
6 years as chair of the National Committee for Vital and Health Statistics,
advising the Secretary of the U.S. Department of Health and Human Services
on health information policy. He received his medical degree in 1974 from
Northwestern University Medical School. He trained in emergency medicine
at the University of Chicago and earned his M.P.H. from the University of
Illinois at Chicago, School of Public Health. Dr. Lumpkin is past president
of the Association of State and Territorial Health Officials, a former member
of the board of trustees of the Foundation for Accountability, former commissioner of the Pew Commission on Environmental Health, former board
member of the National Forum for Health Care Quality Measurement and
Reporting, past board member of the American College of Emergency Physicians, and past president of the Society of Teachers of Emergency Medicine.
He has been the recipient of the Bill B. Smiley Award, Alan Donaldson

Award, and African American History Maker Award, and was named Public Health Worker of the Year.

W. Daniel Manz, B.S., is director of EMS for the Vermont Department of Health. He has been involved in EMS for more than 25 years and worked as an emergency medical technician (EMT), volunteer squad leader, hospital communications technician, EMS regional coordinator, EMS trainer, and state EMS director. Much of his work has been in rural areas, including Maine and Saudi Arabia. Mr. Manz has been active in the National Association of State EMS Directors, serving as its president for 2 years and representing the association on several national projects, including the EMS Agenda for the Future, the Health Care Financing Administration's Negotiated Rule Making process, and the recently completed National EMS Scope of Practice Model. Mr. Manz remains active as a volunteer EMT-Intermediate with the local ambulance service in his community. In his spare time he enjoys running, fishing, and sheep farming.

Milap C. Nahata, M.S., Pharm.D., is professor of pharmacy and chair of the Division of Pharmacy Practice and Administration at the Ohio State University College of Pharmacy. He is also professor of pediatrics and internal medicine at the Ohio State University College of Medicine and Children's Hospital of Columbus. Dr. Nahata earned his master of science and doctor of pharmacy degrees from the Duquesne University School of Pharmacy. He has served as president of the American College of Clinical Pharmacy and the American Association of Colleges of Pharmacy. Dr. Nahata is recognized nationally and internationally for his clinical practice and research endeavors in pediatric pharmacotherapy. His research specialties include the efficacy and safety of various drug therapies in pediatric patients, the pharmacokinetics/pharmacodynamics of drugs in pediatric patients, and health outcome and quality-of-life studies in children and adolescents on pharmacotherapy. His research also focuses on the development of stable and palatable dosage forms of drugs for pediatric patients and he has studied the dosage forms of nearly 50 orally and intravenously administered drugs in children. He has published two books and more than 450 refereed articles in 50 journals. He is editor-in-chief of *The Annals of Pharmacotherapy* and serves on the editorial boards of four journals. Dr. Nahata received the Pharmacist of the Year Award from the Ohio Society of Health-System Pharmacists, the Distinguished Educator Award from the American Association of Colleges of Pharmacy, and the Award for Achievement for Sustained Contributions to the Literature of Health-System Pharmacy from the American Society of Health-System Pharmacists. He is an elected fellow of six national societies and has received five national research awards.

Richard A. Orr, M.D., serves as professor at the University of Pittsburgh School of Medicine, associate director of the Cardiac Intensive Care Unit at the Children's Hospital of Pittsburgh, and medical director of the Children's Hospital Transport Team of Pittsburgh, Pennsylvania. Dr. Orr has devoted much of his career to interfacility transportation problems of infants and children in need of tertiary care. He is a member of many professional organizations and societies and has authored numerous articles regarding the safe and effective air and surface transport of the critically ill and injured pediatric patient. Dr. Orr is also a noted lecturer to the air and ground transport community, both nationally and internationally. He is editor of *Pediatric Transport Medicine*, a unique 700-page book published in 1995. He is the 2001 recipient of the Air Medical Physician Association (AMPA) Distinguished Physician Award and a founding member of AMPA.

Jerry L. Overton, M.A., serves as executive director, Richmond Ambulance Authority, Richmond, Virginia, and has overall responsibility for the Richmond EMS system. His duties extend to planning and administering the high-performance system's design, negotiating and implementing performance-based contracts, maximizing fee-for-service revenues, developing advanced patient care protocols, and employing innovative equipment and treatment modalities. Mr. Overton was previously executive director of the Kansas City, Missouri, EMS system. In addition, he has provided technical assistance to EMS systems throughout the United States and Europe, Russia, Asia, Australia, and Canada. He designed an implementation plan for an emergency medical transport program in Central Bosnia–Herzegovina. Mr. Overton is a faculty member of the Emergency Medical Department of the Medical College of Virginia, Virginia Commonwealth University, and the National EMS Medical Directors Course, National Association of EMS Physicians. He is past president of the American Ambulance Association and serves on the board of directors of the North American Association of Public Utility Models.

John E. Prescott, M.D., is dean of the West Virginia University (WVU) School of Medicine, and received both his B.S. and M.D. degrees at Georgetown University. He completed his residency training in emergency medicine at Brooke Army Medical Center, San Antonio, and was then assigned to Fort Bragg, North Carolina, where he was actively engaged in providing both operational and hospital emergency care in a variety of challenging situations. In 1990 he joined WVU and soon assumed leadership of the Section of Emergency Medicine. During that same year, he founded and became the first director of WVU's Center for Rural Emergency Medicine. In 1993 he became the first chair of WVU's newly established Department of Emergency Medicine. Dr. Prescott is a past recipient of major CDC and private foundation grants. His research and scholarly interests include rural emergency care, injury control and prevention, medical response to disasters and terrorism, and academic and administrative medicine. In 1999 Dr. Prescott became WVU's associate dean for the clinical enterprise and president/chief executive officer of University Health Associates, WVU's physician practice plan. In 2003 he was named senior associate dean; he was appointed dean of the WVU School of Medicine in 2004. He has been a fellow of the American College of Emergency Physicians since 1987 and is the recipient of WVU's Presidential Heroism Award.

Nels D. Sanddal, M.S., REMT-B, is president of the Critical Illness and Trauma Foundation (CIT) in Bozeman, Montana, and is currently on detachment as director of the Rural Emergency Medical Services and Trauma Technical Assistance Center. Mr. Sanddal has been involved in EMS since the 1970s and has held many state, regional, and national positions in organizations furthering EMS causes, including president of the Intermountain Regional EMS for Children Coordinating Council and core faculty for the Development of Trauma Systems Training Programs for the U.S. Department of Transportation. He is a nationally registered EMT-Basic, volunteers with a local fire department, and has been involved with CIT since its inception in 1986. He holds an M.S. in psychology and is currently pursuing a Ph.D. in health services.

C. William Schwab, M.D., F.A.C.S., is professor of surgery and chief of the Division of Traumatology and Surgical Critical Care at the University of Pennsylvania. His surgical practice reflects his expertise in trauma systems, including caring for the severely injured patient and incorporating the most advanced techniques into trauma surgery. He is director of the Firearm and Injury Center at Penn and holds several grants supporting work on reducing firearm and nonfirearm injuries and other repercussions. He has served as a trauma systems consultant to CDC, New York State, and several state health departments. He has established trauma centers and hospital-based aeromedical programs in Virginia, New Jersey, and Pennsylvania. He currently directs a network of three regional trauma centers throughout southeastern Pennsylvania. He has been president of the Eastern Association for the Surgery of Trauma and vice chair of the American College of Surgeons Committee on Trauma and currently serves as president of the American Association for the Surgery of Trauma.

Mark D. Smith, M.D., M.B.A., has led the California HealthCare Foundation in developing research and initiatives aimed at improving California's health care financing and delivery systems since the foundation's formation in 1996. Prior to joining the foundation, he was executive vice president at the Henry J. Kaiser Family Foundation and served as associate director of the AIDS Service and assistant professor of medicine and health policy and management at The Johns Hopkins University. Dr. Smith is a member of the IOM and is on the board of the National Business Group on Health. Previously, he served on the Performance Measurement Committee of the National Committee for Quality Assurance and the editorial board of the *Annals of Internal Medicine*. A board-certified internist, Dr. Smith is a member of the clinical faculty at the University of California, San Francisco, and an attending physician at the AIDS clinic at San Francisco General Hospital.

David N. Sundwall, M.D., was nominated by Governor Jon Huntsman Jr. to serve as executive director of the Utah State Department of Health in January 2005 and was subsequently confirmed for this position by the Utah Senate. In this capacity, he supervises a workforce of almost 1,400 employees and a budget of almost $1.8 billion. Previously, Dr. Sundwall served as president of the American Clinical Laboratory Association (ACLA) from September 1994 until he was appointed senior medical and scientific officer in May 2003. Prior to his position at ACLA, he was vice president and medical director of American Healthcare System (AmHS), at that time the largest coalition of not-for-profit multihospital systems in the country. Dr. Sundwall has extensive experience in federal government and national health policy, including serving as administrator, Health Resources and Services Administration; in the Public Health Service, U.S. Department of Health and Human Services (DHHS); and as assistant surgeon general in the Commissioned Corps of the U.S. Public Health Service (1986–1988). During this period, he had adjunct responsibilities at DHHS, including serving as cochair of the secretary's Task Force on Medical Liability and Malpractice and as the secretary's designee to the National Commission to Prevent Infant Mortality. Dr. Sundwall also served as director, Health and Human Resources Staff (Majority), U.S. Senate Labor and Human Resources Committee (1981–1986). He was in private medical practice in Murray, Utah, from 1973 to 1975. He has held academic appointments at the Uniformed Services University of the Health Sciences, Bethesda, Maryland; Georgetown University School of Medicine, Washington, D.C.; and the University of Utah School of Medicine. He is board certified in internal medicine and family practice. He is licensed to practice medicine in the District of Columbia, is a member of the American Medical Association and the American Academy of Family Physicians, and previously served as volunteer medical staff of Health Care for the Homeless Project.

Donna Ojanen Thomas, R.N., M.S.N., earned her M.S.N. in parent–child nursing from the University of Utah. She currently serves as emergency department director and rapid treatment unit director at Primary Children's Medical Center in Salt Lake City, Utah. She previously served as clinical specialist, responsible for the education and orientation of all emergency department employees. A member of the Emergency Nurses Association (ENA) and one of the original authors of the Emergency Nursing Pediatric Course, Ms. Thomas received the ENA Lifetime Achievement Award in 2002. She has also published extensively in *RN Journal* and *Journal of Emergency Nursing*. She was coeditor of the Core Curriculum for Pediatric Emergency Nursing, which won the 2002 *American Journal of Nursing* Book of the Year Award.

Joseph L. Wright, M.D., M.P.H., is executive director of the Child Health Advocacy Institute at Children's National Medical Center in Washington, D.C. In that capacity, he provides strategic leadership for the organization's advocacy mission and community partnership initiatives. He is professor and vice chair in the Department of Pediatrics, as well as professor of emergency medicine and prevention and community health at The George Washington University Schools of Medicine and Public Health. He has been attending faculty in the Division of Emergency Medicine at Children's Hospital since 1993 and was recently appointed interim executive director for hospital-based specialties at the institution. Dr. Wright is founding director of the Center for Prehospital Pediatrics at Children's and serves as the State EMS Medical Director for Pediatrics within the Maryland Institute for Emergency Medical Services Systems. His major areas of scholarly interest include EMS for children, injury prevention, and the needs of underserved communities. Dr. Wright received the Shining Star award from the Los Angeles-based Starlight Foundation for outstanding community service, was inducted into Delta Omega, the nation's public health honor society; and was elected to membership in Leadership Greater Washington. He has been appointed over the years to several national advisory bodies, including the National Association of Children's Hospitals and Related Institutions and the American Academy of Pediatrics, where he serves as chair of the Subcommittee on Violence.

APPENDIX
C

List of Presentations to the Committee

February 2–4, 2004

Overview of Emergency Care in the U.S. Health System
- Overview of the Emergency Care System
  Arthur L. Kellermann (Emory University School of Medicine)
- Emergency Care Supply and Utilization
  Charlotte S. Yeh (Centers for Medicare and Medicaid Services)
- Rural Issues in Emergency Care
  John E. Prescott (West Virginia University)

Major Emergency Care Issue Areas
- Patient Flow and Emergency Department Crowding
  Brent R. Asplin (University of Minnesota)
- Evolution of the Emergency Department (circa 2004): A Systems
  Perspective
  Eric B. Larson (Group Health Cooperative)
- Mental Health and Substance Abuse Issues
  Michael H. Allen (University of Colorado Health Sciences Center)
- Workforce Education and Training
  Glenn C. Hamilton (Wright State University School of Medicine)
- Information Technology in Emergency Care
  Larry A. Nathanson (Beth Israel Deaconess Medical Center)

Prehospital Care, Public Health, and Emergency Preparedness
- Emergency Care and Public Health
  Daniel A. Pollock (Centers for Disease Control and Prevention)

- Overview of the Issues Facing Prehospital EMS
  Robert R. Bass (Maryland Institute for Emergency Medical Services Systems)
- Emergency Preparedness
  Joseph F. Waeckerle (University of Missouri Baptist Medical Center)

Research Agenda
- Overview of Research in Emergency Care
  E. John Gallagher (Montefiore Medical Center)
- Research Needs for the Future
  Robin M. Weinick (Agency for Healthcare Research and Quality)

June 9–11, 2004

Overview of Emergency Medical Services for Children
- The EMS-C Program: History and Current Challenges
  Jane Ball (The EMSC National Resource Center)
- The 1993 IOM Report: Promise and Progress
  Megan McHugh (IOM Staff)

Issues in Pediatric Emergency Care
- Pediatric Equipment and Care Management
  Marianne Gausche-Hill (Harbor-UCLA Medical Center)
- Special Problems in Pediatric Medication
  Milap Nahata (Ohio State University Schools of Pharmacy and Medicine)
- Training and Skills Maintenance
  Cynthia Wright-Johnson (Maryland Institute for EMS Systems)
- Emergency Research and Data Issues
  David Jaffe (Washington University in St. Louis)

Pediatric Disaster Preparedness
- *George Foltin (New York University Bellevue Hospital Center)*

Organization and Delivery of Emergency Medical Services
- System-Wide EMS and Trauma Planning and Coordination
  Stephen Hise (National Association of State EMS Directors)
- Fire Perspective on EMS
  John Sinclair (International Association of Fire Chiefs)
- Trauma Systems
  Alasdair Conn (Massachusetts General Hospital)
- Critical Care Transport
  Richard Orr (Children's Hospital of Pittsburgh)

History and Organization of EMS in the United States

- EMS System Overview and History
  Robert Bass (Maryland Institute for Emergency Medical Services Systems)
- Overview of Local EMS Systems
  Mike Williams (Abaris Group)
- Issues Facing Rural Emergency Medical Services
  Fergus Laughridge (Emergency Medical Services, Nevada State Health Division)

Prehospital EMS Issue Areas

- EMS Financing and Reimbursement
  Jerry Overton (Richmond Ambulance Authority)
- EMS Quality Improvement and Patient Safety
  Robert A. Swor (William Beaumont Hospital)
- Overview of the EMS Agenda for the Future
  Ted Delbridge (University of Pittsburgh)
- EMS Data Needs
  Greg Mears (University of North Carolina-Chapel Hill)
- Overview of Current EMS Research
  Ron Maio (University of Michigan)

Agency Reaction Panel

- Health Resources and Services Administration, Maternal and Child Health Bureau
  Dave Heppel (Division of Child, Adolescent, and Family Health) and/or Dan Kavanaugh (EMSC-Program)
- National Highway Traffic Safety Administration
  Drew Dawson (EMS Division)
- Agency for Healthcare Research and Quality
  Robin Weinick (Safety Nets and Low Income Populations and Intramural Research)
- Centers for Disease Control and Prevention, National Center for Injury Prevention and Control
  Rick Hunt (Division of Injury and Disability Outcomes and Programs)
- Health Resources and Services Administration, Office of Rural Health Policy
  Evan Mayfield (U.S. Public Health Service and Public Health Analyst)

June 24–25, 2004

Workforce Issues in the Emergency Department

- Issues Facing the Emergency Care Nursing Workforce

Mary Jagim (MeritCare Hospital)
Carl Ray (Bon Secours DePaul Medical Center)
Kathy Robinson (Pennsylvania Department of Health)

Current Initiatives in Patient Flow
- Patient Flow Initiative Implemented at University of Utah
  Jadie Barrie (University of Utah)
  Pamela Proctor (University of Utah)
- Program for Management of Variability in Health Care Delivery
  Eugene Litvak (Boston University Health Policy Institute)

Luncheon Speaker—Medical Technology in Emergency Medicine
- *Michael Sachs (Sg2)*

September 20–21, 2004

Prehospital EMS Issue Areas
- International EMS Systems
  Jerry Overton (Richmond Ambulance Authority)
- Current Status of Federal Emergency Care Legislation and Funding
  Mark Mioduski (Cornerstone Government Affairs)
- Overview of EMS Workforce Issues
  John Becknell (Consultant)
- EMS System Design and Coordination
  Bob Davis (USA Today)

Reimbursement and Funding of Pediatric Emergency Care Services
- Reimbursement Issues in Pediatric Emergency Care
  Steven E. Krug (Northwestern University/Children's Memorial Hospital)
- Current Status of Federal Emergency Care Legislation and Funding
  Mark Mioduski (Cornerstone Government Affairs)

Issues Facing Pediatric Emergency Care
- Funding of Children's Hospitals
  Peter Holbrook (Children's National Medical Center)
- Survey on Pediatric Preparedness
  Marianne Gausche-Hill (Harbor-UCLA Medical Center)

October 4–5, 2004

No open sessions held.

March 2–4, 2005

Public Health Perspectives
- Overview of EMS and Trauma System Issues
  William Koenig (Emergency Medical Services Agency, LA County)
- The Hospital Perspective
  Doug Bagley (Riverside County Regional Medical Center)
- The Safety Net and Community Providers Perspective
  John Gressman (San Francisco Community Clinics Consortium)
- Mental Health and Substance Abuse
  Barry Chaitin (University of California—Irvine)
- The Patient Perspective
  Sandy Schuhmann-Atkins (University of California—Irvine)

On-Call Coverage Issues
- Survey of On-Call Coverage in California
  Mark Langdorf (University of California—Irvine)
- Specialty Physician Perspective—Orthopedics
  Nick Halikis (Little Company of Mary Hospital)
- Specialty Physician Perspective—Neurosurgery
  John Kusske (University of California—Irvine)

Issues in Rural Emergency Care
- The Family Practice Perspective
  *Arlene Brown (Southern New Mexico Family Medicine Residency
    and Family Practice Associates of Ruidoso, PC)*
- Telemedicine in Rural Emergency Care
  Jim Marcin (University of California—Davis)

APPENDIX
D

List of Commissioned Papers

1. **The Role of the Emergency Department in the Health Care Delivery System**
   Consultant: Eva Stahl, Brandeis University

2. **Patient Safety and Quality of Care in Emergency Services**
   Consultant: Jim Adams, Northwestern University

3. **Patient Flow in Hospital-Based Emergency Services**
   Consultant: Brad Prenny, Boston University, Health Policy Institute

4. **Models of Organization, Delivery, and Planning for EMS and Trauma Systems**
   Consultant: Tasmeen Singh, Children's National Medical Center

5. **Information Technology in Emergency Care**
   Consultant: Larry Nathanson, Harvard Medical School

6. **Emergency Care in Rural America**
   Consultant: Janet Williams, University of Rochester

7. **The Emergency Care Workforce**
   Consultant: Jean Moore, State University of New York School of Public Health

8. **The Financing of EMS and Hospital-Based Emergency Services**
   Consultants: John McConnell, Oregon Health and Sciences University; David Gray, Medical University of South Carolina; Richard Lindrooth, Medical University of South Carolina

9. **The Impact of New Medical Technologies on Emergency Care**
   Consultant: Sg2

10. **Mental Health and Substance Abuse in the Emergent Care Setting**
    Consultant: Linda Degutis, DrPH, Yale University

11. **Emergency Care Research Funding**
    Consultant: Roger Lewis, Harbor-UCLA Medical Center

Recommendations and Responsible Entities from the *Future of Emergency Care* Series

HOSPITAL-BASED EMERGENCY CARE: AT THE BREAKING POINT

	Congress	DHHS	DOT	DHS	DOD	States	Hospitals	EMS Agencies	Private Industry	Professional Organizations	Other
Chapter 2: The Evolving Role of Hospital-Based Emergency Care											
2.1 Congress should establish dedicated funding, separate from Disproportionate Share Hospital payments, to reimburse hospitals that provide significant amounts of uncompensated emergency and trauma care for the financial losses incurred by providing those services.	X	X									
2.1a Congress should initially appropriate $50 million for the purpose, to be administered by the Centers for Medicare and Medicaid Services.											
2.1b The Centers for Medicare and Medicaid Services should establish a working group to determine the allocation of these funds, which should be targeted to providers and localities at greatest risk; the working group should then determine funding needs for subsequent years.											
Chapter 3: Building a 21st-Century Emergency Care System											
3.1 The Department of Health and Human Services and the National Highway Traffic Safety Administration, in partnership with professional organizations, should convene a panel of individuals with multidisciplinary expertise to develop evidence-based categorization systems for emergency medical services, emergency departments, and trauma centers based on adult and pediatric service capabilities.		X	X							X	

3.2 The National Highway Traffic Safety Administration, in partnership with professional organizations, should convene a panel of individuals with multidisciplinary expertise to develop evidence-based model prehospital care protocols for the treatment, triage, and transport of patients.

3.3 The Department of Health and Human Services should convene a panel of individuals with emergency and trauma care expertise to develop evidence-based indicators of emergency and trauma care system performance.

3.4 The Department of Health and Human Services should adopt regulatory changes to the Emergency Medical Treatment and Active Labor Act and the Health Insurance Portability and Accountability Act so that the original goals of the laws will be preserved, but integrated systems can be further developed.

3.5 Congress should establish a demonstration program, administered by the Health Resources and Services Administration, to promote coordinated, regionalized, and accountable emergency care systems throughout the country, and appropriate $88 million over 5 years to this program.

	Congress	DHHS	DOT	DHS	DOD	States	Hospitals	EMS Agencies	Private Industry	Professional Organizations	Other
3.6 Congress should establish a lead agency for emergency and trauma care within 2 years of the release of this report. The lead agency should be housed in the Department of Health and Human Services, and should have primary programmatic responsibility for the full continuum of emergency medical services and emergency and trauma care for adults and children, including medical 9-1-1 and emergency medical dispatch, prehospital emergency medical services (both ground and air), hospital-based emergency and trauma care, and medical-related disaster preparedness. Congress should establish a working group to make recommendations regarding the structure, funding, and responsibilities of the new agency, and develop and monitor the transition. The working group should have representation from federal and state agencies and professional disciplines involved in emergency and trauma care.	X	X									

Chapter 4: Improving the Efficiency of Hospital-Based Emergency Care

	Congress	DHHS	DOT	DHS	DOD	States	Hospitals	EMS Agencies	Private Industry	Professional Organizations	Other
4.1 The Centers for Medicare and Medicaid Services should remove the current restrictions on the medical conditions that are eligible for separate clinical decision unit (CDU) payment.	X	X									
4.2 Hospital chief executive officers should adopt enterprisewide operations management and related strategies to improve the quality and efficiency of emergency care.							X				

4.3 Training in operations management and related approaches should be promoted by professional associations; accrediting organizations, such as the Joint Commission on Accreditation of Healthcare Organizations and the National Committee for Quality Assurance; and educational institutions that provide training in clinical, health care management, and public health disciplines.

4.4 The Joint Commission on Accreditation of Healthcare Organizations should reinstate strong standards designed to sharply reduce and ultimately eliminate ED crowding, boarding, and diversion.

4.5 Hospitals should end the practices of boarding patients in the emergency department and ambulance diversion, except in the most extreme cases, such as a community mass casualty event. The Centers for Medicare and Medicaid Services should convene a working group that includes experts in emergency care, inpatient critical care, hospital operations management, nursing, and other relevant disciplines to develop boarding and diversion standards, as well as guidelines, measures, and incentives for implementation, monitoring, and enforcement of these standards.

Chapter 5: Technology and Communication

5.1 Hospitals should adopt robust information and communications systems to improve the safety and quality of emergency care and enhance hospital efficiency.

Chapter 6: The Emergency Care Workforce

6.1 Hospitals, physician organizations, and public health agencies should collaborate to regionalize critical specialty care on-call services.

	Congress	DHHS	DOT	DHS	DOD	States	Hospitals	EMS Agencies	Private Industry	Professional Organizations	Other
6.2 Congress should appoint a commission to examine the impact of medical malpractice lawsuits on the declining availability of providers in high-risk emergency and trauma care specialties, and to recommend appropriate state and federal actions to mitigate the adverse impact of these lawsuits and ensure quality of care.	X										
6.3 The American Board of Medical Specialties and its constituent boards should extend eligibility for certification in critical care medicine to all acute care and primary care physicians who complete an accredited critical care fellowship program.										X	X
6.4 The Department of Health and Human Services, the Department of Transportation, and the Department of Homeland Security should jointly undertake a detailed assessment of emergency and trauma workforce capacity, trends, and future needs, and develop strategies to meet these needs in the future.		X	X	X							
6.5 The Department of Health and Human Services, in partnership with professional organizations, should develop national standards for core competencies applicable to physicians, nurses, and other key emergency and trauma professionals, using a national, evidence-based, multidisciplinary process.		X								X	
6.6 States should link rural hospitals with academic health centers to enhance opportunities for professional consultation, telemedicine, patient referral and transport, and continuing professional education.						X	X				

Chapter 7: Disaster Preparedness

7.1 The Department of Homeland Security, the Department of Health and Human Services, the Department of Transportation, and the states should collaborate with the Veterans Health Administration (VHA) to integrate the VHA into civilian disaster planning and management.

7.2 All institutions responsible for the training, continuing education, and credentialing and certification of professionals involved in emergency care (including medicine, nursing, emergency medical services, allied health, public health, and hospital administration) should incorporate disaster preparedness training into their curricula and competency criteria.

7.3 Congress should significantly increase total preparedness funding in fiscal year 2007 for hospital emergency preparedness in the following areas: strengthening and sustaining trauma care systems; enhancing emergency department, trauma center, and inpatient surge capacity; improving emergency medical services' response to explosives; designing evidence-based training programs; enhancing the availability of decontamination showers, standby intensive care unit capacity, negative pressure rooms, and appropriate personal protective equipment; and conducting international collaborative research on the civilian consequences of conventional weapons terrorism.

Chapter 8: Enhancing the Emergency and Trauma Care Research Base

8.1 Academic medical centers should support emergency and trauma care research by providing research time and adequate facilities for promising emergency care and trauma investigators, and by strongly considering the establishment of autonomous departments of emergency medicine.

	Congress	DHHS	DOT	DHS	DOD	States	Hospitals	EMS Agencies	Private Industry	Professional Organizations	Other
8.2 The Secretary of the Department of Health and Human Services should conduct a study to examine the gaps and opportunities in emergency and trauma care research, and recommend a strategy for the optimal organization and funding of the research effort.	X	X	X	X	X						
8.2a This study should include consideration of training of new investigators, development of multicenter research networks, funding of General Clinical Research Centers that specifically include an emergency and trauma care component, involvement of emergency and trauma care researchers in the grant review and research advisory processes, and improved research coordination through a dedicated center or institute.											
8.2b Congress and federal agencies involved in emergency and trauma care research (including the Department of Transportation, the Department of Health and Human Services, the Department of Homeland Security, and the Department of Defense) should implement the study's recommendations.	X										
8.3 States should ease their restrictions on informed consent to match federal law.											
8.4 Congress should modify Federalwide Assurance (FWA) Program regulations to allow the acquisition of limited, linked, patient outcome data without the existence of an FWA.											

EMERGENCY MEDICAL SERVICES AT THE CROSSROADS

	Congress	DHHS	DOT	DHS	DOD	States	Hospitals	EMS Agencies	Private Industry	Professional Organizations	Other
Chapter 3: Building a 21st-Century Emergency Care System											
3.1 The Department of Health and Human Services and National Highway Traffic Safety Administration, in partnership with professional organizations, should convene a panel of individuals with multidisciplinary expertise to develop evidence-based categorization systems for emergency medical services, emergency departments, and trauma centers based on adult and pediatric service capabilities.		X	X							X	
3.2 The National Highway Traffic Safety Administration, in partnership with professional organizations, should convene a panel of individuals with multidisciplinary expertise to develop evidence-based model prehospital care protocols for the treatment, triage, and transport of patients.			X							X	
3.3 The Department of Health and Human Services should convene a panel of individuals with emergency and trauma care expertise to develop evidence-based indicators of emergency and trauma care system performance.		X									
3.4 Congress should establish a demonstration program, administered by the Health Resources and Services Administration, to promote coordinated, regionalized, and accountable emergency and trauma care systems throughout the country, and appropriate $88 million over 5 years to this program.	X	X									

	Congress	DHHS	DOT	DHS	DOD	States	Hospitals	EMS Agencies	Private Industry	Professional Organizations	Other
3.5 Congress should establish a lead agency for emergency and trauma care within 2 years of the release of this report. This lead agency should be housed in the Department of Health and Human Services, and should have primary programmatic responsibility for the full continuum of emergency medical services and emergency and trauma care for adults and children, including medical 9-1-1 and emergency medical dispatch, prehospital emergency medical services (both ground and air), hospital-based emergency and trauma care, and medical-related disaster preparedness. Congress should establish a working group to make recommendations regarding the structure, funding, and responsibilities of the new agency, and design and monitor the transition to its assumption of the responsibilities outlined above. The working group should include representatives from federal and state agencies and professional disciplines involved in emergency and trauma care.	X	X									
3.6 The Department of Health and Human Services should adopt rule changes to the Emergency Medical Treatment and Active Labor Act and the Health Insurance Portability and Accountability Act so that the original goals of the laws will be preserved, but integrated systems can be further developed.		X									
3.7 The Centers for Medicare and Medicaid Services should convene an ad hoc working group with expertise in emergency care, trauma, and emergency medical services systems to evaluate the reimbursement of emergency medical services, and make recommendations with regard to including readiness costs and permitting payment without transport.		X									

Chapter 4: Supporting a High-Quality EMS Workforce

4.1 State governments should adopt a common scope of practice for emergency medical services personnel, with state licensing reciprocity.

4.2 States should require national accreditation of paramedic education programs.

4.3 States should accept national certification as a prerequisite for state licensure and local credentialing of emergency medical services providers.

4.4 The American Board of Emergency Medicine should create a subspecialty certification in emergency medical services.

Chapter 5: Advancing System Infrastructure

5.1 States should assume regulatory oversight of the medical aspects of air medical services, including communications, dispatch, and transport protocols.

5.2 Hospitals, emergency medical services agencies, public safety departments, emergency management offices, and public health agencies should develop integrated and interoperable communications and data systems.

5.3 The National Coordinator for Health Information Technology should fully involve prehospital emergency medical services leadership in discussions about design, deployment, and financing of the National Health Information Infrastructure.

	Congress	DHHS	DOT	DHS	DOD	States	Hospitals	EMS Agencies	Private Industry	Professional Organizations	Other
Chapter 6: Preparing for Disasters											
6.1 The Department of Health and Human Services, the Department of Transportation, the Department of Homeland Security, and the states should elevate emergency and trauma care to a position of parity with other public safety entities in disaster planning and operations.		X	X	X		X					
6.2 Congress should substantially increase funding for emergency medical services–related disaster preparedness through dedicated funding streams.	X										
6.3 Professional training, continuing education, and credentialing and certification programs for all the relevant professional categories of emergency medical services personnel should incorporate disaster preparedness into their curricula and require the maintenance of competency in these skills.			X			X				X	X
Chapter 7: Optimizing Prehospital Care Through Research											
7.1 Federal agencies that fund emergency and trauma care research should target an increased share of research funding at prehospital emergency medical services research, with an emphasis on systems and outcomes research.		X	X	X	X						X
7.2 Congress should modify Federalwide Assurance (FWA) Program regulations to allow the acquisition of limited, linked patient outcome data without the existence of an FWA.	X										

7.3 The Secretary of the Department of Health and Human Services should conduct a study to examine the research gaps and opportunities in emergency and trauma care research, and recommend a strategy for the optimal organization and funding of the research effort. This study should include consideration of the training of new investigators, the development of multicenter research networks, the involvement of emergency medical services researchers in the grant review and research advisory processes, and improved research coordination through a dedicated center or institute. Congress and federal agencies involved in emergency and trauma care research (including the Department of Transportation, the Department of Health and Human Services, the Department of Homeland Security, and the Department of Defense) should implement the study's recommendations.

EMERGENCY CARE FOR CHILDREN: GROWING PAINS

Chapter 3: Building a 21st-Century Emergency Care System

3.1 The Department of Health and Human Services and the National Highway Traffic Safety Administration, in partnership with professional organizations, should convene a panel of individuals with multidisciplinary expertise to develop evidence-based categorization systems for emergency medical services, emergency departments, and trauma centers based on adult and pediatric service capabilities.

	Congress	DHHS	DOT	DHS	DOD	States	Hospitals	EMS Agencies	Private Industry	Professional Societies	Other
7.3	X	X	X	X	X						
3.1		X	X							X	

	Congress	DHHS	DOT	DHS	DOD	States	Hospitals	EMS Agencies	Private Industry	Professional Societies	Other
3.2 The National Highway Traffic Safety Administration, in partnership with professional organizations, should convene a panel of individuals with multidisciplinary expertise to develop evidence-based model prehospital care protocols for the treatment, triage, and transport of patients, including children.			X							X	
3.3 The Department of Health and Human Services should convene a panel of individuals with emergency and trauma care expertise to develop evidence-based indicators of emergency and trauma care system performance, including the performance of pediatric emergency care.		X									
3.4 Congress should establish a demonstration program, administered by the Health Resources and Services Administration, to promote coordinated, regionalized, and accountable emergency care systems throughout the country, and appropriate $88 million over 5 years to this program.	X	X									
3.5 The Department of Health and Human Services should adopt rule changes to the Emergency Medical Treatment and Active Labor Act and the Health Insurance Portability and Accountability Act so that the original goals of the laws are preserved, but integrated systems may further develop.		X									

3.6 Congress should establish a lead agency for emergency and trauma care within 2 years of the release of this report. The lead agency should be housed in the Department of Health and Human Services, and should have primary programmatic responsibility for the full continuum of emergency medical services and emergency and trauma care for adults and children, including medical 9-1-1 and emergency medical dispatch, prehospital emergency medical services (both ground and air), hospital-based emergency and trauma care, and medical-related disaster preparedness. Congress should establish a working group to make recommendations regarding the structure, funding, and responsibilities of the new agency, and design and monitor the transition to its assumption of the responsibilities outlined above. The working group should have representation from federal and state agencies and professional disciplines involved in emergency and trauma care.

3.7 Congress should appropriate $37.5 million per year for the next 5 years to the Emergency Medical Services for Children program.

Chapter 4: Arming the Emergency Care Workforce with Pediatric Knowledge and Skills

4.1 Every pediatric- and emergency care–related health professional credentialing and certification body should define pediatric emergency care competencies and require practitioners to receive the level of initial and continuing education necessary to achieve and maintain those competencies.

4.2 The Department of Health and Human Services should collaborate with professional organizations to convene a panel of individuals with multidisciplinary expertise to develop, evaluate, and update clinical practice guidelines and standards of care for pediatric emergency care.

	Congress	DHHS	DOT	DHS	DOD	States	Hospitals	EMS Agencies	Private Industry	Professional Societies	Other
4.3 Emergency medical services agencies should appoint a pediatric emergency coordinator, and hospitals should appoint two pediatric emergency coordinators—one a physician—to provide pediatric leadership for the organization.							X	X			
Chapter 5: Improving the Quality of Pediatric Emergency Care											
5.1 The Department of Health and Human Services should fund studies of the efficacy, safety, and health outcomes of medications used for infants, children, and adolescents in emergency care settings in order to improve patient safety.		X									
5.2 The Department of Health and Human Services and the National Highway Traffic Safety Administration should fund the development of medication dosage guidelines, formulations, labeling guidelines, and administration techniques for the emergency care setting to maximize effectiveness and safety for infants, children, and adolescents. Emergency medical services agencies and hospitals should incorporate these guidelines, formulations, and techniques into practice.		X	X				X	X			
5.3 Hospitals and emergency medical services agencies should implement evidence-based approaches to reducing errors in emergency and trauma care for children.							X	X			
5.4 Federal agencies and private industry should fund research on pediatric-specific technologies and equipment for use by emergency and trauma care personnel.		X	X	X					X		

5.5 Emergency medical services agencies and hospitals should integrate family-centered care into emergency care practice.

X

X   X   X

X

Chapter 6: Improving Emergency Preparedness and Response for Children Involved in Disasters

6.1 Federal agencies (the Department of Health and Human Services, the National Highway Traffic Safety Administration, and the Department of Homeland Security), in partnership with state and regional planning bodies and emergency care providers, should convene a panel with multidisciplinary expertise to develop strategies for addressing pediatric needs in the event of a disaster. This effort should encompass the following:

- Development of strategies to minimize parent–child separation and improved methods for reuniting separated children with their families.
- Development of strategies to improve the level of pediatric expertise on Disaster Medical Assistance Teams and other organized disaster response teams.
- Development of disaster plans that address pediatric surge capacity for both injured and noninjured children.
- Development of and improved access to specific medical and mental health therapies, as well as social services, for children in the event of a disaster.
- Development of policies to ensure that disaster drills include a pediatric mass casualty incident at least once every 2 years.

Chapter 7: Building the Evidence Base for Pediatric Emergency Care

	Congress	DHHS	DOT	DHS	DOD	States	Hospitals	EMS Agencies	Private Industry	Professional Societies	Other
7.1 The Secretary of Health and Human Services should conduct a study to examine the gaps and opportunities in emergency care research, including pediatric emergency care, and recommend a strategy for the optimal organization and funding of the research effort. This study should include consideration of the training of new investigators, development of multicenter research networks, involvement of emergency and trauma care researchers in the grant review and research advisory processes, and improved research coordination through a dedicated center or institute. Congress and federal agencies involved in emergency and trauma care research (including the Department of Transportation, Department of Health and Human Services, Department of Homeland Security, and Department of Defense) should implement the study's recommendations.		X	X	X	X						
7.2 Administrators of state and national trauma registries should include standard pediatric-specific data elements and provide the data to the National Trauma Data Bank. Additionally, the American College of Surgeons should establish a multidisciplinary pediatric specialty committee to continuously evaluate pediatric-specific data elements for the National Trauma Data Bank and identify areas for pediatric research.											X

Index

A

Accidental Death and Disability: The Neglected Disease of Modern Society, 17, 36–37, 105
Accountability
  fragmentation of EMS system and, 135
  importance of, 5, 115
  model EMS systems, 121, 123, 124, 125
  new lead agency for EMS system and, 138, 140
  obstacles to, 5, 115
  performance measurement and, 5
  recommendation for, 117
  strategies for enhancing, 116
Accreditation
  disaster drill requirements, 238
  EMS system components, 116–117
  pediatric emergency care, 162–163
Adolescent patients, 211–212
Advanced life support (ALS)
  field stabilization *vs.* transport, 112–113
  pediatric, 158
  role of emergency medical technicians, 152
  in rural areas, 79–80
  shortcomings of pediatric care capabilities, 50–51

training for, 154, 155, 164–165
Adverse events
  current state of pediatric emergency care, 193–194
  language difference as cause of, 210
  mandated reporting, 198
  in prescription or administration of drugs, 196–197
  recommendations for reducing, 198, 212
  risk in EDs, 188–190
  risks for children in emergency care, 190–193
  strategies for reducing, 197–198
Agency for Healthcare Research and Quality, 27, 132, 141, 195, 197, 201, 227, 249, 261
Airbags, 254–255
Ambulance services
  appropriateness of dispatch, 63–64
  diversion, 71–72, 115, 129
  origins and development, 37
  payer mix, 82
  pediatric utilization, 62, 63–64
  response times, 75
  shortcomings of pediatric care capabilities, 50–51
  See also Transport of patients
American Academy of Pediatrics, 39, 227, 247, 265, 268